Biological Activities and Potential Applications of Phytotoxins

Biological Activities and Potential Applications of Phytotoxins

Guest Editor

Marco Masi

MDPI

Basel • Beijing • Wuhan • Barcelona • Belgrade • Novi Sad • Cluj • Manchester

Guest Editor
Marco Masi
University of Naples Federico II
Naples
Italy

Editorial Office
MDPI AG
Grosspeteranlage 5
4052 Basel, Switzerland

This is a reprint of the Special Issue, published open access by the journal *Toxins* (ISSN 2072-6651), freely accessible at: https://www.mdpi.com/journal/toxins/special_issues/applications_phytotoxins.

For citation purposes, cite each article independently as indicated on the article page online and as indicated below:

Lastname, A.A.; Lastname, B.B. Article Title. *Journal Name* **Year**, *Volume Number*, Page Range.

ISBN 978-3-7258-2699-5 (Hbk)
ISBN 978-3-7258-2700-8 (PDF)
https://doi.org/10.3390/books978-3-7258-2700-8

Contents

Marco Masi
Biological Activities and Potential Applications of Phytotoxins
Reprinted from: *Toxins* **2024**, *16*, 444, https://doi.org/10.3390/toxins16100444 1

Gabriele Soriano, Claudia Petrillo, Marco Masi, Mabrouka Bouafiane, Aminata Khelil, Angela Tuzi, et al.
Specialized Metabolites from the Allelopathic Plant *Retama raetam* as Potential Biopesticides
Reprinted from: *Toxins* **2022**, *14*, 311, https://doi.org/10.3390/toxins14050311 4

Gabriele Soriano, Antonietta Siciliano, Mónica Fernández-Aparicio, Antonio Cala Peralta, Marco Masi, Antonio Moreno-Robles, et al.
Iridoid Glycosides Isolated from *Bellardia trixago* Identified as Inhibitors of *Orobanche cumana* Radicle Growth
Reprinted from: *Toxins* **2022**, *14*, 559, https://doi.org/10.3390/toxins14080559 16

Eleonora Barilli, Pierluigi Reveglia, Francisco J. Agudo-Jurado, Vanessa Cañete García, Alessio Cimmino, Antonio Evidente and Diego Rubiales
Comparative Analysis of Secondary Metabolites Produced by *Ascochyta fabae* under In Vitro Conditions and Their Phytotoxicity on the Primary Host, *Vicia faba*, and Related Legume Crops
Reprinted from: *Toxins* **2023**, *15*, 693, https://doi.org/10.3390/toxins15120693 29

Davide Palmieri, David Segorbe, Manuel S. López-Berges, Filippo De Curtis, Giuseppe Lima, Antonio Di Pietro and David Turrà
Alkaline pH, Low Iron Availability, Poor Nitrogen Sources and CWI MAPK Signaling Are Associated with Increased Fusaric Acid Production in *Fusarium oxysporum*
Reprinted from: *Toxins* **2023**, *15*, 50, https://doi.org/10.3390/toxins15010050 46

Francisco J. R. Mejías, Alexandra G. Durán, Nuria Chinchilla, Rosa M. Varela, José A. Álvarez, José M. G. Molinillo, et al.
In Silico Evaluation of Sesquiterpenes and Benzoxazinoids Phytotoxins against M^{pro}, RNA Replicase and Spike Protein of SARS-CoV-2 by Molecular Dynamics. Inspired by Nature
Reprinted from: *Toxins* **2022**, *14*, 599, https://doi.org/10.3390/toxins14090599 56

Alessia Staropoli, Paola Cuomo, Maria Michela Salvatore, Gaetano De Tommaso, Mauro Iuliano, Anna Andolfi, et al.
Harzianic Acid Activity against *Staphylococcus aureus* and Its Role in Calcium Regulation
Reprinted from: *Toxins* **2023**, *15*, 237, https://doi.org/10.3390/toxins15040237 74

Alexandra G. Durán, Nuria Chinchilla, Ana M. Simonet, M. Teresa Gutiérrez, Jorge Bolívar, Manuel M. Valdivia, et al.
Biological Activity of Naphthoquinones Derivatives in the Search of Anticancer Lead Compounds
Reprinted from: *Toxins* **2023**, *15*, 348, https://doi.org/10.3390/toxins15050348 88

Marina Murillo-Pineda, Juan M. Coto-Cid, María Romero, Jesús G. Zorrilla, Nuria Chinchilla, Zahara Medina-Calzada, et al.
Effects of Sesquiterpene Lactones on Primary Cilia Formation (Ciliogenesis)
Reprinted from: *Toxins* **2023**, *15*, 632, https://doi.org/10.3390/toxins15110632 101

Marco Masi, Jesús García Zorrilla and Susan Meyer
Bioactive Metabolite Production in the Genus *Pyrenophora* (Pleosporaceae, Pleosporales)
Reprinted from: *Toxins* **2022**, *14*, 588, https://doi.org/10.3390/toxins14090588 116

Hisashi Kato-Noguchi
Defensive Molecules Momilactones A and B: Function, Biosynthesis, Induction and Occurrence
Reprinted from: *Toxins* **2023**, *15*, 241, https://doi.org/10.3390/toxins15040241 . . . . **136**

Jin Han, Shaoyong Zhang, Jun He and Tianze Li
Piperine: Chemistry and Biology
Reprinted from: *Toxins* **2023**, *15*, 696, https://doi.org/10.3390/toxins15120696 . . . . **154**

toxins

MDPI

Editorial

Biological Activities and Potential Applications of Phytotoxins

Marco Masi

Department of Chemical Sciences, Complesso Universitario Monte Sant'Angelo, University of Naples, Federico II, Via Cintia 4, 80126 Napoli, Italy; marco.masi@unina.it

Specialized metabolites, also known as secondary metabolites, produced by plants and microbes possess several biological activities [1]. Among them, phytotoxins are substances which are poisonous or toxic for plants [2]. They seem to play an important role in plant–pathogen interactions when produced by phytopathogenic fungi or bacteria, while plant-produced phytotoxins—including allelochemicals—seem to be involved in plant–plant interactions [3]. These compounds belong to different classes of natural substances and the determination of their chemical structure, or their identification, are fundamental for understanding their function [4]. Most of these phytotoxins have shown interesting potential applications in agriculture or medicine [5]. However, many biological activities of these compounds have not been investigated, limiting their potential practical use. They can serve as efficient tools to design safe biopesticides, avoiding the use of synthetic pesticides that are able to cause long-term impact of residues in agricultural products with a risk to human and animal health [3,6]. They can also be used for the development of new, more effective drugs to overcome problems of antibiotic resistance being the reservoir of new mechanisms of action [7].

This Special Issue is focused on the isolation and characterization of new bioactive phytotoxins or on the evaluation of the biological activities of known phytotoxins to further investigate their potential applications in different fields. This collection comprises eleven papers with eight research articles [Contributions 1–8] and three reviews [Contributions 9–11].

Some research articles investigated the production of phytotoxins by plants as potentialbiopesticides for the control of parasitic plants and fungal phytopathogens that can cause devastating losses to crop yields in several parts of the world [Contributions 1–2]. Among them, *Orobanche cumana* is an obligate holoparasitic plant with strong effects in sunflower crops, while the fungus *Stemphylium vesicarium* has pathogenic effects on many hosts, especially on pear. In the first research article [Contributions 1], the authors investigated the production of specialized metabolites from the allelopathic plant *Retama raetam* and their activity against *S. vesicarium* and *O. cumana*. Six compounds belonging to isoflavones and flavones subgroups have been isolated from the *R. raetam* dichloromethane extract and identified using spectroscopic and optical methods. Among them, laburnetin and ephedroidin resulted in being the most promising metabolites for the control of these pests [Contributions 1]. The allelopathic effects of specialized metabolites produced by the plant *Bellardia trixago* on the growth of *O. cumana* seedlings were described in the second research article contribution [Contributions 2]. Five iridoid glycosides were isolated together with benzoic acid from the ethyl acetate extract of aerial green organs of this plant by bio-guided purification. Among them, melampyroside was found to be the most abundant constituent in the extract (44.3% w/w), as well as the most phytotoxic iridoid on *O. cumana* radicle, showing a 72.6% inhibition in radicle growth. The ecotoxicological profile of melampyroside was evaluated, providing useful information for the generation of green bioherbicides for the control of parasitic plants [Contributions 2].

Phytotoxins produced by phytopathogenic fungi were also investigated. The third article contribution to the Special Issue [Contributions 3] reports a comparative analysis of secondary metabolites produced by the phytopathogenic fungus *Ascochyta fabae* under

Citation: Masi, M. Biological Activities and Potential Applications of Phytotoxins. *Toxins* **2024**, *16*, 444. https://doi.org/10.3390/toxins16100444

Received: 4 October 2024
Accepted: 14 October 2024
Published: 16 October 2024

in vitro conditions and their phytotoxicity on the primary host, *Vicia faba*, and related legume crops. The produced metabolites were analyzed by NMR and LC-HRMS methods, resulting in the dereplication of seven metabolites, which varied with cultural substrates The phytotoxicity of the pure metabolites was assessed at different concentrations on their primary hosts and related legumes. Among them, ascosalitoxin and benzoic acid resulted in being the most phytotoxic, and thus are expected to play an important role in necrosis appearance [Contributions 3]. Fusaric acid (FA) is one of the first secondary metabolites isolated from phytopathogenic fungi belonging to the genus *Fusarium*, and the fourth article contribution [Contributions 4] provides novel insights on this matter. Specifically the authors evaluated the effect of different nitrogen sources, iron content, extracellular pH and cellular signaling pathways on the production of FA siderophores by the pathogen *Fusarium oxysporum* [Contributions 4].

The antiviral, anticancer, anti-inflammatory and antibiotic properties of some fungal and plant phytotoxins were also studied. In particular, the fifth research article contribution [Contributions 5] to this Special Issue focuses on the evaluation of natural sesquiterpenes and benzoxazinoids, along with their easily accessible derivatives, against the main protease, RNA replicase and spike glycoprotein of SARS-CoV-2 by molecular docking [Contributions 5]. The sixth research article contribution [Contribution 6] investigates the activity of harzianic acid, a bioactive metabolite derived from fungi of the genus *Trichoderma* against the Gram-positive bacterium *Staphylococcus aureus* and its role in calcium regulation [Contribution 6]. Naphthoquinones are a valuable source of secondary metabolites that have been well known for their dye properties since ancient times. In the seventh research article contribution [Contribution 7], the authors investigated the biological activity of some naphthoquinone's derivatives in the search of anticancer lead compounds. Their results encourage further studies on the development of new anticancer drugs for more directed therapies and reduced side effects with the naphthoquinone skeleton [Contribution 7]. Sesquiterpene lactones (SLs) are plant-derived metabolites with a broad spectrum of biological effects, including anti-tumor and anti-inflammatory effects, and are thus promising candidates for drug development. In their herein-presented work, the eighth article contribution [Contribution 8] to this Special Issue, the authors evaluated the effects of selected SLs (grosheimin, costunolide, and three cyclocostunolides) on primary cilia biogenesis and stability in human retinal pigment epithelial (RPE) cells [Contribution 8].

The first review contribution [Contribution 9] provides an overview on the bioactive metabolite production in the genus *Pyrenophora* (Pleosporaceae, Pleosporales). The toxic metabolites discovered from three well-studied species (namely, *P. tritici-repentis*, *P. teres* and *P. semeniperda*) are presented, along with a few reports from additional species, and their isolation, structure determination, and biological activities are discussed [Contribution 9]. The second review [Contribution 10] is focused on momilactones A and B, two labdane-related diterpenoids, mainly identified in rice and several other *Poaceae* species. Their functions biosynthesis, induction and occurrence in plant species are reported [Contribution 10]. The third review [Contribution 11] is related to the chemistry and biology of piperine. This plant-derived piperamide, isolated from black pepper (*Piper nigrum* L.), possesses several biological activities and potential applications in different fields. The recent progress in its studies, mechanisms of action and structural modifications are summarized to pave the way for future development and utilization of this compound and its derivatives as potent drugs and pesticides [Contribution 11].

Funding: This research received no external funding.

Conflicts of Interest: The author declares no conflicts of interest.

List of Contributions:

1. Soriano, G.; Petrillo, C.; Masi, M.; Bouafiane, M.; Khelil, A.; Tuzi, A.; Isticato, R.; Fernández-Aparicio, M.; Cimmino, A. Specialized metabolites from the allelopathic plant *Retama raetam* as potential biopesticides. *Toxins* **2022**, *14*, 311.
2. Soriano, G.; Siciliano, A.; Fernández-Aparicio, M.; Cala Peralta, A.; Masi, M.; Moreno-Robles, A; Guida, M.; Cimmino, A. Iridoid glycosides isolated from *Bellardia trixago* identified as inhibitors of *Orobanche cumana* radicle growth. *Toxins* **2022**, *14*, 559.
3. Barilli, E.; Reveglia, P.; Agudo-Jurado, F.J.; Cañete García, V.; Cimmino, A.; Evidente, A.; Rubiales, D. Comparative analysis of secondary metabolites produced by *Ascochyta fabae* under in vitro conditions and their phytotoxicity on the primary host, *Vicia faba*, and related legume crops. *Toxins* **2023**, *15*, 693.
4. Palmieri, D.; Segorbe, D.; López-Berges, M.S.; De Curtis, F.; Lima, G.; Di Pietro, A.; Turrà, D. Alkaline pH, low iron availability, poor nitrogen sources and CWI MAPK signaling are associated with increased fusaric acid production in *Fusarium oxysporum*. *Toxins* **2023**, *15*, 50.
5. Mejías, F.J.; Durán, A.G.; Chinchilla, N.; Varela, R.M.; Álvarez, J.A.; Molinillo, J.M.; García-Cozar, F.; Macías, F.A. In Silico evaluation of sesquiterpenes and benzoxazinoids phytotoxins against Mpro, RNA replicase and spike protein of SARS-CoV-2 by molecular dynamics. Inspired by nature. *Toxins* **2022**, *14*, 599.
6. Staropoli, A.; Cuomo, P.; Salvatore, M.M.; De Tommaso, G.; Iuliano, M.; Andolfi, A.; Tenore, G.; Capparelli, R.; Vinale, F. Harzianic acid activity against *Staphylococcus aureus* and its role in calcium regulation. *Toxins* **2023**, *15*, 237.
7. Durán, A.G.; Chinchilla, N.; Simonet, A.M.; Gutiérrez, M.T.; Bolívar, J.; Valdivia, M.M.; Molinillo J.M.G.; Macías, F.A. Biological activity of naphthoquinones derivatives in the search of anticancer lead compounds. *Toxins* **2023**, *15*, 348.
8. Murillo-Pineda, M.; Coto-Cid, J.M.; Romero, M.; Zorrilla, J.G.; Chinchilla, N.; Medina-Calzada, Z.; Varela, R.M., Juárez-Soto, A.; Macías, F.A.; Reales, E. Effects of sesquiterpene lactones on primary cilia formation (ciliogenesis). *Toxins* **2023**, *15*, 632.
9. Masi, M.; Zorrilla, J.G.; Meyer, S. Bioactive metabolite production in the genus *Pyrenophora* (Pleosporaceae, Pleosporales). *Toxins* **2022**, *14*, 588.
10. Kato-Noguchi, H. Defensive molecules momilactones A and B: Function, biosynthesis, induction and occurrence. *Toxins* **2023**, *15*, 241.
11. Han, J.; Zhang, S.; He, J.; Li, T. Piperine: Chemistry and biology. *Toxins* **2023**, *15*, 696.

References

1. Oladipo, A.; Enwemiwe, V.; Ejeromedoghene, O.; Adebayo, A.; Ogunyemi, O.; Fu, F. Production and functionalities of specialized metabolites from different organic sources. *Metabolites* **2022**, *12*, 534. [CrossRef]
2. Gunthardt, B.F.; Hollender, J.; Hungerbuhler, K.; Scheringer, M.; Bucheli, T.D. Comprehensive toxic plants–phytotoxins database and its application in assessing aquatic micropollution potential. *J. Agric. Food Chem.* **2018**, *66*, 7577–7588. [CrossRef] [PubMed]
3. Cimmino, A.; Masi, M.; Evidente, M.; Superchi, S.; Evidente, A. Fungal phytotoxins with potential herbicidal activity: Chemical and biological characterization. *Nat. Prod. Rep.* **2015**, *32*, 1629–1653. [CrossRef] [PubMed]
4. Dewick, P.M. *Medicinal Natural Products*, 3rd ed.; John Wiley and Sons Ltd.: Chicester, UK, 2009.
5. Chen, H.; Singh, H.; Bhardwaj, N.; Bhardwaj, S.K.; Khatri, M.; Kim, K.H.; Peng, W. An exploration on the toxicity mechanisms of phytotoxins and their potential utilities. *Crit. Rev. Environ. Sci. Technol.* **2022**, *52*, 395–435. [CrossRef]
6. Walia, S.; Saha, S.; Tripathi, V.; Sharma, K.K. Phytochemical biopesticides: Some recent developments. *Phytochem. Rev.* **2017**, *16*, 989–1007. [CrossRef]
7. Gorlenko, C.L.; Kiselev, H.Y.; Budanova, E.V.; Zamyatnin, A.A., Jr.; Ikryannikova, L.N. Plant secondary metabolites in the battle of drugs and drug-resistant bacteria: New heroes or worse clones of antibiotics? *Antibiotics* **2020**, *9*, 170. [CrossRef] [PubMed]

toxins

MDPI

Article

Specialized Metabolites from the Allelopathic Plant *Retama raetam* as Potential Biopesticides

Gabriele Soriano [1], Claudia Petrillo [2,*], Marco Masi [1,*], Mabrouka Bouafiane [3,4], Aminata Khelil [3], Angela Tuzi [1], Rachele Isticato [2], Mónica Fernández-Aparicio [5,†] and Alessio Cimmino [1,†]

1 Department of Chemical Sciences, University of Naples Federico II, 80126 Naples, Italy; gabriele.soriano@unina.it (G.S.); angela.tuzi@unina.it (A.T.); alessio.cimmino@unina.it (A.C.)
2 Department of Biology, University of Naples Federico II, 80126 Naples, Italy; isticato@unina.it
3 Laboratoire de Protection des Ecosystèmes en Zones Arides et Semi-Arides, Universit'e Kasdi Merbah-Ouargla, Ouargla 30000, Algeria; bouafiane-mabrouka@univ-eloued.dz (M.B.); aminatakhelil@yahoo.fr (A.K.)
4 Department of Agronomy, Faculty of Life and Natural Sciences, University of El Oued, El Oued 39000, Algeria
5 Department of Plant Breeding, Institute for Sustainable Agriculture (IAS), CSIC, Avenida Menéndez Pidal s/n, 14004 Córdoba, Spain; monica.fernandez@ias.csic.es
* Correspondence: claudia.petrillo@unina.it (C.P.); marco.masi@unina.it (M.M.)
† These authors contributed equally to this work.

Abstract: To cope with the rising food demand, modern agriculture practices are based on the indiscriminate use of agrochemicals. Although this strategy leads to a temporary solution, it also severely damages the environment, representing a risk to human health. A sustainable alternative to agrochemicals is the use of plant metabolites and plant-based pesticides, known to have minimal environmental impact compared to synthetic pesticides. *Retama raetam* is a shrub growing in Algeria's desert areas, where it is commonly used in traditional medicine because of its antiseptic and antipyretic properties. Furthermore, its allelopathic features can be exploited to effectively control phytopathogens in the agricultural field. In this study, six compounds belonging to isoflavones and flavones subgroups have been isolated from the *R. raetam* dichloromethane extract and identified using spectroscopic and optical methods as alpinumisoflavone, hydroxyalpinumisoflavone, laburnetin, licoflavone C, retamasin B, and ephedroidin. Their antifungal activity was evaluated against the fungal phytopathogen *Stemphylium vesicarium* using a growth inhibition bioassay on PDA plates. Interestingly, the flavonoid laburnetin, the most active metabolite, displayed an inhibitory activity comparable to that exerted by the synthetic fungicide pentachloronitrobenzene, in a ten-fold lower concentration. The allelopathic activity of *R. raetam* metabolites against parasitic weeds was also investigated using two independent parasitic weed bioassays to discover potential activities on either suicidal stimulation or radicle growth inhibition of broomrapes. In this latter bioassay, ephedroidin strongly inhibited the growth of *Orobanche cumana* radicles and, therefore, can be proposed as a natural herbicide.

Keywords: biocontrol; *Retama raetam*; *Stemphylium vesicarium*; *Orobanche cumana*; laburnetin; ephedroidin

Key Contribution: The inhibitory effects of six natural compounds with potential application as biopesticides from the allelopathic plant *R. raetam* were evaluated in vitro against the fungal phytopathogen *Stemphylium vesicarium* and on parasitic weed plants. Laburnetin emerged as the only metabolite active against the fungus, whereas ephedroidin strongly inhibited the growth of *O. cumana* radicles.

Citation: Soriano, G.; Petrillo, C.; Masi, M.; Bouafiane, M.; Khelil, A.; Tuzi, A.; Isticato, R.; Fernández-Aparicio, M.; Cimmino, A. Specialized Metabolites from the Allelopathic Plant *Retama raetam* as Potential Biopesticides. *Toxins* **2022**, *14*, 311. https://doi.org/10.3390/toxins14050311

Received: 8 April 2022
Accepted: 25 April 2022
Published: 28 April 2022

1. Introduction

Since the second half of the 20th century, the agricultural practices have been based on the uncontrolled use of chemical pesticides, and herbicides, to cope with the rising crop demands of an ever-growing human population [1,2]. As a consequence of the massive use of agrochemicals, harmful effects such as environmental pollution, human health threats, insect resistance to pesticides, parasitoids, and pollinators loss occurred [3–5]. Therefore, researchers are seeking alternative and eco-friendly solutions. Within this framework, plants are receiving increasing attention as remarkable sources of bioactive substances, due to their ability to synthesize an impressive variety of low molecular weight metabolites, often exploited as biocontrol agents in the agricultural field [4,6–8]. Interestingly, the release of these compounds can either be constitutive, or induced in response to a pathogenic attack [9], and their biosynthesis is closely related to the growth stage of the plant [10].

Plant diseases represent a considerable threat to agricultural production due to phytopathogenic fungi [11]. One of the most relevant fungal diseases is the brown spot of pear caused by *Stemphylium vesicarium* (Wallr.) E.G. Simmons, which every year leads to important economic losses in the European pear production areas. *S. vesicarium* has pathogenic effects on many other hosts, such as garlic, onion, and asparagus [12]. So far, the most effective method to control *S. vesicarium* spread is the preventive application of chemical fungicides such as dithiocarbamates or strobilurins [13].

Moreover, a large number of parasitic plants, such as broomrape (*Orobanche* and *Phelipanche* spp.), are adapted to infect crops in agriculture environments, depicting a serious threat to crop productivity by inducing severe yield losses [14]. For many crops, single methods of parasitic weed control are limited or non-existing, and thus integrated pest management systems appear the best solution to find effective, long-lasting, widely applicable, and environmentally benign methods for parasitic weed control. The identification of plant species as sources of allelopathic molecules against the parasitic weed lifecycle acting as either inducers of suicidal germination or inhibitors of radicle growth provide alternative methods for their use in integrated methods of parasitic weed control [15,16].

Retama spp. are perennial and unarmed shrubs from the Fabaceae family. They have been used traditionally for the treatment of different diseases in many parts of the Mediterranean Basin, especially in North Africa and the Middle East. In fact, they showed several biological activities, including antibacterial [17], anti-inflammatory [18], antioxidant [19], anti-proliferative [20], anti-ulcer [19], anti-viral [21], and hepatoprotective activities [22,23].

Among them, *Retama raetam* is mainly distributed in North Africa, including Morocco, Algeria, Tunisia, Libya, Egypt, Asia, and certain Middle Eastern countries, and widely used in the folk medicine, as a powder, an infusion, or decoction, to treat different diseases [10]. Within the potential applications, *R. raetam* has been employed to treat several disorders, including sore throat, skin diseases, fever, and inflammation [24], and it also displayed strong antioxidant, antimicrobial, hepatoprotective, and hypoglycemic activity [10]. According to most authors, *R. raetam* properties may be associated with its abundance in flavonoids, isoflavonoids, and alkaloids [24], which have also been related to the inhibition of a range of root pathogens and pests, ranging from bacteria to fungi and insects [25]. Furthermore, as reported by Chouikh et al. [26], this plant is an extraordinary source of various phenolic compounds, which are known to possess a strong antioxidant effect on free radicals and antibacterial effects. A recent study has shown that natural flavonoids from *R. raetam* exhibit important interaction with the active site of α-glucosidase, inspiring the development of a new drug with anti-diabetic activity [27].

Despite the numerous studies cited above, the antifungal activity against the fungal pathogen *S. vesicarium* has not been investigated. Moreover, the plant studied was collected in the Souf region located in the north-east of the Algerian Saharan desert, an extremely arid zone of great importance among medicinal plants [28–31]. Recently, researchers have highlighted the effectiveness of aqueous extracts of some Saharan plant species, including *R. raetam,* on seed germination or seedling growth of target species [32]. This result suggests that the plant can be a source of allelochemicals able to inhibit the radicle growth of parasitic weeds [15].

Thus, the main purpose of the present study was to further investigate the potential of the crude organic extract obtained from the *R. raetam* aerial part as a source of biopoesticides. Bioactivity-guided purification was performed using anti-fungal bioassays against the phytopathogenic fungus *S. vesicarium*. This is a traditional method used in natural product discovery that allows researchers to isolate the pure bioactive compounds from a complex mixture, such as plants' organic extracts [33–36]. In particular, following the identification of a crude extract with promising biological activity, the next step is its (often multiple) consecutive bioactivity-guided fractionation until the pure bioactive compounds are isolated [37].

This manuscript reports the isolation of six metabolites identified by spectroscopic and chemical methods. Their potential antifungal activity against the phytopathogen *S. vesicarium* and the herbicidal activity against broomrapes (as inductors of suicidal germination and inhibitors of radicle growth), are also discussed.

2. Results and Discussion

The dried aerial parts of *R. raetam* were extracted as detailed in the Materials and Methods Section. Bioactivity-guided purification was performed using anti-fungal bioassays against the phytopathogenic fungus *S. vesicarium*. The active CH_2Cl_2 extract was fractionated by CC, yielding 13 fractions (F1–13) with variable chemical profiles, which were evaluated for their antifungal activity against *S. vesicarium* (Figure 1).

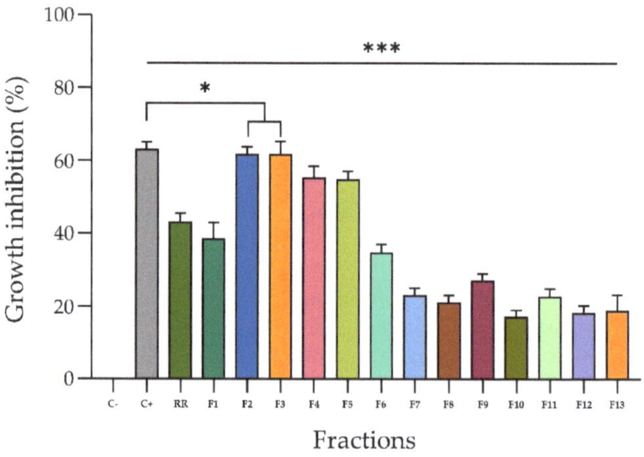

Figure 1. Inhibitory effect of the CH_2Cl_2 crude extract (RR) and the thirteen fractions obtained from the preliminary purification of RR, on the mycelium of *S. vesicarium*, at a concentration of 2 mg/mL (crude extract) and 250 µg/mL (fractions), respectively. The negative control was absolute methanol (C−), and the positive control was 200 µg/mL of PCNB. The fungal growth inhibition is represented as the percentage reduction of the fungal mycelia diameter in the treated plate compared to that in the control plate. All experiments were performed in triplicate with three independent trials. Data are presented as means ± standard deviation (n = 3) compared to the control. *** $p < 0.0001$ and * $p < 0.05$.

Interestingly, the activity exhibited by the fractions F2–F5 (~60%) was stronger than that displayed by the total crude extract (~43%) and comparable to the commercial fungicide pentachloronitrobenzene (PCNB), used as a positive control (Figure 1). These latter fractions were further purified by combined column and TLCs (Scheme S1) to afford six pure metabolites (**1–6**, Figure 2), as described in the Materials and Methods Section. The first investigation of their ^{1}H NMR and ESI MS spectra (Figures S1–S14) showed that they are isoflavones and flavones with different substitutions. They were identified by comparing their ^{1}H NMR and MS data with those reported in the literature as alpinumisoflavone

(**1**) [38–40], hydroxyalpinumisoflavone (**2**) [41], laburnetin (**3**) [42], licoflavone C (**4**) [43], retamasin B (**5**) [44], and ephedroidin (**6**) [41].

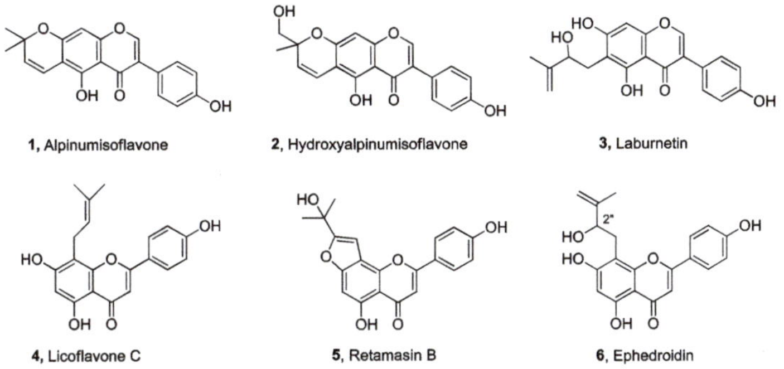

Figure 2. Chemical structures of specialized metabolites (**1–6**) isolated from *Retama raetam*.

The structure of alpinumisoflavone (**1**) was confirmed by X-ray diffractometric analysis. An ORTEP view is reported in Figure 3. The X-ray crystal structure is reported here to undoubtedly identify the compound **1** as alpinumisoflavone [45]. Alpinumisoflavone consists of three nearly coplanar fused rings, and one attached out-of-plane twisted phenyl ring. In the tricyclic ring system, a liner junction of A/B/C rings is observed. It should be noted that compound **1** showed a different junction between the dimethylpyran ring (A) and the chromenone moiety (B/C), with respect to the analog derrone (Figure 4) previously isolated from *R. raetam* flowers [46].

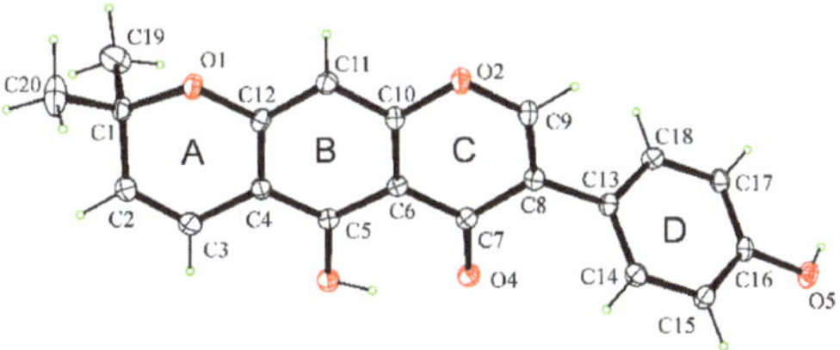

Figure 3. ORTEP view of alpinumisoflavone (**1**) with thermal ellipsoids drawn at the 30% probability level.

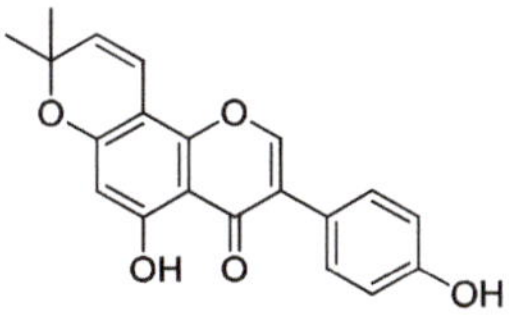

Figure 4. Structure of derrone, previously isolated from *R. raetam*.

Although compounds **2**, **3**, and **6** have chiral centers, their absolute configurations were not determined so far. Due to the limited available amounts of these compounds, a modified Mosher method [47] was applied only to compound **6** to determine the absolute configuration of its secondary hydroxylated carbon (C-2″). When compound **6** was treated with S-MTPA chloride, its ester derivative showed two sets of signals with an enantiomeric ratio of 50:50, indication that **6** is an enantiomeric mixture of 2″(*S*)-**6** and 2″(*R*)-**6**. The same result was obtained when **6** was treated with *R*-MTPA chloride. An optical rotation value of zero $[\alpha]_D^{25}$ 0 (c 0.4, MeOH) was also obtained. This result was not unexpected because a similar prenylated xantone, named (±)-graciesculenxanthone C, isolated from

Garcinia esculenta showed an enantiomeric ratio of 60:40 when it was treated with *S*- and *R*-MTPA chloride [48].

Thus, the six compounds (**1–6**) isolated from *R. raetam* were spot-inoculated on PDA plates to test their antifungal activity against the fungal phytopathogen *S. vesicarium*. As shown in Figure 5, only laburnetin (**3**) exhibited quite a strong activity when spot-inoculated (50 µg/mL), inhibiting the growth of *S. vesicarium* by around 55%, confirming the antagonistic effect displayed by the most active fractions, which inhibited *S. vesicarium* mycelium's growth by around 60% (Figure 1). Interestingly, the commercial fungicide PCNB, used at a concentration of 0.5 mg/mL, exhibited an antagonistic effect comparable to the one exerted by laburnetin used at a 10-fold lower concentration (50 µg/mL) (Figure 5b), demonstrating how natural compounds could represent an effective alternative to chemicals in the agricultural field. The other compounds instead displayed a fungal inhibition of around 25% (**1**, **6**), 20% (**2**, **4**), and 17% (**5**) (Figure 5b). Considering the results obtained it is possible to ascribe to laburnetin the main role in the antagonistic effect exhibited by *R. raetam* extract against the fungus *S. vesicarium*.

a

b

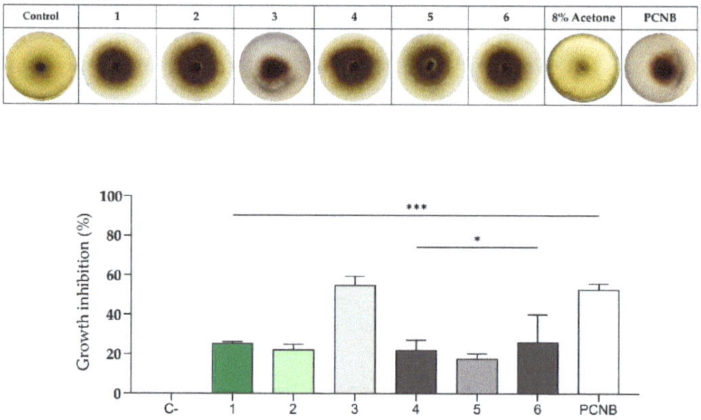

Figure 5. Effects of alpinumisoflavone (**1**), hydroxyalpinumisoflavone (**2**), laburnetin (**3**), licoflavone C (**4**), retamasin B (**5**), and ephedroidin (**6**) against *S. vesicarium*. The plot shows the fungal growth inhibition exerted by the tested compounds at a concentration of 50 µg/mL. (**a**) Representative photos of the biological assay for in vitro inhibition of mycelial growth of *S. vesicarium*. 8% Acetone and 0.5 mg/mL PCNB were used as negative and positive controls, respectively. (**b**) Fungal growth inhibition reported as the percentage of the reduction in the diameter of the fungal mycelium in the treated plate compared to that in the control plate. *** $p < 0.0001$ and * $p < 0.05$.

The isoflavonoid laburnetin (**3**) has already been isolated from the *Genista* genus [41], as well as from other plants, and its antimicrobial activity was demonstrated [49]. To the best of our knowledge, here, the antifungal activity of this compound against *S. vesicarium* is being reported for the first time, showing that laburnetin could be proposed as a natural antagonist for the control of this phytopathogen that infests several important cultivated species.

R. raetam is an allelopathic plant species collected in the Saharan ecosystem from the Souf region in southeastern Algeria. Allelochemicals involved in plant–plant interactions are a potential source for alternative agrochemicals to solve the negative effects caused by synthetic herbicides. Thus, the six metabolites (**1–6**) were tested on two independent parasitic weed bioassays to discover potential activities of *R. raetam* metabolites on either suicidal stimulation or radicle growth inhibition of broomrapes. First, the germination induction effect of alpinumisoflavone, ephedroidin, hydroxyalpinoisolflavone, laburnetin, licoflavone C, and retamasin B was tested on seeds of four parasitic weed species, *Orobanche crenata*

O. cumana, *O. minor*, and *Phelipanche ramosa*, using in vitro germination bioassays. The synthetic germination stimulant GR24 used as a positive control induced germination levels of 53.2% ± 1.7%, 64.6% ± 1.8%, 91.7% ± 1.7%, and 94.2% ± 0.4% in *O. crenata*, *O. cumana*, *O. minor*, and *P. ramosa*, respectively. Null germination was observed when seeds of the broomrape species were treated with the negative control (distilled water) or with compounds **1–6**. The results obtained in the germination bioassay indicate that none of the metabolites isolated from the stem of *R. raetam* act as suicidal germination inducers of the broomrape species studied. Field application of inductors of suicidal germination of broomrape seeds in the absence of a specific host is a control strategy for obligate root parasitic weeds. In fact, the subsequent parasitic growth after germination leads to the death of the parasite due to nutrient starvation in the absence of host-derived nutrients [50].

In a second parasitic weed bioassay, the six purified compounds (**1–6**) were tested at 100 µM as potential inhibitors of radicle growth of *O. crenata*, *O. cumana*, *O. minor*, and *P. ramosa*. Among the compounds tested, low to negligible activity was found in all compounds tested except for ephedroidin (**6**), which strongly inhibited the normal development of *O. cumana* radicles in comparison with *O. cumana* control radicles (Figure 6A). Ephedroidin induced a strong toxic effect, observed as darkening in the *O. cumana* radicle and an average length inhibition of 80.8% ± 1.6% in comparison with radicles control (Figure 6B,C). Similar toxic effects on broomrape radicles were previously described for cytochalasans [51].

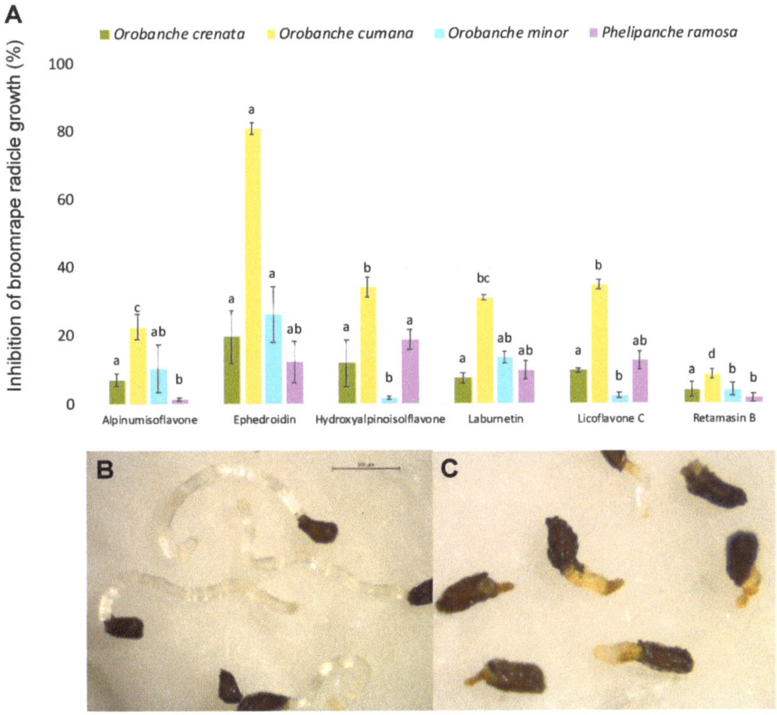

Figure 6. (**A**) Inhibition of broomrape radicle growth induced by alpinumisoflavone, ephedroidin, hydroxyalpinoisolflavone, laburnetin, licoflavone C, and retamasin B, expressed as a percentage with respect to the control GR24. (**B**,**C**) Photographs illustrating the effects of ephedroidin in radicles of *Orobanche cumana*: (**B**) control, (**C**) 100 µM ephedroidin. Analysis of variance was applied to angular transformed replicate data. For each broomrape species, bars with different letters are significantly different according to the Tukey test ($p = 0.05$). Error bars represent standard error.

Ephedroidin (**6**) is a flavanoid previously isolated together with laburnetin (**3**) from the *Genista ephedroides* [41] and from *R. raetam* [52]. Recently, ephedroidin resulted to be the most active in inhibiting nitric oxide synthase (iNOS) and nuclear factor kappa B (NF-κB) as well as in decreasing oxidative stress, when compared with other flavonoids isolated from the same source [44]. Our results demonstrated that ephedroidin strongly inhibited the radical development of *O. cumana* seeds and can be proposed as a natural herbicide against this dangerous parasitic weed.

3. Conclusions

Bio-guided purification of *R. raetam* CH_2Cl_2 extract allowed us to isolate six metabolites, identified by spectroscopic and chemical methods as alpinumisoflavone, hydroxyalpinumisoflavone, laburnetin, licoflavone C, retamasin B, and efedroidin. In particular, the isoflavonoid laburnetin showed antifungal activity against the phytopathogen *S. vesicarium* 10-fold higher than that of the commercial fungicide PCNB. The flavonoid ephedroidin exhibited a strong inhibition of broomrape seed germination, suggesting their application as potential biopesticides against these noxious biotic stresses. Finally, the structure of alpinumisoflavone was confirmed by X-ray diffractometric analysis, which showed a different junction with respect to the analog derrone, previously isolated from the *R. raetam* plant. These data prompted further studies aimed to formulate the active compounds and test them in greenhouse and field trials. However, analyses on their ecotoxicological profile are needed before the practical application as biopesticides.

4. Materials and Methods

4.1. General Experimental Procedures

A JASCO P-1010 digital polarimeter was used to measure the optical rotations. A Bruker (Karlsruhe, Germany) spectrometer working at 400/100 MHz was used to record $^1H/^{13}C$ NMR spectra in $CDCl_3$ or CD_3OD, which were also used as internal standards. The LC/MS TOF system (Agilent 6230B, HPLC 1260 Infinity) (Milan, Italy) was used to record ESI mass spectra. Analytical and preparative Thin-Layer Chromatography (TLC) was performed on silica gel plates (Kieselgel 60, F_{254}, 0.25 and 0.5 mm, respectively) (Merck Darmstadt, Germany). The spots were visualized by exposure to UV light (254 nm) and/or iodine vapors and/or by spraying first with 10% H_2SO_4 in MeOH, and then with 5% phosphomolybdic acid in EtOH, followed by heating at 110 °C for 10 min. Column chromatography (CC) was performed using silica gel (Kieselgel 60, 0.063–0.200 mm) (Merck Darmstadt, Germany). All the solvents were supplied by Sigma-Aldrich (Milan, Italy). The balance model used is Analytical ES 225SM-DR (Precisa, Dietikon, Switzerland).

4.2. Plant Material

Aerial parts of *R. raetam* were collected between December 2017 and February 2018, corresponding to the flowering phase of the plant. This study was carried out in the Souf region and is located in the north-east of Algerian Sahara, between 33° and 34° north latitude, and 6° and 8° longitude. Sea level = 40 m [32]. The plant material was then carefully rinsed with distilled water to remove dust particles and dried in the air for a few days at room temperature; finally, it was ground in a blender.

Seeds of parasitic weeds were collected from mature plants of *O. crenata* infecting pea in Spain, *O. cumana* infecting sunflower in Spain, *O. minor* infecting red clover in France and *Phelipanche ramosa* infecting oilseed rape in France. Dry parasitic seeds were separated from capsules using winnowing combined with a sieve of 0.6 mm-mesh size and then stored dry in the dark at room temperature until use for this work.

4.3. Fungal Strain

The phytopathogen *S. vesicarium* was isolated from pears showing brown spot disease symptoms, sampled in Benevento, Campania, Italy, in 2019, as previously reported [1]. The strain was stored on Potato Dextrose Agar (PDA) plates in the culture collection of Agriges s.r.l., San Salvatore Telesino, Benevento, Italy (40.93345, 14.65799, 401 m.a.s.l.).

4.4. Extraction and Purification of Secondary Metabolites

Plant material (273.7 g) was extracted (1 × 500 mL) by H_2O/MeOH (1/1, *v/v*), 1% NaCl, under stirred conditions at room temperature for 24 h, the suspension was centrifuged, and the supernatant was extracted by *n*-hexane (3 × 300 mL) and successively with CH_2Cl_2 (3 × 300 mL) and, after removing methanol under reduced pressure, with EtOAc (3 × 200 mL). The residue (6.7 g) of CH_2Cl_2 organic extract was purified by CC eluted with CH_2Cl_2/*i*-PrOH (9/1, *v/v*), yielding thirteen homogeneous fractions (F1–F13). The most active fractions (F2–F5, Figure 1) were further purified. In particular, the residue (70.2 mg) of F2 was purified by CC eluted with CH_2Cl_2/MeOH (97/3, *v/v*), yielding seven groups of homogeneous fractions (F2.1–F2.7). The residue (21.2 mg) of fraction F2.3 was further purified by TLC eluted with CH_2Cl_2/MeOH (97/3, *v/v*), yielding alpinumisoflavone (**1**, 12.9 mg). The residues of F3–F4 were combined (for a total amount of 235.6 mg) and then purified by CC eluted with $CHCl_3$/*i*-PrOH (95/5, *v/v*), yielding seven fractions. The residue of the fourth fraction of the latter column were further purified by two successive steps on TLC eluted with $CHCl_3$/MeOH (95/5, *v/v*) and EtOAc/*n*-hexane (4/6, *v/v*), yielding hydroxyalpinumisoflavone (**2**, 3.2 mg), laburnetin (**3**, 1.3 mg), and licoflavone C (**4**, 3.1 mg). The residue (98.2 mg) of F5 was purified by CC eluted with CH_2Cl_2/MeOH (95/5, *v/v*), yielding four fractions. The residue of the second fraction of this latter column was further purified by TLC eluted three times with acetone/*n*-hexane (4/6, *v/v*), yielding four metabolites. They were identified as retamasin B (**5**, 3.3 mg), ephedroidin (**6**, 10.1 mg), and further amounts of laburnetin (**3**, 1.0 mg, total of 2.3 mg) and licoflavone C (**4**, 1.1 mg, total of 4.2 mg).

Alpinumisoflavone (**1**): ^{1}H and ^{13}C NMR data are in agreement with those previously reported [38,39]. ESI MS (+) *m/z*: 695 $[2M + Na]^+$, 337 $[M + H]^+$.
Hydroxyalpinumisoflavone (**2**): ^{1}H NMR data are in agreement with those previously reported [41]. ESI MS (+) *m/z*: 727 $[2M + Na]^+$, 333 $[M + H]^+$.
Laburnetin (**3**): ^{1}H and ^{13}C NMR data are in agreement with those previously reported [42]. ESI-MS (+), *m/z*: 355 $[M + H]^+$.
Licoflavone C (**4**): ^{1}H and ^{13}C NMR data are in agreement with those previously reported [43]. ESI-MS (+), *m/z*: 339 $[M + H]^+$.
Retamasin B (**5**): ^{1}H and ^{13}C NMR data are in agreement with those previously reported [44]. ESI-MS (+), *m/z*: 727 $[2M + Na]^+$, 353 $[M + H]^+$.
Ephedroidin (**6**): $[\alpha]_D^{25}$ 0 (c 0.4, MeOH), ^{1}H and ^{13}C NMR data are in agreement with those previously reported [41]. ESI-MS (+), *m/z*: 355 $[M + H]^+$.

4.5. X-ray Crystal Structure Analysis of Compound **1**

Single crystals of compound **1** suitable for X-ray analysis were obtained by slow evaporation from a mixture of MeOH:H_2O (9.0:1.0). X-ray diffraction data were collected on a Bruker-Nonius KappaCCD diffractometer (Bruker-Nonius, Delft, The Netherlands) (graphite mono-chromated MoKα radiation, λ = 0.71073 Å). The structure was solved by direct methods (SIR97 program) [53] and anisotropically refined by the full-matrix least-squares method on F^2 against all independent measured reflections (SHELXL-2018/3 program) [54]. H atoms of hydroxy groups were located in different Fourier maps and freely refined. All the other hydrogen atoms were introduced in calculated positions and refined according to the riding model. Platon TwinRotMap check suggests 2-axis (0 0 1) [1 0 4] twinning with basf 0.10, and refinement was performed using the HKLF5 data file. The figure of the ORTEP view was generated using the ORTEP-3 program [55].

Crystallographic Data of **1**: $C_{20}H_{16}O_5$; M_r= 336.33; monoclinic, space group $P2_1/c$; a = 13.774(4) Å, b = 5.940(3)Å, c = 19.936(5) Å, β = 99.673(15)°; V = 1607.9(10) Å^3; T = 173 K; Z = 4; D_c = 1.389 g cm^{-3}; μ = 0.100 mm^{-1}, F (000) = 704. Independent reflections: 9456. The final R_1 values were 0.0569, wR_2 = 0.1129 ($I > 2\sigma(I)$). Goodness of fit on F^2 = 1.081. Largest diff. peak and hole = 0.203 and −0.252 e/$Å^3$.

4.6. Antifungal Assay

The extract obtained from *R. raetam* aerial parts was tested against the phytopathogen *S. vesicarium*, as described by Yusoff et al. [56], with some modifications. The crude extract and the following fractions were dissolved in MeOH and mixed with 5 mL of cooled PDA to obtain a final concentration of 2 mg/mL and 250 µg/mL, respectively. The mix was then poured into Petri dishes and left to dry. Fungal plugs (6 × 6 mm diameter) cut from the growing edge of *S. vesicarium* mycelium were placed in the center of the plates and grown for 6/7 days at 28 ± 2 °C. Plates containing the fungal plugs alone were used as a control. As a positive control, fungicidal pentachloronitrobenzene ≥ 94% (PCNB) (Sigma-Aldrich, Saint-Louis, MO, USA) dissolved in toluene was used. Toluene and MeOH were used as negative controls. The in vitro antifungal bioassays of the purified metabolites, **1** laburnetin, **2** licoflavone C, **3** alpinumisoflavone, **4** hydroxyalpinumisoflavone, **5** raetamsin B, and **6** ephedroidin, were performed according to the method previously described in [57], with some modifications. The metabolites and PCNB dissolved in 8% acetone and toluene, respectively, were placed at the four opposite sides of each Petri dish, 1 cm away from the fungal plug at the center of the plate, at a final concentration of 50 µg/mL. Acetone and toluene were used as negative controls. The plates were incubated for 6/7 days at 28 ± 2 °C. The percentage of inhibition of the fungal growth was calculated using the following formula:

$$\% = [(Rc - Ri)/Rc] \times 100 \quad (1)$$

where *Rc* is the radial growth of the test fungi in the control plates (mm), and *Ri* is the radial growth of the fungi in the presence of different compounds tested (mm). The results show the antifungal activity of different compounds analyzed by ANOVA using Tukey's test. The experiments were performed in triplicate.

4.7. Broomrape Assays

Allelopathic effects of alpinumisoflavone, ephedroidin, hydroxyalpinoisolflavone, laburnetin, licoflavone C, and retamasin B were tested on broomrape suicidal germination and radicle growth in two independent bioassays conducted according to previous protocols [51].

Seeds of four broomrape species, *Orobanche crenata*, *Orobanche cumana*, *Orobanche minor*, and *Phelipanche ramosa*, were surface-sterilized by immersion in 0.5% (*w/v*) NaOCl and 0.02% (*v/v*) Tween 20, for 5 min, rinsed thoroughly with sterile distilled water, and dried in a laminar airflow cabinet. First, broomrape seeds were submitted to a conditioning period using a warm stratification, as follows. Approximately 100 seeds of each broomrape species were placed separately on 9 mm-diameter glass fiber filter paper disks (GFFP) (Whatman International Ltd., Maidstone, UK), moistened with 50 µL of sterile distilled water, and placed in incubators at 23 °C for 10 days inside Parafilm-sealed Petri dishes, to allow seed conditioning.

Then, GFFP disks containing conditioned broomrape seeds were transferred onto a sterile sheet of filter paper and transferred to new 9 cm sterile Petri dishes. For the assay of suicidal germination, induction stock solutions of each metabolite respectively dissolved in methanol were individually diluted in sterile distilled water up to an equivalent concentration of 100 µM. For the assay of radicle growth inhibition, stock solutions of each metabolite respectively dissolved in methanol were individually diluted to 100 µM using an aqueous solution of GR24. For each assay, triplicate aliquots of each sample were applied to GFFP discs containing conditioned broomrape seeds. Treated seeds were incubated in the dark at 23 °C for 7 days and the percent of germination and radicle growth was determined for each GFFP disc, as described previously [51], using a stereoscopic microscope (Leica S9i, Leica Microsystems GmbH, Wetzlar, Germany). For germination induction assays, the germination was determined by counting the number of germinated seeds on 100 seeds for each GFFP disk. For the characteristic of radicle growth, the value used was the average of 10 randomly selected radicles per GFFP disc [58]. The percentage of germination induction of each metabolite was then calculated relative to the average germination of control seeds (seeds treated with water), and the percentage of radicle growth inhibition of each treatment was then calculated relative to the average radicle growth of control treatment (radicles treated with GR24) [41].

4.8. Data Analysis

Statistical analyses were performed using GraphPad Prism 8 software, and data were expressed as the mean ± SD. Differences among groups were compared by the ANOVA test. Differences were considered statistically significant at $p < 0.05$.

Supplementary Materials: The following supporting information can be downloaded at: https://www.mdpi.com/article/10.3390/toxins14050311/s1, Scheme S1:Extraction and bioguided purification of compounds 1–6 from R. raetam aerial parts; Figure S1: ^{1}H NMR spectrum of alpinumisoflavone, 1 (acetone-*d6*, 400 MHz); Figure S2: ^{13}C NMR spectrum of alpinumisoflavone, 1 (acetone-*d6*, 100 MHz); Figure S3: ESI MS spectrum of alpinumisoflavone, 1 recorded in positive modality; Figure S4: ^{1}H NMR spectrum of hydroxyalpinumisoflavone, 2 (MeOD, 500 MHz); Figure S5: ESI MS spectrum of hydroxyalpinumisoflavone, 2 recorded in positive modality; Figure S6: H NMR spectrum of laburnetin, 3 (MeOD, 500 MHz); Figure S7: ESI MS spectrum of laburnetin, 3 recorded in positive modality; Figure S8: ^{1}H NMR spectrum of licoflavone C, 4 (acetone-*d6*, 500 MHz); Figure S9: ESI MS spectrum of licoflavone C, 4 recorded in positive modality; Figure S10: ^{1}H NMR spectrum of retamasin B, 5 (acetone-*d6*, 400 MHz); Figure S11: ^{13}C NMR spectrum of retamasin B, 5 (acetone-*d6*, 100 MHz); Figure S12: ^{13}C NMR spectrum of retamasin B, 5 (acetone-*d6*, 100 MHz); Figure S13: ^{1}H NMR spectrum of ephedroidin, 6 (acetone-*d6*, 500 MHz); Figure S14: ESI MS spectrum of ephedroidin, 6 recorded in positive modality.

Author Contributions: Resources, M.B., A.K., R.I., M.F.-A. and A.C.; conceptualization, C.P., M.M., M.F.-A. and A.C.; investigation, G.S., C.P., A.T., and M.F.-A.; formal analysis, C.P. and M.F.-A.; writing—original draft preparation, G.S., C.P., M.M. and A.C.; writing—review and editing, G.S., C.P., M.M., M.B., A.K., A.T., R.I., M.F.-A. and A.C.; supervision, A.C.; funding acquisition, G.S. and M.F.-A. All authors have read and agreed to the published version of the manuscript.

Funding: Financial support is acknowledged to G.S. from a Ph.D. grant funded by INPS (Istituto Nazionale Previdenza Sociale), and to M.F.-A. from the Spanish Ministry of Science and Innovation (grants PID2020-114668RB-I00 and RYC-2015-18961).

Institutional Review Board Statement: Not applicable.

Informed Consent Statement: Not applicable.

Data Availability Statement: Not applicable.

Conflicts of Interest: The authors declare no conflict of interest.

References

1. Petrillo, C.; Castaldi, S.; Lanzilli, M.; Selci, M.; Cordone, A.; Giovannelli, D.; Isticato, R. Genomic and physiological characterization of Bacilli isolated from salt-pans with plant growth promoting features. *Front. Microbiol.* **2021**, *12*, 715678–715693. [CrossRef] [PubMed]
2. Evidente, A.; Cimmino, A.; Masi, M. Phytotoxins produced by pathogenic fungi of agrarian plants. *Phytochem. Rev.* **2019**, *18*, 843–870. [CrossRef]
3. Castillo-Sánchez, L.E.; Jiménez-Osornio, J.J.; Delgado-Herrera, M.A. Secondary metabolites of the Annonaceae, Solanaceae and Meliaceae families used as biological control of insects. *Trop. Subtrop. Agroecosyst.* **2010**, *12*, 445–462.
4. Walia, S.; Saha, S.; Tripathi, V.; Sharma, K.K. Phytochemical biopesticides: Some recent developments. *Phytochem. Rev.* **2017**, *16*, 989–1007. [CrossRef]
5. Cimmino, A.; Masi, M.; Evidente, M.; Superchi, S.; Evidente, A. Fungal phytotoxins with potential herbicidal activity: Chemical and biological characterization. *Nat. Prod. Rep.* **2015**, *32*, 1629–1653. [CrossRef]
6. Ivanescu, B.; Burlec, A.F.; Crivoi, F.; Rosu, C.; Corciova, A. Secondary metabolites from *Artemisia* genus as biopesticides and innovative nano-based application strategies. *Molecules* **2021**, *26*, 3061. [CrossRef] [PubMed]

7. Bohinc, T.; Horvat, A.; Ocvirk, M.; Kosir, I.; Rutnik, K.; Trdan, S. The first evidence of the insecticidal potential of plant powders from invasive alien plants against rice weevil under laboratory conditions. *Appl. Sci.* **2020**, *10*, 7828. [CrossRef]
8. Lengai, G.M.W.; Muthomi, J.W.; Mbega, E.R. Phytochemical activity and role of botanical pesticides in pest management for sustainable agricultural crop production. *Sci. Afr.* **2020**, *7*, e00239. [CrossRef]
9. Freiesleben, S.H.; Jager, A.K. Correlation between plant secondary metabolites and their antifungal mechanisms—A review. *Med. Aromat. Plants* **2014**, 3, 1000154–1000160.
10. Saada, M.; Wasli, H.; Jallali, I.; Kboubi, R.; Girard-Lalancette, K.; Mshvildadze, V.; Ksouri, R.; Legault, J.; Cardoso, S.M. Bio-guided fractionation of *Retama raetam* (Forssk.) webb & berthel polar extracts. *Molecules* **2021**, *26*, 5800–5816.
11. Kim, Y.M.; Lee, C.H.; Kim, H.G.; Lee, H.S. Anthraquinones isolated from Cassia tora (Leguminosae) seed show an antifungal property against phytopathogenic fungi. *J. Agric. Food Chem.* **2004**, *52*, 6096–6100. [CrossRef]
12. Llorente, I.; Moragrega, C.; Ruz, L.; Montesinos, E. An update on control of brown spot of pear. *Trees* **2012**, *26*, 239–245. [CrossRef] [PubMed]
13. Brunelli, R.; Rovesti, R.; Di Marco, S.; Ponti, I. Attivita di diversifungicide contro la maculatura bruna del pero. *Riv. Frutticolt. Ortofloricolt.* **1986**, *1*, 51–54.
14. Fernández-Aparicio, M.; Flores, F.; Rubiales, D. The effect of Orobanche crenata infection severity in faba bean, field pea and grass pea productivity. *Front. Plant Sci.* **2016**, *7*, 1049–1057. [CrossRef]
15. Cimmino, A.; Masi, M.; Rubiale, D.; Evidente, A.; Fernández-Aparicio, M. Allelopathy for parasitic plant management. *Nat. Prod. Commun.* **2018**, *13*, 289–294. [CrossRef]
16. Fernández-Aparicio, M.; Delavault, P.; Timko, M.P. Management of infection by parasitic weeds: A Review. *Plants* **2020**, *9*, 1184. [CrossRef] [PubMed]
17. Hammouche-Mokranea, N.; León-Gonzálezb, A.J.; Navarroc, I.; Boulilaa, F.; Benallaouad, S.; Martín-Corderob, C. Phytochemical profile and antibacterial activity of *Retama raetam* and *R. sphaerocarpa* cladodes from Algeria. *Nat. Prod. Commun.* **2017**, *12*, 1857–1860. [CrossRef]
18. González-Mauraza, H.; Martín-Cordero, C.; Alarcón-de-la-Lastra, C.; Rosillo, M.A.; León-González, A.J.; Sánchez-Hidalgo, M. Anti-inflammatory effects of *Retama monosperma* in acute ulcerative colitis in rats. *J. Physiol. Biochem.* **2014**, *70*, 163–172. [CrossRef]
19. El-toumy, S.A.; Mohamed, S.M.; Hassan, E.M.; Mossa, A.T.H. Phenolic metabolites from *Acacia nilotica* flowers and evaluation of its free radical scavenging activity. *Am. J. Sci.* **2011**, *7*, 287–295. [CrossRef]
20. Belayachi, L.; Aceves-Luquero, C.; Merghoub, N.; Bakri, Y.; de Mattos, S.F.; Amzazi, S.; Villalonga, P. *Retama monosperma n*-hexane extract induces cell cycle arrest and extrinsic pathway-dependent apoptosis in Jurkat cells. *BMC Complement. Altern. Med.* **2014**, *14*, 38–49. [CrossRef]
21. Hayet, E.; Maha, M.; Samia, A.; Mata, M.; Gros, P.; Raida, H.; Ali, M.; Ali, M.; Gutmann, L.; Mighri, Z.; et al. Antimicrobial, antioxidant, and antiviral activities of *Retama raetam* (Forssk.) Webb flowers growing in Tunisia. *World J. Microbiol. Biotechnol.* **2008**, *24*, 2933–2940. [CrossRef]
22. Omara, E.A.; Nada, S.A.; El-Toumy, S.A. Evaluation of hepatoprotective activity of the *Retama raetam* seeds on carbon tetrachloride-induced liver damage in rats. *Planta Med.* **2009**, *75*, 29. [CrossRef]
23. Koriem, K.M.M.; Arbid, M.S.; El-Gendy, N.F.I. The protective role of *Tropaeolum majus* on blood and liver toxicity induced by diethyl maleate in rats. *Toxicol. Mech. Methods* **2010**, *20*, 579–586. [CrossRef]
24. León-González, A.J.; Navarro, I.; Acero, N.; Mingarro, M.D.; Martín-Cordero, C. Genus Retama: A review on traditional uses, phytochemistry, and pharmacological activities. *Phytochem. Rev.* **2018**, *17*, 701–731. [CrossRef]
25. Hassan, S.; Mathesius, U. The role of flavonoids in root–rhizosphere signalling: Opportunities and challenges for improving plant–microbe interactions. *J. Exp. Bot.* **2012**, *63*, 3429–3444. [CrossRef]
26. Chouikh, A.; Fatma, A. Phytochemical properties, antibacterial and anti-free radical activities of the phenolic extracts of *Retama raetam* (Forssk) Webb. & Berthel. collected from Algeria Desert. *Ovidius Univ. Ann. Chem.* **2021**, *32*, 33–39.
27. Saada, M.; Falleh, H.; Catarino, M.D.; Cardoso, S.M.; Ksouri, R. Plant growth modulates metabolites and biological activities in Retama raetam (Forssk.) Webb. *Molecules* **2018**, *23*, 2177. [CrossRef]
28. Ould El Hadj, M.; Hadj-Mahammed, M.; Zabeirou, H. Place des Plantes Spontanées dans la Médicine Traditionnelle de la Région de Ouargla (Sahara Septentrional Est). *Courr. Savoir* **2003**, 47–51. Available online: http://archives.univ-biskra.dz/handle/123456789/395 (accessed on 1 April 2022).
29. Atmani, D.; Chaher, N.; Berboucha, M.; Ayouni, K.; Lounis, H.; Boudaoud, H.; Debbache, N.; Atmani, D. Antioxidant capacity and phenol content of selected Algerian medicinal plants. *Food Chem.* **2009**, *112*, 303–309. [CrossRef]
30. Benlamdini, N.; Elhafian, M.; Rochdi, A.; Zidane, L. Étude floristique et ethnobotanique de la flore médicinale du Haut Atlas oriental (Haute Moulouya). *J. Appl. Biosci.* **2014**, *78*, 6771–6787. [CrossRef]
31. Ramdane, F.; Mahfoud Hadj, M.; Ould Hadj, M.; Chanai, A.; Hammoudi, R.; Hillali, N.; Mesrouk, H.; Bouafia, I.; Bahaz, C Ethnobotanical study of some medicinal plants from Hoggar, Algeria. *J. Med. Plants Res.* **2015**, *9*, 820–827.
32. Bouafiane, M.; Khelil, A.; Cimmino, A.; Kemassi, A. Prediction and evaluation of allelopathic plants species in Algerian Saharan ecosystem. *Perspect. Plant Ecol. Evol. Syst.* **2021**, *53*, 125647. [CrossRef]
33. Masi, M.; Roscetto, E.; Cimmino, A.; Catania, M.R.; Surico, G.; Evidente, A. Farnesane-type sesquiterpenoids with antibiotic activity from *Chiliadenus lopadusanus*. *Antibiotics* **2021**, *10*, 148. [CrossRef] [PubMed]

34. Cimmino, A.; Roscetto, E.; Masi, M.; Tuzi, A.; Radjai, I.; Gahdab, C.; Paolillo, R.; Guarino, A.; Catania, M.R.; Evidente, A. Sesquiterpene lactones from *Cotula cinerea* with antibiotic activity against clinical isolates of *Enterococcus faecalis*. *Antibiotics* **2021**, *10*, 819. [CrossRef] [PubMed]
35. Wang, W.; Jiang, L.; Zhu, Y.; Mei, L.; Tao, Y.; Liu, Z. Bioactivity-guided isolation of cyclooxygenase-2 inhibitors from *Saussurea obvallata* (DC.) Edgew. Using affinity solid phase extraction assay. *J. Ethnopharmacol.* **2022**, *284*, 114785. [CrossRef] [PubMed]
36. Ahmed, S.R.; El-sherei, M.M.; Michel, C.G.; Musa, A.; Al-Sanea, M.M.; Qasim, S. Botanical description, bioactivity guided isolation and in silico mode of action of anti-diabetic constituents of *Pterocarpus dalbergioides* flowers. *S. Afr. J. Bot.* **2022**, *147*, 163–175. [CrossRef]
37. Atanasov, A.G.; Zotchev, S.B.; Dirsch, V.M.; Supuran, C.T. Natural products in drug discovery: Advances and opportunities. *Nat. Rev. Drug Discov.* **2021**, *20*, 200–216. [CrossRef]
38. Jackson, B.; Owen, P.J.; Sceihnmann, F. Extractives from poisonous British plants. Part I. The structure of alpinumisoflavone, a new pyranoisoflavone from *Laburnum alpinum* J. Presl. *J. Chem. Soc. C* **1971**, *20*, 3389–3392. [CrossRef]
39. Olivares, M.E.; Lwande, W.; Delle Monache, F.; Marini Bettolo, G.B. A pyrano-isoflavone from seeds of *Milletia thonningii*. *Phyrochemistry* **1982**, *21*, 1763–1765. [CrossRef]
40. Han, X.H.; Hong, S.S.; Hwang, J.S.; Jeong, S.H.; Hwang, J.H.; Lee, H.M.; Lee, M.K.; Lee, D.; Ro, J.S.; Hwang, B.Y. Monoamine oxidase inhibitory constituents from the fruits of *Cudrania tricuspidate*. *Arch. Pharm. Res.* **2005**, *28*, 1324–1327. [CrossRef]
41. Pistelli, L.; Bertoli, A.; Giachi, I.; Manunta, A. Flavonoids from *Genista ephedroides*. *J. Nat. Prod.* **1998**, *61*, 1404–1406. [CrossRef] [PubMed]
42. Sato, H.; Tahara, S.; Ingham, J.L.; Dziedzic, S.Z. Isoflavones from pods of *Laburnum anagyroides*. *Phytochemistry* **1995**, *39*, 673–676. [CrossRef]
43. Kajiyama, K.; Demizu, S.; Hiraga, Y. New prenylflavones and dibenzoylmethane from *Glycyrrhiza inflata*. *J. Nat. Prod.* **1992**, *55*, 1197–1203. [CrossRef]
44. Xu, W.H.; Al-Rehaily, A.J.; Yousaf, M.; Ahmad, M.S.; Khan, S.I.; Khan, I.A. Two new flavonoids from *Retama raetam*. *Helv. Chim. Acta* **2015**, *98*, 561–568. [CrossRef]
45. Harrison, J.J.E.K.; Tabuchi, Y.; Ishida, H.; Kingsford-Adaboh, R. Alpinumisoflavone. *Acta Crystallogr. E* **2008**, *64*, 713. [CrossRef] [PubMed]
46. Edziri, H.; Mastouri, M.; Mahjoub, M.A.; Mighri, Z.; Mahjoub, A.; Verschaeve, L. Antibacterial, antifungal and cytotoxic activities of two flavonoids from *Retama raetam* flowers. *Molecules* **2012**, *17*, 7284–7293. [CrossRef]
47. Cimmino, A.; Masi, M.; Evidente, M.; Superchi, S.; Evidente, A. Application of Mosher's method for absolute configuration assignment to bioactive plants and fungi metabolites. *J. Pharm. Biomed.* **2017**, *144*, 59–89. [CrossRef] [PubMed]
48. Zheng, D.; Zhang, H.; Jiang, J.-M.; Chen, Y.-Y.; Wan, S.-J.; Lin, Z.-X.; Xu, H.-X. Prenylated xanthones and biphenyls from *Garcinia esculenta* with antistaphylococcal activity. *Nat. Prod. Res.* **2021**, *35*, 2137–2144. [CrossRef]
49. Kuete, V.; Ngameni, B.; Simo, C.C.F.; Tankeu, R.K.; Ngadjui, B.T.; Meyer, J.J.M.; Lall, N.; Kuiate, J.R. Antimicrobial activity of the crude extracts and compounds from *Ficus chlamydocarpa* and *Ficus cordata* (Moraceae). *J. Ethnopharmacol.* **2008**, *120*, 17–24. [CrossRef]
50. Zwanenburg, B.; Mwakaboko, A.S.; Kannan, C. Suicidal germination for parasitic weed control. *Pest Man. Sci.* **2016**, *72*, 2016–2025. [CrossRef] [PubMed]
51. Cimmino, A.; Fernandez-Aparicio, M.; Andolfi, A.; Basso, S.; Rubiales, D.; Evidente, A. Effect of fungal and plant metabolites on broomrapes (*Orobanche* and *Phelipanche* spp.) seed germination and radicle growth. *J. Agric. Food Chem.* **2014**, *62*, 10485–10492. [CrossRef]
52. Kassem, M.; Mosharrafa, S.A.; Saleh, N.A.; Abdel-Wahab, S.M. Two new flavonoids from *Retama raetam*. *Fitoterapia* **2000**, *71*, 649–654. [CrossRef]
53. Altomare, A.; Burla, M.C.; Camalli, M.; Cacarano, G.L.; Giacovazzo, C.; Guagliardi, A.; Moliterni, A.G.G.; Polidori, G.; Spagna, R. SIR97: A new tool for crystal structure determination and refinement. *J. Appl. Crystallogr.* **1999**, *32*, 115–119. [CrossRef]
54. Sheldrick, G.M. Crystal structure refinement with SHELXL. *Acta Crystallogr. Sect. C Struct. Chem.* **2015**, *71*, 3–8. [CrossRef] [PubMed]
55. Farrugia, L.J. WinGX and ORTEP for Windows: An Update. *J. Appl. Crystallogr.* **2012**, *45*, 849–854. [CrossRef]
56. Yusoff, S.F.; Haron, F.; Muda, M.; Asib, N.S.Z.; Ismail, S. Antifungal activity and phytochemical screening of *Vernonia amygdalina* extract against *Botrytis cinerea* causing gray mold disease on tomato fruits. *Biology* **2020**, *9*, 286. [CrossRef] [PubMed]
57. Puopolo, G.; Masi, M.; Raio, A.; Andolfi, A.; Zoina, A.; Cimmino, A.; Evidente, A. Insights on the susceptibility of plant pathogenic fungi to phenazine-1-carboxylic acid and its chemical derivatives. *Nat. Prod. Res.* **2013**, *27*, 956–966. [CrossRef] [PubMed]
58. Westwood, J.H.; Foy, C.L. Influence of nitrogen on germination and early development of broomrape (*Orobanche* spp.). *Weed Sci.* **1999**, *47*, 2–7. [CrossRef]

toxins

Article

Iridoid Glycosides Isolated from *Bellardia trixago* Identified as Inhibitors of *Orobanche cumana* Radicle Growth

Gabriele Soriano [1], Antonietta Siciliano [2], Mónica Fernández-Aparicio [3,*], Antonio Cala Peralta [1,4], Marco Masi [1,*], Antonio Moreno-Robles [5], Marco Guida [2] and Alessio Cimmino [1]

1 Department of Chemical Sciences, University of Naples Federico II, Complesso Universitario Monte S. Angelo, Via Cintia 4, 80126 Naples, Italy
2 Department of Biology, University of Naples Federico II, Complesso Universitario Monte Sant'Angelo, Via Cintia 4, 80126 Naples, Italy
3 Department of Plant Breeding, Institute for Sustainable Agriculture (IAS), CSIC, Avenida Menéndez Pidal s/n, 14004 Córdoba, Spain
4 Allelopathy Group, Department of Organic Chemistry, School of Science, Institute of Biomolecules (INBIO), University of Cádiz, C/República Saharaui 7, 11510 Cádiz, Spain
5 Department of Electronics and Computer Engineering, University of Córdoba, Campus de Rabanales, 14071 Córdoba, Spain
* Correspondence: monica.fernandez@ias.csic.es (M.F.-A.); marco.masi@unina.it (M.M.)

Abstract: *Orobanche cumana* is an obligate holoparasitic plant with noxious effects in sunflower crops. *Bellardia trixago* is a facultative hemiparasitic plant that infects ruderal plants without noxious significance in agriculture and is known to produce a wide spectrum of bioactive metabolites. The objective of this study was to evaluate the allelopathic effects of *B. trixago* on the growth of *O. cumana* seedlings. Three different extracts using solvents of increasing polarity (*n*-hexane, dichloromethane and ethyl acetate) were prepared from the flowers, aerial green organs and roots of two populations, a white-flowered and a yellow-flowered population of *B. trixago*, both collected in southern Spain. Each extract was studied using allelopathic screenings on *O. cumana* which resulted in the identification of allelopathic activity of the ethyl acetate extracts against *Orobanche* radicles. Five iridoid glycosides were isolated together with benzoic acid from the ethyl acetate extract of aerial green organs by bio-guided purification. These compounds were identified as bartsioside, melampyroside, mussaenoside gardoside methyl ester and aucubin. Among them, melampyroside was found to be the most abundant constituent in the extract (44.3% *w*/*w*), as well as the most phytotoxic iridoid on *O. cumana* radicle, showing a 72.6% inhibition of radicle growth. This activity of melampyroside was significantly high when compared with the inhibitory activity of benzoic acid (25.9%), a phenolic acid with known allelopathic activity against weeds. The ecotoxicological profile of melampyroside was evaluated using organisms representing different trophic levels of the aquatic and terrestrial ecosystems, namely producers (green freshwater algae *Raphidocelis subcapitata* and macrophyte *Lepidium sativum*), consumers (water flea *Daphnia magna* and nematode *Caenorhabditis elegans*) and decomposers (bacterium *Aliivibrio fischeri*). The ecotoxicity of melampyroside differed significantly depending on the test organism showing the highest toxicity to daphnia, nematodes and bacteria, and a lower toxicity to algae and macrophytes. The findings of the present study may provide useful information for the generation of green alternatives to synthetic herbicides for the control of *O. cumana*.

Keywords: parasitic weed; melampyroside; allelopathy; ecotoxicity; sustainable crop protection

Key Contribution: Five iridoid glycosides and benzoic acid were isolated from the ethyl acetate extract of aerial vegetative organs from plants of a white-flowered *Bellardia trixago* population Bartsioside, melampyroside and mussaenoside were identified for the first time as inhibitors of *Orobanche cumana* radicle growth. Melampyroside was found to be the most phytotoxic compound and could be considered as a promising biocontrol agent for *O. cumana* considering the absence of relevant toxic effects observed in a preliminary ecotoxicological study.

Citation: Soriano, G.; Siciliano, A.; Fernández-Aparicio, M.; Cala Peralta, A.; Masi, M.; Moreno-Robles, A.; Guida, M.; Cimmino, A. Iridoid Glycosides Isolated from *Bellardia trixago* Identified as Inhibitors of *Orobanche cumana* Radicle Growth. *Toxins* **2022**, *14*, 559. https://doi.org/10.3390/toxins14080559

Received: 15 July 2022
Accepted: 14 August 2022
Published: 17 August 2022

1. Introduction

Approximately 1% of all angiosperms are parasites with the ability to infect other plants. Some parasitic plants are facultative parasites, capable of living autotrophically but shifting to a parasitic life form when a host is available, while others are obligated parasites requiring the infection of another plant shortly after germination. Some parasitic plants are hemiparasites with the ability to photosynthesize, while others are holoparasitic plants without photosynthetic competence, relying on their host for photoassimilates. Parasitic plants are distributed among 28 dicotyledonous families, and among them, the Orobanchaceae contains examples of parasitic species from all cases of host dependency [1,2]. Orobanchaceae contains facultative hemiparasitic plants, such as the non-weedy *Bellardia trixago* L. (syn. *Bartsia trixago* L.) with a Mediterranean origin that parasitizes the roots of ruderal species [3,4]. Orobanchaceae also contains obligate holoparasitic weeds from *Orobanche* genus from which control is limited or non-existent [5].

Among *Orobanche* species, *Orobanche cumana* Wallr. is one of the most noxious biotic stresses for sunflower crops [6]. Sunflower infection by *O. cumana* occurs in southern and eastern Europe, in the Mediterranean basin and in Asia [7]. Both types of sunflower, the oilseed type and the confectionary type, are severely affected by *O. cumana* [8]. The most feasible crop protection measures against the infection of *Orobanche* species are the cultivation of resistant varieties and chemical control [1,9]. However, for the specific sunflower problem caused by *O. cumana*, the resistant varieties are not durable, since their bred resistance is overcome by new races of *O. cumana* [10]. On the other hand, the chemical solution to control *O. cumana* is the use of imidazolinone herbicides that inhibit the enzyme acetohydroxy acid synthase [8,11]. However, the capacity to evolve imidazolinone-resistance in weeds, and the lack of alternative chemical methods for *O. cumana* threatens the sustainability of chemical control of *O. cumana* in sunflower [12]. Characterization of novel modes of allelopathic action against *O. cumana* in previously known natural compounds is an alternative solution to provide efficacy and sustainability in strategies for parasitic weed management [13].

B. trixago is a source of several bioactive compounds [14–17] but the screening of *B. trixago* as source of herbicidal compounds has not been performed before. Different *B. trixago* extracts have been screened for insecticidal activity [18,19]. Formisano et al. [19] demonstrated variation in insecticidal activity among different parts of *B. trixago* plants, with root extracts being significantly more active than extracts from aerial parts. In addition, Barrero et al. [16] demonstrated that qualitative and quantitative differences exist in the plant chemical composition among different populations of *B. trixago*. Here, we report the isolation and identification of iridoid glycosides—bartsioside, melampyroside and mussaenoside—with inhibitory activity on *O. cumana* radicle growth. Furthermore, the ecotoxicity of melampyroside (the most phytotoxic compound isolated) was assessed considering aquatic and terrestrial ecosystems as well as different trophic levels to reveal its toxicity and safety to environment and human health in order to be used as potent biocontrol agent.

2. Results and Discussion

Three different organs (flowers, aerial vegetative green organs and roots) of two *B. trixago* populations (a white-flowered and yellow-flowered population) were extracted by maceration with a hydroalcoholic solution and then employing three different solvents of increasing polarity (*n*-hexane, dichloromethane and ethyl acetate) in sequential order as described in the Materials and Methods section. The allelopathic activity of the resulting *B. trixago* extracts was analysed at 100 μg/mL using radicle growth bioassays on *O. cumana* (Figure 1). The inhibition of radicle growth was significantly affected by the *B. trixago* population and by the solvent used for the extraction, but not by the plant organ (ANOVA, $p = 0.022$, $p < 0.001$ and $p = 0.347$ respectively). Significant effects on radicle growth inhibition were observed by the interaction of *B. trixago* population × plant organ (ANOVA, $p = 0.002$), by the interaction *B. trixago* population × solvent used for the extraction (ANOVA, $p < 0.007$) and also by the interaction plant organ × solvent used for the extraction (ANOVA, $p < 0.009$). Previously, quantitative and qualitative variations in the chemical profiles have been reported among different populations of *B. trixago* [16] and among different plant organs of *B. trixago* plants [19]. Formisano et al. [19] located the insecticidal activity in the roots of one *B. trixago* population collected in Italy, whereas aerial parts of plants of the same population were less active.

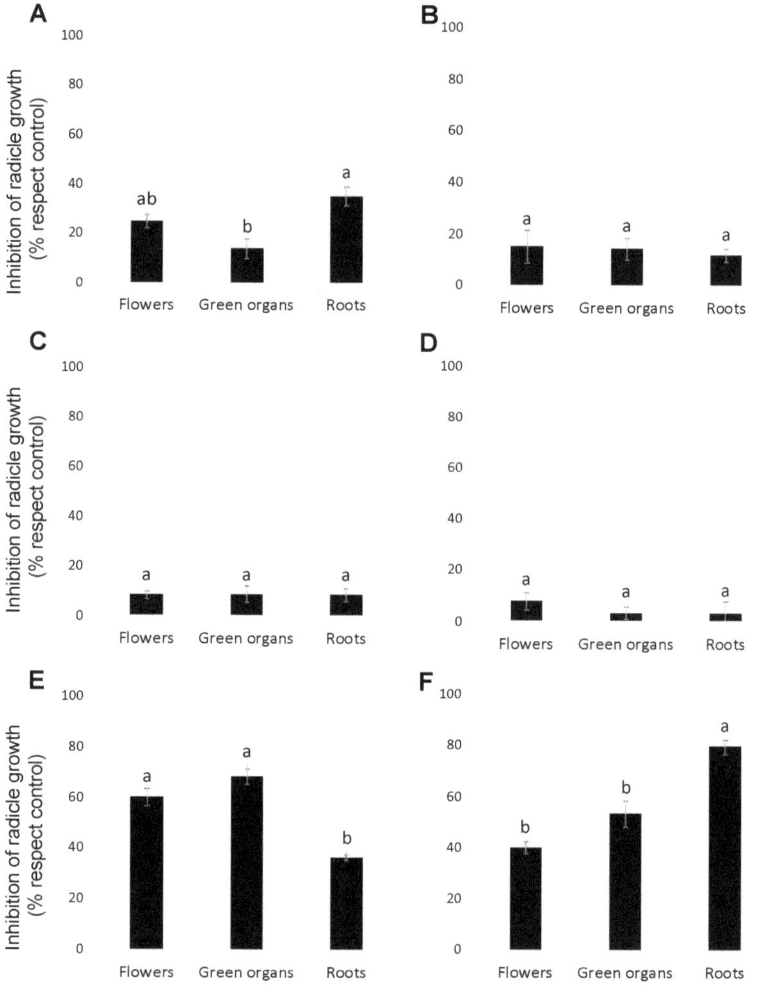

Figure 1. Allelopathic effects on *Orobanche cumana* radicle growth induced by extracts prepared from sequential extractions with *n*-hexane (**A**,**B**), dichloromethane (**C**,**D**), and ethyl acetate (**E**,**F**) of three types of *Bellardia trixago* organs: flowers, aerial green organs and roots of two *Bellardia trixago* populations—a white-flowered population (**A**,**C**,**E**) and yellow-flowered population (**B**,**D**,**F**). In each figure, bars with different letters are significantly different according to the Tukey test ($p = 0.05$). Error bars represent the standard error of the mean.

In both populations studied, the main inhibitory activity was obtained with the ethyl acetate (EtOAc) extraction (Figure 1E,F). In the white-flowered population, the strongest inhibitory activity was found in the EtOAc extract of the aerial parts, mainly in the green vegetative organs followed by the EtOAc extract of the flowers (68.31 ± 2.9% and 60.1 ± 3.4%

inhibition, respectively, in comparison with control). In the yellow-flowered *B. trixago* population, the strongest *Orobanche* inhibition activity was found in the EtOAc extract of roots (inhibition average of 79.5 ± 2.9%), followed by the EtOAc extracts of aerial parts of plants, both green organs and flowers (53.5 ± 5.1% and 40.1 ± 2.5% inhibition, respectively, in comparison with control). As a result of the allelopathic screening, a preliminary qualitative evaluation of the chromatographic profiles of all EtOAc extracts was performed. This evaluation revealed the common presence of a main compound and a common pattern of secondary metabolites among the different populations and plant organs (data not showed). This fact and also the larger amount of vegetative green tissues available in the laboratory allowed the selection of EtOAc extract of green organs of the white-flowered population as the source for the isolation and characterization of inhibitors of *O. cumana* radicle growth.

Thus, an amount of 189.0 g of lyophilized green organs of the white population were extracted following the procedure described in the Materials and Methods section. The sample yielded 1.45 g (0.77%) of EtOAc organic extract which was fractionated by different steps of purification by column chromatography and preparative TLCs, as reported in Scheme S1, obtaining six pure compounds which were identified as benzoic acid (**1**, 10.8 mg), bartsioside (**2**, 13.9 mg), aucubin (**3**, 12.4 mg), melampyroside (**4**, 642.3 mg), gardoside methyl ester (**5**, 2.0 mg), and mussaenoside (**6**, 6.1 mg) (Figure 2). The structures of these compounds were confirmed by NMR spectroscopy and MS, and by comparison with the data reported in the literature. Optical rotation allowed us to unequivocally identify the stereochemistry of the compounds by comparing with the values of the natural iridoids, which is a well-established family of natural products among which absolute stereochemistry was previously reported by chiroptical methods and X Ray [20,21]. Compounds **1** [16] and **2**–**6** were previously isolated from *B. trixago* [17,22] and other iridoid-containing plants [23–30].

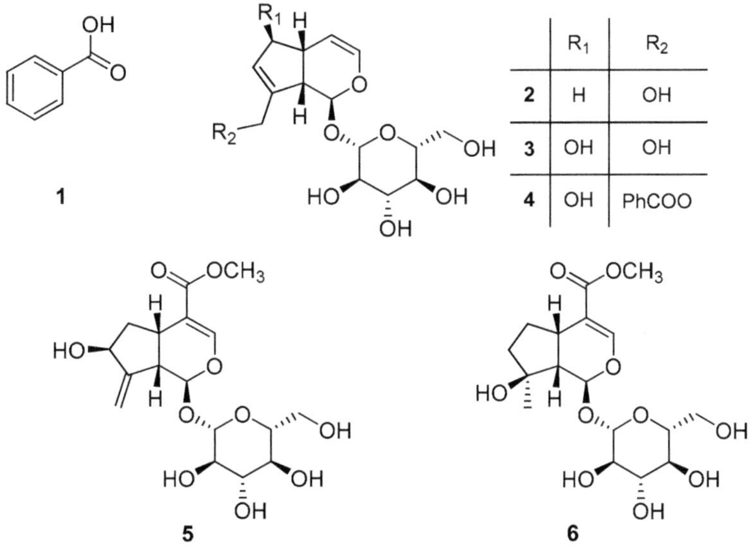

Figure 2. Chemical structures of benzoic acid (**1**), bartsioside (**2**), aucubin (**3**), melampyroside (**4**), gardoside methyl ester (**5**), and mussaenoside (**6**).

The allelopathic effects of compounds **1**–**6** were assayed at 100 μg/mL on *O. cumana* radicles (Figure 3). Compounds **3** and **5** showed no significant inhibitory activity in the growth of *O. cumana* radicles in comparison with radicles treated with the control. On the other hand, compound **4** showed the strongest inhibition of radicle growth (72.6 ± 0.9%), followed by the inhibition activity induced by compounds **2** and **6** (61.1 ± 1.5% and 65.9 ± 2.9%, respectively). This is the first time that the inhibitory activity of *Orobanche* radicle growth has been reported in compounds **2**, **4** and **6**. Their activity was significantly higher than the activity of compound **1**, a phenolic acid with recognized weedicide activity [31]. Compound **1** showed low but significant inhibitory activity on *O. cumana* radicle (25.9 ± 0.3%), which agrees with the moderate inhibitory activity observed by a previously study on the radicles of the legume-specific parasitic plant *Orobanche crenata* [32]. Compound **1** has been previously described as a growth-regulating agent, affecting plant growth in a dose-dependent manner on different plants [33–35]. Previous reports describe formulations including **1** in a combination with other components as an herbicide or growth-regulating agent [36–38].

Compound **4** was firstly reported as an iridoid in *Melampyrum silvaticum* L. [39] while compounds **2**, **3**, **5** and **6** were first isolated from *B. trixago* [15], *Aucuba japonica* Thunb. [40], *Melampyrum arvense* L. [28] and *Mussaenda parviflora* Miq. [41], respectively. In the recent literature, it has been reported that compound **4** has anti-inflammatory activity [42], along with other iridoids not reported herein, which linked to a study on the potential activity of *Odontites vulgaris* against rheumatoid arthritis. In an even earlier study [43] including other iridoids and compound **4**, the latter was also found to be cardioactive in Wistar rats.

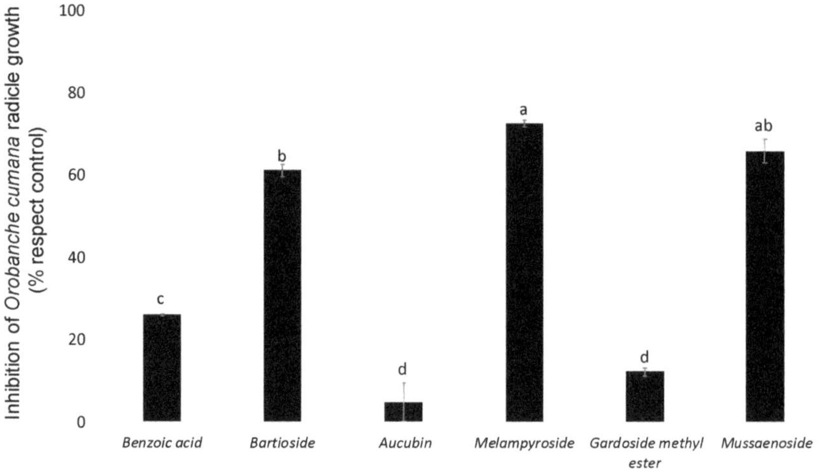

Figure 3. Inhibition of *Orobanche cumana* radicle growth induced by benzoic acid (**1**), bartioside (**2**), aucubin (**3**), melampyroside (**4**), gardoside methyl ester (**5**) and mussaenoside (**6**) at 100 μg/mL. Bars with different letters are significantly different according to the Tukey test (p = 0.05). Error bars represent the standard error of the mean.

Despite the similar chemical structures of **3** and **4**, differences in their biological activities have been reported before. Compounds **4**, **1** and **3**, isolated from *M. arvense*, were reported to display antiprotozoal effects on different species, showing a certain degree of species-specificity [24]. Among the most active compounds **2**, **4** and **6** on *O. cumana* growth, compound **4** induced some degree of phytotoxicity observed as darkening in the *O. cumana* radicles (Figure 4). Compounds **3**, **4** and **6** were tested for antioxidant activity in previous reports [23,44]. Although no DPPH scavenging activity was found for these compounds, interestingly, through a β-carotene bleaching assay [23], compound **6** was found to be an antioxidant, **4** a pro-oxidant (by inducing a faster than spontaneous oxidation of β-carotene) and **3** was inactive. The pro-oxidation effect of **4** could damage the tissue of the plant explaining phytotoxicity; however, whether and how the pro-oxidant activity and the lack of antioxidant activity of **3** might be related with the observed (or not) inhibition of growth is unclear.

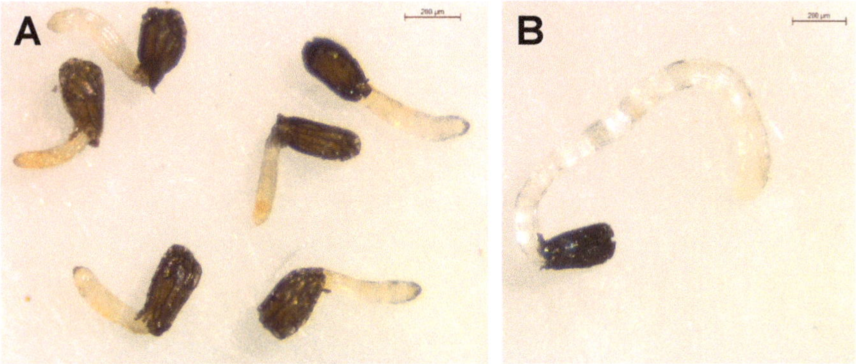

Figure 4. Growth of *Orobanche cumana* radicles treated with melampyroside (**4**) at 100 µg/mL (**A**) and control (**B**).

CLog*P* was calculated for the isolated compounds in an effort to correlate the observed inhibitory activity of compounds **1–6** (Table 1). Negative values were obtained for all the compounds except **1**, indicating a preference for the aqueous media instead of the organic. A good solubility in water is needed in order to favor the transport phenomena for the compound to reach the active site; however, a very low lipophilicity might jeopardize the ability of such to traverse through the cell membrane [45,46]. Thus, the compounds with the highest absolute CLog*P* values (over ∣2∣) have the least bioactivity (**3** and **5**), while the most active ones **4** (−1.153), **6** (−1.849) and **2** (−1.941) have lower CLog*P* values. In the case of compound **4**, the less affinity to water is joined to the presence of the benzoyl group which may have a positive effect on the bioactivity by release of this group by enzymatic transformation to benzoic acid inside the cell. As mentioned above, it has been reported that standalone benzoic acid has phytotoxic properties. The much lower activity of compound **1** when compared with **4** might be caused by two factors: their lipophilicity (CLog*P*: +1.885) and a possible synergistic effect with **4** after metabolization.

Table 1. Calculated Log*P* for compounds (**1–6**).

	1	**2**	**3**	**4**	**5**	**6**
CLog*P*	1.885	−1.941	−4.028	−1.153	−2.133	−1.849

The ecotoxicological tests are considered a valuable tool for preliminary toxicity screening of compounds, especially plant extracts [47]. The ecotoxicity of compound **4** was determined in three aquatic and two terrestrial organisms with different concentrations starting from 100 µg/mL, namely the effective concentration used for *O. cumana*. The influence of compound **4** on the observed effect in *R. subcapitata*, *L. sativum*, *D. magna*, *C. elegans* and *A. fischeri*, was shown in Figure 5.

The results of ecotoxicity showed significant differences in the sensitivity of tested organisms. The differences were reflected in the sensitivity of the plant species and the other organisms to compound **4**. While melampyroside showed the highest toxicity to daphnia (24 h EC_{50} = 33.26 µg/mL), nematodes (24 h EC_{50} = 57.23 µg/mL) and bacteria (EC_{50} 30′ = 76.05 µg/mL), it was less toxic for plant species, such as algae and macrophytes with 72 h $EC_{50} \geq 100$ µg/mL. It is noteworthy that, when compared the effect in *L. sativum* by concentration, the difference was not statistically significant from 5 µg/mL to 100 µg/mL, and the growth observed with these treatments was not significantly different from the growth of control group (Figure 5B). One explanation for this different species-specific sensitivity to melampyroside may be related to the non-absorption of this compound by some plants suggesting a selectivity of melampyroside to inhibit radicle growth of *O. cumana* [48].

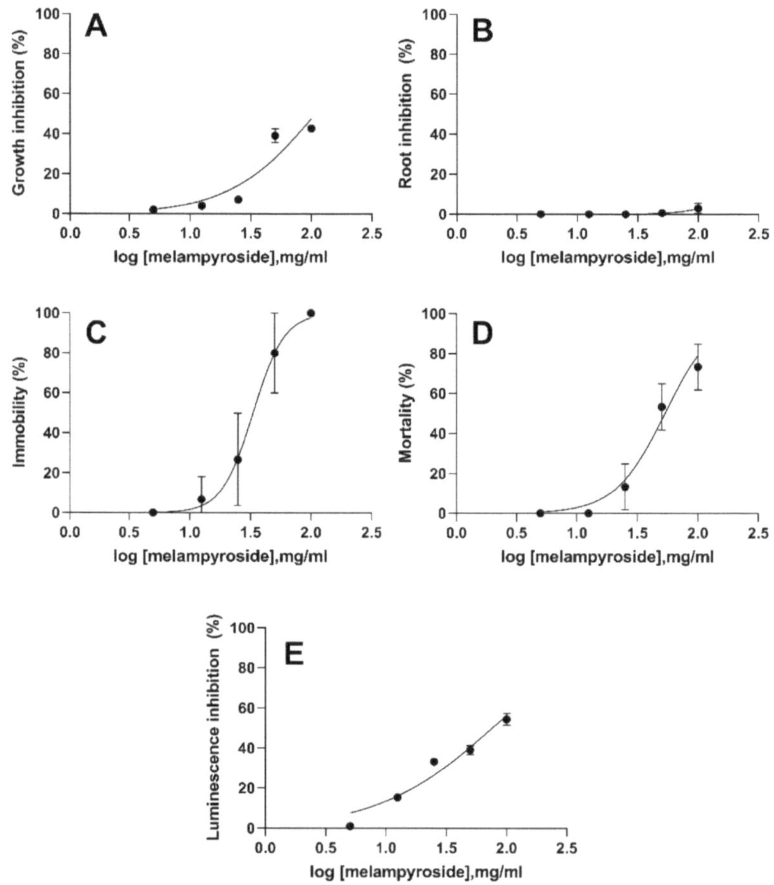

Figure 5. Concentration–response curves of melampyroside (**4**) for *R. subcapitata* (**A**), *L. sativum* (**B**), *D. magna* (**C**), *C. elegans* (**D**) and *A. fischeri* (**E**). Error bars correspond to 95% confidence intervals. Dotted lines represent the fitting to the effect equation.

Considering the EU-Directive 93/67/ECC (EC, 1996) [49] (whereby EC_{50} values < 1.0 µg/mL were considered highly toxic; 1.0–10 µg/mL are considered toxic, 10–100 µg/mL were classified as slightly toxic and above 100 µg/mL were non-toxic), the response of the investigated organisms revealed that compound **4** had little or no toxicity. In contrast to other compounds that are exceedingly toxic, melampyroside could be considered as potential antiparasitic weed agent with an optimal toxicity/selectivity ratio [50,51].

3. Conclusions

Ethyl acetate extracts from different organs of *B. trixago* exhibited significant levels of growth inhibition on radicles of *O. cumana* at extract concentration as low as 100 µg/mL. Subsequently, we isolated and identified the active compounds contained in the ethyl acetate extract of aerial vegetative organs. We found three iridoid glycosides bartsioside (**2**), melampyroside (**4**) and mussaenoside (**6**) with growth inhibition activity in the radicles of *O. cumana*. The radicle of *Orobanche* species is a parasitic organ that grows towards the host and upon host contact, it allows infection. The use of allelochemicals to inhibit the normal growth of *Orobanche* radicles inhibits crop infection and, as a consequence, the death of this parasitic weed. Ecotoxicological tests carried out on compound **4** (the most abundant and phytotoxic iridoid isolated from ethyl acetate extract) showed little or no toxicity according to the EU Directive 93/67/ECC [49]. Plant species-specific phytotoxicity is a desirable trait in the development of novel molecules with herbicidal action to satisfy the principle of pesticide selectivity recommended for integrated pest management [52]. Future studies should determine, at the molecular level, the mode of action of the active iridoid glycosides on the radicles of *O. cumana*.

4. Materials and Methods

4.1. General Experimental Procedures

A JASCO P-1010 digital polarimeter (Tokyo, Japan) was used to measure the optical rotations. ^{1}H NMR spectra were recorded at 400/100 MHz on a Bruker 400 Anova Advance (Karlsruhe, Germany) spectrometer or at 500/125 MHz on a Varian Inova 500 (Palo Alto, CA, USA). The spectra were recorded using $CDCl_3$ or CD_3OD and the same solvents were used as internal standards. Column chromatography (CC) was performed using silica gel (Kieselgel 60, 0.063–0.200 mm, Merck, Darmstadt, Germany). Thin-layer chromatography (TLC) was performed on analytical and preparative silica gel plates (Kieselgel 60, F_{254}, 0.25 and 0.5 mm, respectively, Merck, Darmstadt, Germany). The spots were visualized via exposure to UV light (254 nm) and/or iodine vapours and/or by spraying first with 10% H_2SO_4 in MeOH and then with 5% phosphomolybdic acid in EtOH, followed by heating at 110 °C for 10 min. Electrospray ionization mass spectra (ESIMS) were performed using the LC/MS TOF system AGILENT 6230B (Agilent Technologies, Milan, Italy), HPLC 1260 Infinity. Sigma-Aldrich Co. (St. Louis, MO, USA) supplied all the reagents and the solvents.

4.2. Plant Material

Plants of two populations of *Bellardia trixago*—a white-flowered population and yellow-flowered population—were harvested at the phenological stage of flowering in spring of 2021 in Cordoba, southern Spain (coordinates 37.856 N, 4.806 W, datum WGS84). *Bellardia trixago* plants were immediately carried to the laboratory, and the plants were separated into three compartments: flowers, aerial green organs (stems and leaves) and roots. Each compartment was immediately frozen with liquid nitrogen, stored at −80 °C, subsequently lyophilized and the dry material stored in the dark at 4 °C until use. *Orobanche* seeds were collected from mature plants of *O. cumana* infecting sunflowers in southern Spain. Dry parasitic seeds were separated from capsules using winnowing combined with a sieve of 0.6 mm mesh size and then stored dry in the dark at room temperature until use for this work.

4.3. Extractions of Bellardia trixago *Organs*

A total of 3.0 g of each *B. trixago* organs were extracted, following a previously reported protocol often used for the extraction of plant material [53,54], in order to perform a preliminary activity screening against parasitic plants. In particular, the flowers, green organs and roots of each population were extracted separately by H_2O/MeOH (1/1, *v*/*v*), under stirred conditions at room temperature for 24 h. The hydroalcoholic suspensions were centrifuged at 7000 rpm and extracted with *n*-hexane (3 × 50 mL), CH_2Cl_2 (3 × 50 mL), and after removing methanol under reduced pressure, with EtOAc (3 × 50 mL). The yield of each extract is reported in SI (Table S1).

4.4. Isolation and Identification of Metabolites from Bellardia trixago *Green Organs of the White-Flowered Population*

White green organs (189.0 g) were extracted (1 × 500 mL) by H_2O/MeOH (1/1, *v*/*v*), under stirred conditions at room temperature for 24 h, the suspension centrifuged, and the supernatant extracted by *n*-hexane (3 × 300 mL) and successively with CH_2Cl_2 (3 × 300 mL) and, after removing methanol under reduced pressure, with EtOAc (3 × 200 mL). The residue (1.45 g) of EtOAc organic extract was purified by CC eluted with CH_2Cl_2/MeOH

(8.5/1.5, *v/v*) yielding nine homogeneous fractions (F1-9), as reported in Scheme S1. The residue (54.6 mg) of F3 was purified by TLC eluted with EtOAc/MeOH/H_2O (9/0.75/0.25, *v/v/v*), yielding six groups of homogeneous fractions (F3.1-F3.6). F3.1 was identified as benzoic acid (**1**, 10.8 mg) and F3.5 as melampyroside (**4**, 8.4 mg). The residue (584.7 mg) of fraction F4 yielded pure melampyroside (**4**). The residue (77.9 mg) of F5 was purified by TLC eluted by CH_2Cl_2/EtOAc/MeOH (2/2/1, *v/v/v*), yielding two homogeneous fractions The first fraction of the latter purification yielded a further amount of melampyroside (**4**, 20.4 mg, for a total of 613.5 mg). The residue (498.4 mg) of F6 was purified by CC eluted with CH_2Cl_2/EtOAc/MeOH (2/2/1, *v/v/v*), yielding seven fractions (F6.1-F6.7) The residue (36.5 mg) of F6.4 was further purified by reverse-phase TLC eluted with MeCN/H_2O (4/6, *v/v*), yielding gardoside methyl ester (**5**, 2.0 mg), bartsioside (**2**, 13.9 mg), and mussaenoside (**6**, 6.1 mg). The residue (64.7 mg) of F7 was purified by TLC eluted with EtOAc/MeOH/H_2O (8.5/1/0.5, *v/v/v*) giving further amount of mussaenoside (**6**, 2.3 mg, for a total of 8.4 mg) and aucubin (**3**, 12.4 mg).

Benzoic acid (**1**): ^{1}H NMR spectrum (Figure S1) was in agreement with data previously reported [55]. ESI MS (-) *m/z*: 121 $[M-H]^-$.
Bartsioside (**2**): $[\alpha]_D{}^{22}$-71.9 (c 0.64, MeOH) [lit. [56]: $[\alpha]_D{}^{25}$-86.4 (c 0.5 MeOH)]. ^{1}H NMR spectrum (Figure S2) was in agreement with data previously reported [57]. ESI-MS (+), *m/z*: 330 $[M+H]^+$.
Aucubin (**3**): $[\alpha]_D{}^{22}$-89.8 (c 1.0, MeOH) [lit. [27]: $[\alpha]_D{}^{26}$-92.8 (c 0.27, MeOH)]. ^{1}H NMR spectrum (Figure S3) was in agreement with data previously reported [17,58,59]. ESI-MS (+), *m/z*: 347 $[M+H]^+$.
Melampyroside (**4**): $[\alpha]_D{}^{22}$-69.6 (c 0.79, MeOH) [lit. [27]: $[\alpha]_D{}^{26}$-52.9 (c 0.31, MeOH)] ^{1}H and ^{13}C NMR spectra (Figures S4 and S5) were in agreement with data previously reported [11,49], while its NOESY spectrum is reported in Figure S6. ESI MS (+) *m/z*: 451 $[M+H]^+$.
Gardoside methyl ester (**5**): $[\alpha]_D{}^{22}$-49.8 (c 0.20, MeOH) [lit. [28]: $[\alpha]_D{}^{20}$-46 (c 0.3, MeOH)] ^{1}H NMR spectrum (Figure S7) was in agreement with data previously reported [11,22] ESI-MS (+), *m/z*: 389 $[M+H]^+$.
Mussaenoside (**6**): $[\alpha]_D{}^{22}$-81.3 (c 0.30, MeOH) [lit. [27]: $[\alpha]_D{}^{26}$-77.9 (c 0.32, MeOH)]. ^{1}H NMR spectrum (Figure S8) was in agreement with data previously reported [17,59–61] ESI-MS (+), *m/z*: 391 $[M+H]^+$.

4.5. Bioactivity on Parasitic Weed Seeds

Allelopathic effects of each *B. trixago* extracts and isolated compounds were tested on *Orobanche* radicle growth according to previous protocols [62]. Seeds of *Orobanche cumana*, were surface-sterilized by immersion in 0.5% (*w/v*) NaOCl and 0.02% (*v/v*) Tween 20, for 5 min, rinsed thoroughly with sterile distilled water, and dried in a laminar airflow cabinet. Approximately 100 seeds of *Orobanche* seeds were placed separately on 9 mm diameter glass fiber filter paper disks (GFFP) (Whatman International Ltd., Maidstone UK), moistened with 50 µL of sterile distilled water, and placed in incubators at 23 °C for 10 days inside Parafilm-sealed Petri dishes, to allow seed conditioning. Then, GFFP disks containing conditioned *Orobanche* seeds were transferred onto a sterile sheet of filter paper and transferred to new 9 cm sterile Petri dishes. Stock solutions of each *B. trixago* extract and isolated metabolite were respectively dissolved in dimethyl sulfoxide and subsequently individually diluted to 100 µg/mL using an aqueous solution of GR24 (10^{-6} M). The final concentration of dimethyl sulfoxide was 2% in all test treatments. For each assay, 50 µL aliquots of each sample were applied to GFFP discs containing conditioned *Orobanche* seeds Triplicate aliquots of a treatment only containing GR24 and 2% dimethyl sulfoxide was used as a control. Treated seeds were incubated in the dark at 23 °C for 7 days and radicle growth was determined for each GFFP disc, using a stereoscopic microscope (Leica S9i Leica Microsystems GmbH, Wetzlar, Germany). For the characteristic of radicle growth the value used was the average of 10 randomly selected radicles per GFFP disc [63]. The percentage of radicle growth inhibition of each treatment was then calculated relative to the average radicle growth of control treatment.

4.6. Molecular Modelling

CLog*P* were calculated using ChemOffice v20.1 (PerkinElmer, Waltham, MA, USA) by means of the appropriate tool in ChemDraw Professional [64].

4.7. Ecotoxicity Analysis on Melampyroside

The ecotoxicological tests were carried out on green freshwater algae *Raphidocelis subcapitata*, macrophyte *Lepidium sativum*, water flea *Daphnia magna*, nematode *Caenorhabditis elegans* and bacterium *Aliivibrio fischeri* to expand the range of endpoints due to differences in species sensitivity and exposure. Testing on *R. subcapitata* was performed using as endpoint the algal growth inhibition after 72 h of exposure and was based on ISO 8692:2012 [65]. The algal density was determined by spectrophotometric analysis (DR5000, Hach Lange GbH, Weinheim, Germany). Ecotoxicity tests were carried out in triplicate, at 25 ± 1 °C with constant illumination of 6700 lux. Testing on *L. sativum* was performed according to ISO 11269-1:2012 [66] considering germination and root elongation as endpoint after 72 h. Seeds (n = 10) were exposed in triplicate in Petri dishes and incubated at 25 ± 1 °C in darkness. Daphnia magna test was conducted according to UNI EN ISO 6341:2013 [67] and the endpoint evaluated was the immobilization after 24 h. Daphnids (less than 24 h old) were exposed to the samples at 20 ± 2 °C, in darkness without feeding. Testing on *C. elegans* was carried out, with a few modifications, according to the ASTM E2172-01 Standard Method (2014) using the 24 h mortality endpoint. The test was performed using age-synchronous adult nematodes exposed at 20 °C to compound **4**, without feeding. Testing on *A. fischeri* was based on ISO 11348-3:2007 [68] and the inhibition of the bioluminescence of the bacterium after 30 min of exposure was measured as endpoint. The test was performed using Microtox® Model 500 (M500) analyzer with osmotic adjustment solution (OAS) at 15 ± 1 °C.

4.8. Data Analyses

All bioassays were performed using a completely randomized design. Percentage data in *Orobanche* assays were approximated to normal frequency distribution by means of angular transformation and subjected to analysis of variance (ANOVA) using SPSS software for Windows (SPSS Inc., Chicago, IL, USA). The significance of mean differences among treatments was evaluated by the Tukey test. The null hypothesis was rejected at the level of 0.05. Results of ecotoxicological tests were given as the mean of effect ± standard error. Median effect concentrations EC_{50}, EC_{20} and EC_5 were calculated as mean values and relative 95% confidence limit values for compound **4**. Statistical analysis was carried out via XLSTAT and GraphPad Prism 2.5. (Systat Software, San Jose, CA, USA).

Supplementary Materials: The following are available online at https://www.mdpi.com/article/10.3390/toxins14080559/s1, Table S1: Extract weights of organic extracts obtained from different *Bartsia trixago* organs; Scheme S1: Purification scheme of EtOAc extract of *B. trixago* white green organs; Figure S1: ^{1}H NMR spectrum of benzoic acid, **1** ($CDCl_3$, 400 MHz); Figure S2: ^{1}H NMR spectrum of bartsioside, **2** (MeOD, 500 MHz); Figure S3: ^{1}H NMR spectrum of aucubin, **3** (MeOD, 400 MHz); Figure S4: ^{1}H NMR spectrum of melampyroside, **4** (MeOD, 400 MHz); Figure S5: ^{13}C NMR spectrum of melampyroside, **4** (MeOD, 100 MHz); Figure S6: NOESY spectrum of melampyroside, **4** (MeOD, 400 MHz); Figure S7: ^{1}H NMR spectrum of gardoside methyl ester, **5** (MeOD, 400 MHz). Figure S8: ^{1}H NMR spectrum of mussaenoside, **6** (MeOD, 500 MHz).

Author Contributions: Conceptualisation, M.F.-A., M.M., and A.C.; formal analysis, A.S., M.F.-A., and A.C.P.; writing—original draft preparation, G.S., A.S., M.F.-A., A.C.P., and M.M.; data curation, G.S., A.S., M.F.-A., A.C.P., A.M.-R.; writing—review and editing, G.S., A.S., M.F.-A., A.C.P., M.M.; M.G., and A.C.; Supervision, A.C.; Funding acquisition, M.F.-A. All authors have read and agreed to the published version of the manuscript.

Funding: This research was funded by the Spanish Agencia Estatal de Investigación (projects PID2020-114668RB-I00 and RYC-2015-18961). Authors wish to express gratitude for the Ph.D. grant to Gabriele Soriano funded by INPS (Istituto Nazionale Previdenza Sociale), and for the Galileo grant from Córdoba University-Diputación to Antonio Moreno-Robles.

Institutional Review Board Statement: Not applicable.

Informed Consent Statement: Not applicable.

Data Availability Statement: The data presented in this study are available on request from the corresponding author.

Acknowledgments: We thank the "CSIC Interdisciplinary Thematic Platform (PTI) Optimization of Agricultural and Forestry Systems (PTI-AGROFOR)", the "Consejería de Transformación Económica, Industria, Conocimiento y Universidades de la Junta de Andalucía, project ID: QUAL21 023 IAS" and "Máster Universitario en Agroalimentación, Córdoba University, Spain". A.C.P. expresses his sincere gratitude to the "Plan Propio—UCA 2022-2023" (REF. EST2022-087), the "Consejería de Economía, Conocimiento, Empresas y Universidad de la Junta de Andalucía" and the "Programa Operativo Fondo Social Europeo de Andalucía 2014–2020" for their financial support.

Conflicts of Interest: The authors declare no conflict of interest.

References

1. Parker, C.; Riches, C.R. *Parasitic Weeds of the World: Biology and Control*; CAB International: Wallingford, UK, 1993; ISBN 9780851988733.
2. Westwood, J.H.; Yoder, J.I.; Timko, M.P.; dePamphilis, C.W. The evolution of parasitism in plants. *Trends Plant Sci.* **2010**, *15*, 227–235. [CrossRef] [PubMed]
3. Press, M.C.; Parsons, A.N.; Mackay, A.W.; Vincent, C.A.; Cochrane, V.; Seel, W.E. Gas exchange characteristics and nitrogen relations of two Mediterranean root hemiparasites: *Bartsia trixago* and *Parentucellia viscosa*. *Oecologia* **1993**, *95*, 145–151. [CrossRef] [PubMed]
4. Uribe-Convers, S.; Tank, D.C. Phylogenetic revision of the genus *Bartsia* (Orobanchaceae): Disjunct distributions correlate to independent lineages. *Syst. Bot.* **2016**, *41*, 672–684. [CrossRef]
5. Fernández-Aparicio, M.; Sillero, J.C.; Rubiales, D. Resistance to broomrape species (*Orobanche* spp.) in common vetch (*Vicia sativa* L.). *Crop. Prot.* **2009**, *28*, 7–12. [CrossRef]
6. Molinero-Ruiz, L.; Delavault, P.; Pérez-Vich, B.; Pacureanu-Joita, M.; Bulos, M.; Altieri, E.; Domínguez, J. History of the race structure of *Orobanche cumana* and the breeding of sunflower for resistance to this parasitic weed: A review. *Span. J. Agric. Res* **2015**, *13*, e10R01. [CrossRef]
7. Parker, C. Observations on the current status of *Orobanche* and *Striga* problems worldwide. *Pest Manag. Sci.* **2009**, *65*, 453–459. [CrossRef]
8. Eizenberg, H.; Hershenhorn, J.; Ephrath, J.E. Factors affecting the efficacy of *Orobanche cumana* chemical control in sunflower. *Weed Res.* **2008**, *49*, 308–315. [CrossRef]
9. Joel, D.M.; Hershenhorn, J.; Eizenberg, H.; Aly, R.; Ejeta, G.; Rich, P.J.; Ransom, J.K.; Sauerborn, J.; Rubiales, D. Biology and management of weedy root parasites. In *Horticultural Reviews*; Janick, J., Ed.; John Wiley & Sons: New York, NY, USA, 2007; Volume 33, pp. 267–350.
10. Labrousse, P.; Arnaud, M.C.; Griveau, Y.; Fer, A.; Thalouarn, P. Analysis of resistance criteria of sunflower recombined inbred lines against *Orobanche cumana* Wallr. *Crop Prot.* **2004**, *23*, 407–413. [CrossRef]
11. Aly, R.; Goldwasser, Y.; Eizenber, H.; Hershenhorn, J.; Golan, S.; Kleifeld, Y. Broomrape (*Orobanche cumana*) control in sunflower (*Helianthus annuus*) with imazapic. *Weed Technol.* **2009**, *15*, 306–3009. [CrossRef]
12. Lerner, F.; Pfenning, M.; Picard, L.; Lerchl, J.; Hollenbach, E. Prohesadione calcium is herbicidal to the sunflower root parasite *Orobanche cumana*. *Pest Manag. Sci.* **2021**, *77*, 1893–1902. [CrossRef]
13. Fernández-Aparicio, M.; Delavault, P.; Timko, M.P. Management of infection by parasitic weeds: A Review. *Plants* **2020**, *9*, 1184. [CrossRef] [PubMed]
14. Tomas-Barberan, F.A.; Cole, M.D.; Garcia-Viguera, C.; Tomas-Lorente, F.; Guirado, A. Epicuticular flavonoids from *Bellardia trixago* and their antifungal fully methylated derivatives. *Int. J. Crude Drug Res.* **1990**, *28*, 57–60. [CrossRef]
15. Bianco, A.; Guiso, M.; Iavarone, C.; Trogolo, C. Iridoids. XX. Bartsioside, structure and configuration. *Gazz. Chim. Ital.* **1976**, *106*, 725–732.
16. Barrero, A.F.; Sánchez, J.F.; Cuenca, F.G. Dramatic variation in diterpenoids of different populations of *Bellardia trixago*. *Phytochemistry* **1988**, *27*, 3676–3678. [CrossRef]
17. Ersöz, T.; Yalçin, F.N.; Taşdemir, D.; Sticher, O.; Çaliş, İ. Iridoid and lignan glucosides from *Bellardia trixago* (L.) All. *Turk. J. Med. Sci.* **1998**, *28*, 397–400.

18. Pascual-Villalobos, M.J.; Robledo, A. Screening for anti-insect activity in Mediterranean plants. *Ind. Crops Prod.* **1998**, *8*, 183–194. [CrossRef]
19. Formisano, C.; Rigano, D.; Senatore, F.; Simmonds, M.S.J.; Bisio, A.; Bruno, M.; Rosselli, S. Essential oil composition and antifeedant properties of *Bellardia trixago* (L.) All. (sin. *Bartsia trixago* L.) (Scrophulariaceae). *Biochem. Syst. Ecol.* **2008**, *36*, 454–457. [CrossRef]
20. Weinges, K.; Ziegler, H.J. Chemie und Stereochemie der Iridoide, XIV. Aucubin und Scandosid aus Catalpol. *Liebigs Ann. Chem.* **1990**, *1990*, 715–717. [CrossRef]
21. Tietze, L.F.; Niemeyer, U.; Marx, P.; Glüsenkamp, K.H.; Schwenen, L. Iridoide—XIII: Bestimmung der absoluten konfiguration und konformation isomerer iridoidglycoside mit hilfe chiroptischer methoden. *Tetrahedron* **1980**, *36*, 735–739. [CrossRef]
22. Venditti, A.; Ballero, M.; Serafini, M.; Bianco, A. Polar compounds from *Parentucellia viscosa* (L.) Caruel from Sardinia. *Nat. Prod. Res.* **2015**, *29*, 602–606. [CrossRef]
23. Cuendet, M.; Potterat, O.; Hostettmann, K. Iridoid glucosides, phenylpropanoid derivatives and flavanoids from *Bartsia alpina*. *Pharm. Biol.* **1999**, *37*, 318–320. [CrossRef]
24. Kirmizibekmez, H.; Atay, I.; Kaiser, M.; Brun, R.; Cartagena, M.M.; Carballeira, N.M.; Yesilada, E.; Tasdemir, D. Antiprotozoal activity of *Melampyrum arvense* and its metabolites. *Phytother. Res.* **2011**, *25*, 142–146. [CrossRef] [PubMed]
25. Takeda, Y.; Tamura, K.; Matsumoto, T.; Terao, H.; Tabata, M.; Fujita, T.; Honda, G.; Sezik, E.; Yesiladat, E. 6′-*O*-benzoylshanzhiside methyl ester from *Rhinanthus angustifolius* subsp. *grandiflorus*. *Phytochemistry* **1993**, *33*, 623–625. [CrossRef]
26. Bianco, A.; Bolli, D.; Passacantilli, P. 6-*O*-β-Glucopyranosylaucubin, a new irodoid from *Odontites verna*. *Planta Med.* **1982**, *44*, 97–99. [CrossRef]
27. Takeda, Y.; Fujita, T. Iridoid glucosides of *Melampyrum laxum*. *Planta Med.* **1981**, *41*, 192–194. [CrossRef] [PubMed]
28. Damtoft, S.; Hansen, S.B.; Jacobsen, B.; Jensen, S.R.; Nielsen, B.J. Iridoid glucosides from *Melampyrum*. *Phytochemistry* **1984**, *23*, 2387–2389. [CrossRef]
29. Bianco, A.; Passacantilli, P.; Righi, G.; Nicoletti, M. Iridoid glucosides from *Parentucellia viscosa*. *Phytochemistry* **1985**, *24*, 1843–1845. [CrossRef]
30. Petitto, V.; Serafini, M.; Ballero, M.; Foddai, S.; Stanzione, A.; Nicoletti, M. Iridoids from *Euphrasia genargentea*, a rare Sardinian endemism. *Nat. Prod. Res.* **2009**, *23*, 431–435. [CrossRef]
31. Khanh, T.D.; Anh, L.H.; Nghia, L.T.; Trung, K.H.; Hien, P.B.; Trung, D.M.; Xuan, T.D. Allelopathic responses of rice seedlings under some different stresses. *Plants* **2018**, *7*, 40. [CrossRef] [PubMed]
32. Fernández-Aparicio, M.; Cimmino, A.; Evidente, A.; Rubiales, D. Inhibition of *Orobanche crenata* seed germination and radicle growth by allelochemicals identified in cereals. *J. Agric. Food Chem.* **2013**, *61*, 9797–9803. [CrossRef]
33. Zhang, W.; Lu, L.-Y.; Hu, L.-Y.; Cao, W.; Sun, K.; Sun, Q.-B.; Siddikee, A.; Shi, R.-H.; Dai, C.-C. Evidence for the involvement of auxin, ethylene and ROS signaling during primary root inhibition of *Arabidopsis* by the allelochemical benzoic acid. *Plant Cell Physiol.* **2018**, *59*, 1889–1904. [CrossRef] [PubMed]
34. Ma, H.; Chen, Y.; Chen, J.; Zhang, Y.; Zhang, T.; He, H. Comparison of allelopathic effects of two typical invasive plants: *Mikania micrantha* and *Ipomoea cairica* in Hainan island. *Sci. Rep.* **2020**, *10*, 11332. [CrossRef] [PubMed]
35. Baziramakenga, R.; Leroux, G.D.; Simard, R.R. Effects of benzoic and cinnamic acids on membrane permeability of soybean roots. *J. Chem. Ecol.* **1995**, *21*, 1271–1285. [CrossRef]
36. Earl, D.F. Method of Treating Plants. U.S. Patent US2723909A, 21 August 1952.
37. Pang, J. One Kind Greening Momordica Grosvenori Herbicide and Preparation Method Thereof. Chinese Patent CN107372626A, 14 August 2017.
38. Jin, X.; Lin, Y.; Li, Y.; Lin, D.; Lin, J.; Lin, Z. Organic Crop Herbicide Containing Organic Acid and Mineral Oil and Preparation Method Thereof. Chinese Patent CN113925063A, 14 January 2022.
39. Ahn, B.Z.; Pachaly, P. Melampyrosid, ein neus iridoid aus *Melampyrum silvaticum* L. *Tetrahedron* **1974**, *30*, 4049–4054. [CrossRef]
40. Karrer, P.; Schmid, H. Über die Konstitution des Aucubins. *Helv. Chim. Acta* **1946**, *29*, 525–552. [CrossRef]
41. Takeda, Y.; Nishimura, H.; Inouye, H. Two new iridoid glucosides from *Mussaenda parviflora* and *Mussaenda shikokiana*. *Phytochemistry* **1977**, *16*, 1401–1404. [CrossRef]
42. Ji, M.; Wang, C.; Yang, T.; Meng, X.; Wang, X.; Li, M. Integrated phytochemical analysis based on UPLC–MS/MS and network pharmacology approaches to explore the effect of *Odontites vulgaris* Moench on rheumatoid arthritis. *Front. Pharmacol.* **2021**, *12*, 707687. [CrossRef]
43. Pennacchio, M.; Syah, Y.M.; Ghisalberti, E.L.; Alexander, E. Cardioactive iridoid glycosides from *Eremophila* species. *Phytomedicine* **1997**, *4*, 325–330. [CrossRef]
44. Çaliş, I.; Kirmizibekmez, H.; Taşdemir, D.; Ireland, C.M. Iridoid glycosides from *Globularia davisiana*. *Chem. Pharm. Bull.* **2002**, *50*, 678–680. [CrossRef]
45. Liu, X.; Testa, B.; Fahr, A. Lipophilicity and its relationship with passive drug permeation. *Pharm. Res.* **2011**, *28*, 962–977. [CrossRef]
46. Zhang, R.; Qin, X.; Kong, F.; Chen, P.; Pan, G. Improving cellular uptake of therapeutic entities through interaction with components of cell membrane. *Drug Deliv.* **2019**, *26*, 328–342. [CrossRef] [PubMed]
47. Afolayan, A.J.; Ohikhena, F.U.; Wintola, O.A. Toxicity assessment of different solvent extracts of the medicinal plant, *Phragmanthera capitata* (Sprengel) Balle on brine shrimp (*Artemia salina*). *Int. J. Pharmacol.* **2016**, *12*, 701–710.

48. Page, S.W. Antiparasitic drugs. In *Small Animal Clinical Pharmacology*; Maddison, J.E., Page, S.W., Church, D.B., Eds.; Elsevier: Amsterdam, The Netherlands, 2008; pp. 198–260.
49. European Commission (EC). *Technical Guidance Document in Support of the Commission Directive 93/67/EEC on Risk Assessment for New Notified Substances and Commission Regulation (EC) No 1488/94 on Risk Assessment for Existing Substances*; Parts 1–4; Office for Official Publications of the EC: Luxembourg, 1996.
50. Koko, W.S.; Jentzsch, J.; Kalie, H.; Schobert, R.; Ersfeld, K.; Al Nasr, I.S.; Biersack, B. Evaluation of the antiparasitic activities of imidazol-2-ylidene-gold (I) complexes. *Arch. Pharm.* **2020**, *353*, e1900363. [CrossRef] [PubMed]
51. Wright, C.W.; Phillipson, J.D. Natural products and the development of selective antiprotozoal drugs. *Phytother. Res.* **1990**, *4*, 127–139. [CrossRef]
52. Barzman, M.; Bàrberi, P.; Birch, A.N.E.; Boonekamp, P.; Dachbrodt-Saaydeh, S.; Graf, B.; Sattin, M. Eight principles of integrated pest management. *Agron. Sustain. Dev.* **2015**, *35*, 1199–1215. [CrossRef]
53. Cimmino, A.; Roscetto, E.; Masi, M.; Tuzi, A.; Radjai, I.; Gahdab, C.; Paolillo, R.; Guarino, A.; Catania, M.R.; Evidente, A. Sesquiterpene lactones from *Cotula cinerea* with antibiotic activity against clinical isolates of *Enterococcus faecalis*. *Antibiotics* **2021**, *10*, 819. [CrossRef]
54. Soriano, G.; Petrillo, C.; Masi, M.; Bouafiane, M.; Khelil, A.; Tuzi, A.; Isticato, R.; Fernández-Aparicio, M.; Cimmino, A. Specialized metabolites from the allelopathic plant *Retama raetam* as potential biopesticides. *Toxins* **2022**, *14*, 311. [CrossRef]
55. Cui, L.-Q.; Liu, K.; Zhang, C. Effective oxidation of benzylic and alkane C–H bonds catalyzed by sodium o-iodobenzenesulfonate with Oxone as a terminal oxidant under phase-transfer conditions. *Org. Biomol. Chem.* **2011**, *9*, 2258–2265. [CrossRef]
56. Delicato, A.; Masi, M.; de Lara, F.; Rubiales, D.; Paolillo, I.; Lucci, V.; Falco, G.; Calabro, V.; Evidente, A. *In vitro* characterization of iridoid and phenylethanoid glycosides from *Cistanche phelypaea* for nutraceutical and pharmacological applications. *Phytother. Res.* **2022**, 1–12. [CrossRef]
57. Andrzejewska-Golec, E.; Ofterdinger-Daegel, S.; Calis, I.; Światek, L. Chemotaxonomic aspects of iridoids occurring in *Plantago* subg. *Psyllium (Plantaginaceae)*. *Plant Syst. Evol.* **1993**, *185*, 85–89. [CrossRef]
58. Chaudhuri, R.K.; Afifi-Yazar, F.Ü.; Sticher, O.; Winkler, T. ^{13}C NMR spectroscopy of naturally occurring iridoid glucosides and their acylated derivatives. *Tetrahedron* **1980**, *36*, 2317–2326. [CrossRef]
59. Chu, H.-B.; Tan, N.-H.; Zhang, Y.-M. Chemical constituents from *Pedicularis rex* C. B. Clarke. *Z. Naturforsch. B* **2007**, *62*, 1465–1470 [CrossRef]
60. Otsuka, H.; Watanabe, E.; Yuasa, K.; Ogimi, C.; Takushi, A.; Takeda, Y. A verbascoside iridoid glucoside conjugate from *Premna corymbosa* var. *abtusifolia*. *Phytochemistry* **1993**, *32*, 983–986. [CrossRef]
61. Gardner, D.R.; Narum, J.; Zook, D.; Stermitz, F.R. New iridoid glucosides from Castilleja and Besseya: 6-Hydroxyadoxoside and 6-isovanillylcatapol. *J. Nat. Prod.* **1987**, *50*, 485–489. [CrossRef]
62. Fernández-Aparicio, M.; Moral, A.; Kharrat, M.; Rubiales, D. Resistance against broomrapes (*Orobanche* and *Phelipanche* spp.) in faba bean (*Vicia faba*) based in low induction of broomrape seed germination. *Euphytica* **2012**, *186*, 897–905. [CrossRef]
63. Westwood, J.H.; Foy, C.L. Influence of nitrogen on germination and early development of broomrape (*Orobanche* spp.). *Weed Sci.* **1999**, *47*, 2–7. [CrossRef]
64. Cala, A.; Zorrilla, J.G.; Rial, C.; Molinillo, J.M.G.; Varela, R.M.; Macías, F.A. Easy access to alkoxy, amino, carbamoyl, hydroxy, and thiol derivatives of sesquiterpene lactones and evaluation of their bioactivity on parasitic weeds. *J. Agric. Food Chem.* **2019**, *67*, 10764–10773. [CrossRef]
65. *ISO 8692:2012*; Water Quality—Fresh Water Algal Growth Inhibition Test with Unicellular Green Algae. ISO: Geneva, Switzerland, 2012.
66. *ISO 11269-1:2012*; Soil Quality—Determination of the Effects of Pollutants on Soil Flora—Part 1: Method for the Measurement of Inhibition of Root Growth. ISO: Geneva, Switzerland, 2012.
67. *UNI EN ISO 6341:2013*; Water Quality—Determination of the Inhibition of the Mobility of *Daphnia magna* Straus (Cladoc-Era, Crustacea)—Acute Toxicity Test. Ente Nazionale Italiano di Unificazione (UNI): Milan, Italy, 2013.
68. *ISO 11348-3:2007*; Water Quality—Determination of the Inhibitory Effect of Water Samples on the Light Emission of *Vibrio fischeri* (Luminescent Bacteria Test)—Part 3: Method Using Freeze-Dried Bacteria. ISO: Geneva, Switzerland, 2007.

toxins

MDPI

Article

Comparative Analysis of Secondary Metabolites Produced by *Ascochyta fabae* under In Vitro Conditions and Their Phytotoxicity on the Primary Host, *Vicia faba*, and Related Legume Crops

Eleonora Barilli [1,*,†], Pierluigi Reveglia [1,†], Francisco J. Agudo-Jurado [1], Vanessa Cañete García [1], Alessio Cimmino [2], Antonio Evidente [2,3] and Diego Rubiales [1,*]

1 Institute for Sustainable Agriculture, Spanish National Research Council (CSIC), 14004 Córdoba, Spain; preveglia@ias.csic.es (P.R.); q92agjuf@uco.es (F.J.A.-J.); q22cagav@uco.es (V.C.G.)
2 Department of Chemical Science, University of Naples Federico II (UNINA), 80126 Naples, Italy; alessio.cimmino@unina.it (A.C.); evidente@unina.it (A.E.)
3 Institute of Sciences of Food Production, National Research Council, 70126 Bari, Italy
* Correspondence: ebarilli@ias.csic.es (E.B.); diego.rubiales@ias.csic.es (D.R.)
† These authors contributed equally to this work.

Abstract: Ascochyta blight, caused by *Ascochyta fabae*, poses a significant threat to faba bean and other legumes worldwide. Necrotic lesions on stems, leaves, and pods characterize the disease. Given the economic impact of this pathogen and the potential involvement of secondary metabolites in symptom development, a study was conducted to investigate the fungus's ability to produce bioactive metabolites that might contribute to its pathogenicity. For this investigation, the fungus was cultured in three substrates (Czapek-Dox, PDB, and rice). The produced metabolites were analyzed by NMR and LC-HRMS methods, resulting in the dereplication of seven metabolites, which varied with the cultural substrates. Ascochlorin, ascofuranol, and (*R*)-mevalonolactone were isolated from the Czapek-Dox extract; ascosalipyrone, benzoic acid, and tyrosol from the PDB extract; and ascosalitoxin and ascosalipyrone from the rice extract. The phytotoxicity of the pure metabolites was assessed at different concentrations on their primary hosts and related legumes. The fungal exudates displayed varying degrees of phytotoxicity, with the Czapek-Dox medium's exudate exhibiting the highest activity across almost all legumes tested. The species belonging to the genus *Vicia* spp. were the most susceptible, with faba bean being susceptible to all metabolites, at least at the highest concentration tested, as expected. In particular, ascosalitoxin and benzoic acid were the most phytotoxic in the tested condition and, as a consequence, expected to play an important role on necrosis's appearance.

Keywords: fungal metabolites; Ascochyta blight; legumes; phytotoxins

Key Contribution: Frist report from *Ascochyta fabae* of ascochlorin; ascofuranol; (*R*)-mevalonolactone ascosalipyrone; benzoic acid; tyrosol; ascosalitoxin and ascosalipyrone as phytotoxic metabolites affecting *Vicia* species.

Citation: Barilli, E.; Reveglia, P.; Agudo-Jurado, F.J.; Cañete García, V.; Cimmino, A.; Evidente, A.; Rubiales, D. Comparative Analysis of Secondary Metabolites Produced by *Ascochyta fabae* under In Vitro Conditions and Their Phytotoxicity on the Primary Host, *Vicia faba*, and Related Legume Crops. *Toxins* **2023**, *15*, 693. https://doi.org/10.3390/toxins15120693

Received: 8 November 2023
Revised: 4 December 2023
Accepted: 6 December 2023
Published: 9 December 2023

1. Introduction

Cold-weather legumes are a valuable source of premium plant-based protein suitable for human consumption and livestock feed. They play an essential role in crop rotation on arable lands, helping to minimize the requirement for fertilizer usage and acting as effective interim crops [1–6]. However, as for any crop, legumes can be affected by a number of diseases, out of which Ascochyta blights are one of the most important groups of necrotic fungal diseases globally present in all legume cultivation areas [7]. Different *Ascochyta* species cause Ascochyta blight diseases in a host-specific manner in many instances: *Ascochyta fabae* Speg., *Ascochyta lentis* Vassiljevsky, *Ascochyta pisi* Lib., *Ascochyta pinodes*

(Berk. & Blox.) Jones, *Ascochyta rabiei* (Pass) Labr., and *Ascochyta viciae-villosae* Ondrej are pathogens of faba bean (*Vicia faba* L.), lentil (*Lens culinaris* Medik.), pea (*Pisum sativum* L.), chickpea (*Cicer arietinum* L.), and hairy vetch (*Vicia villosa* Roth), respectively [7–11].

Ascochyta blight management remains problematic, mainly due to the reduced levels of plant resistance available and also because the use of fungicides is uneconomic, forcing the integration of genetic resistance with cultural practices [12,13]. Symptoms generally emerge in the above-ground sections of the plants when exposed to a high percentage of humidity and moderate temperature, resulting in necrotic lesions on both leaves and stems [14,15]. Leaves with multiple lesions tend to fade prematurely, particularly in the lower sections of the plants. On diseased stems, these fungi induce extensive necrotic lesions, which can result in stem breakage and the demise of plant portions situated above the affected area. The infection can also spread through contaminated grains and pods, posing a risk to subsequent crops, as their use can have detrimental effects on the growth of emerging plants. In this study, we focus on the Ascochyta blight of faba bean which is widespread and can cause significant damage by breaking stems, leaf lesions, and seed depreciation. Disease control through crop rotation, clean seed, and chemical treatment is not wholly effective [4] and only moderate levels of genetic resistance are available [16,17], reinforcing the need to understand pathogenicity factors as targets both for resistance breeding and for designing alternative management strategies.

A histological examination revealed that cellular damage and collapse occurred prior to direct fungal contact aimed at breaking down host tissues for nutrient acquisition [18]. To achieve this, necrotrophic fungi can suppress plant defences by releasing harmful substances, primarily enzymes that catalyze the breakdown of structural components and other vital compounds, as well as phytotoxins that induce cell damage and modifications. Nevertheless, the phytotoxic compounds produced by *Ascochyta* associated with legumes are often host specific or exhibit toxicity toward various plants, including their respective hosts. The precise roles of these compounds in the pathogenic process remain unknown [19].

Several metabolites with cytotoxic capacity involved in the pathogenesis process have been found in different *Ascochyta* species. In detail, a range of polyketide-derived secondary metabolites were isolated from the organic extracts of *A. lentis*, *A. pinodes*, and *A. pisi* and chemically characterized by 1D and 2D NMR spectroscopy and mass spectrometry.

Previously, only one metabolite named ascochitine, an *o*-quinone methide, has been identified in *A. fabae* [20]. However, pathogenicity studies have shown that ascochitine is not crucial for causing disease in faba beans, and there is no apparent correlation between the amount of ascochitine and the aggressiveness of *A. fabae* isolates [21]. This finding suggests that other phytotoxic metabolites may be produced by *A. fabae* that play a role in pathogenicity.

To obtain new insight on the interaction between *A. fabae* with its host plants and to obtain new insights into the role of secondary metabolites involved in pathogenicity, we conducted a comprehensive study to isolate and characterize the phytotoxic secondary metabolites produced by *A. fabae* under in vitro conditions. *A. fabae* was grown here in three common culture media to explore their influence on secondary metabolite production. Crude organic extracts from the cultures were subjected to bioassays on the primary host (faba bean) and related legumes of the genera *Vicia*, *Lens*, and *Pisum*. Following this, the organic extracts were purified using chromatographic methods, and spectroscopic techniques, essentially NMR, were employed to dereplicate and characterize the most abundant secondary metabolites fully. Finally, the phytotoxicity of the purified compounds was assessed to gain valuable insights into their roles in fungal pathogenesis.

2. Results

Ascochyta fabae isolate Af-CO99-01 was grown in vitro in three different substrates (two liquid media, Czapek-Dox and PDB, and one solid rice culture, as detailed in the Section 4) to explore the production of secondary metabolites. After extraction, the phytotoxicity of the three corresponding organic residues on the primary host, faba bean, and other related legumes of economic importance was assayed at different concentrations.

2.1. Bioassays of Fungal Organic Extract

The three organic extracts exhibited varying degrees of phytotoxicity, which depended on the fungal growth medium, the applied concentration, and the specific plant species. All three fungal extracts displayed significantly higher phytotoxicity (assessed as foliar damaged area, mm^2) compared to the controls. The faba bean was the legume crop with the most significant damage, regardless of the culture media employed. Both narbon and common vetches were also significantly damaged, while disease symptoms were generally lower on lentil and pea leaves (Figure 1, Table 1, Supplementary Table S1).

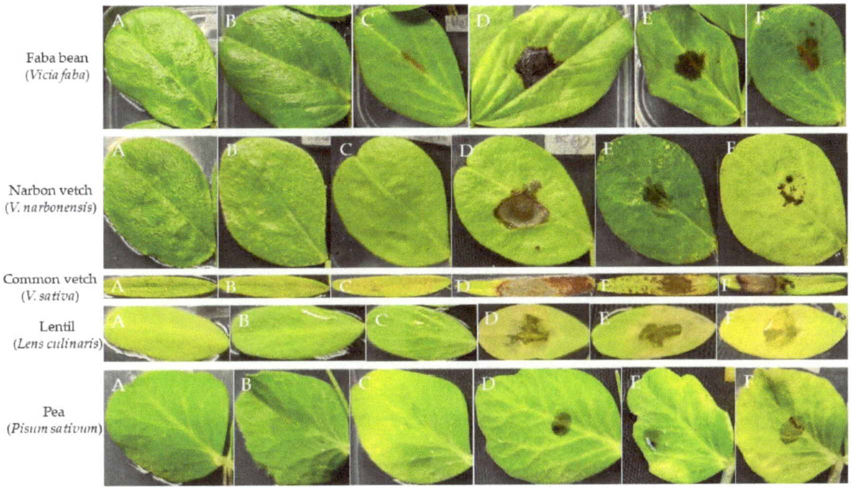

Figure 1. Symptoms developed on detached leaves of several legume hosts as a consequence of the following treatments: (**A**) uninoculated, (**B**) water, (**C**) methanol (MeOH 5%), (**D**) *A. fabae* extract at 2 mg/mL from Czapek-Dox medium, (**E**) *A. fabae* extract at 2 mg/mL from PDB medium and, (**F**) *A. fabae* extract at 2 mg/mL from rice substrate.

Table 1. Differences by host specie on disease severity (necrotic area, mm^2) caused by *Ascochyta fabae* fungal exudates from different culture media (Czapek-Dox, PDB, and rice). Values are the general average of all concentrations tested. Negative controls (blank untreated, water and MeOH 5%) were also included. The experiment was repeated four times.

	Host Plant									
Treatment	**Faba Bean**		**Narbon Vetch**		**Common Vetch**		**Lentil**		**Pea**	
Blank	0 ± 0	d	0 ± 0	c	0 ± 0	c	0 ± 0	c	0 ± 0	c
Water	0 ± 0	d	1.8 ± 1.6	c	0.2 ± 0.1	c	0 ± 0	c	0.3 ± 0.2	c
MeOH	3.4 ± 1.5	c	7.3 ± 3.3	bc	0.2 ± 0.05	c	0.5 ± 0.3	c	0.4 ± 0.2	c
Czapek-Dox	110.6 ± 3.9	a	96.4 ± 8.8	a	27.9 ± 5.5	ab	19.9 ± 5.2	a	29.2 ± 3.2	a
PDB	95.6 ± 5.4	b	45.2 ± 4.7	b	30.2 ± 7.3	a	1.0 ± 0.6	c	7.5 ± 2.6	b
Rice	81.6 ± 2.6	b	38.9 ± 5.1	b	17.1 ± 5.1	b	9.1 ± 3.4	b	9.9 ± 2.1	b

Values, per column and treatment, followed by different letters differ significantly at $p < 0.01$.

Regardless of the host species, the fungal exudate from the Czapek-Dox medium caused higher disease symptoms, followed by exudates from PDB and rice culture (Figure 2, Table 1, Supplementary Table S1). In addition, dose-dependent differences were also observed, especially for the exudate from the Czapek-Dox medium on faba bean, narbon vetch, and pea, as well as for exudate from PDB on faba bean, being the higher dose applied (2 mg/mL) the most phytotoxic. Other treatments did not show a dose-dependent effect.

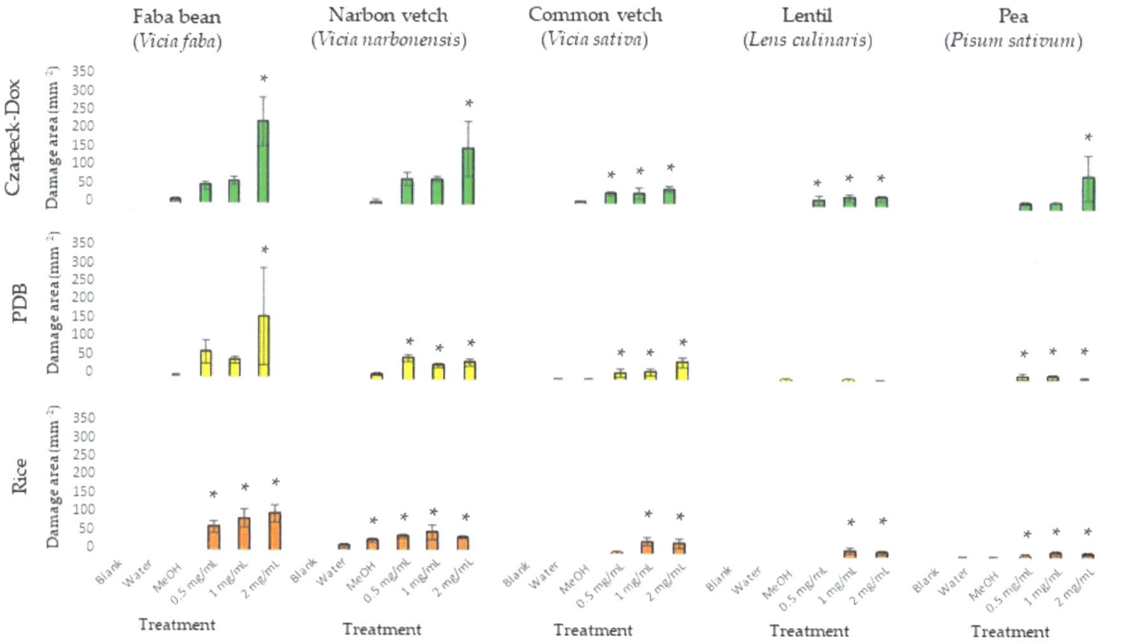

Figure 2. Diseased area (mm^2) measured on detached leaves of 5 legume crops treated with exudates from the fungus *Ascochyta faba* growth in vitro on 3 different culture media as: Czapek-Dox (green), potato dextrose broth = PDB (yellow) and rice (orange) at concentrations of 0.5, 1, and 2 mg/mL. Negative controls (blank untreated, water and MeOH 5%) were also included. The experiment was repeated four times. Asterisk (*) indicates values significantly different from control MeOH 5%.

Given the phytotoxicity exhibited by all three fungal exudates, with the Czapek-Dox extract being the most active among all legume species tested, a comprehensive analysis was conducted to determine the specific metabolite composition displayed by each exudate. The objective of this analysis was to elucidate the distinct metabolic profiles inherent to each exudate. This investigation was undertaken to elucidate potential commonalities or disparities within the exudates, shedding light on the underlying factors contributing to the different phytotoxic effects observed.

2.2. *Identification of Secondary Metabolites from Culture Filtrates of A. fabae Cultures*

Due to the different phytotoxicity displayed by the organic extracts derived from the Czapek-Dox, PDB, and rice cultures observed on both host and no-host legume crops, their purification was carried out using chromatographic techniques, as detailed in the materials and methods section. The predominant metabolites synthesized by the fungus in each culture medium were identified through a comprehensive analysis of NMR spectroscopy and high-resolution LC/MS spectra.

From the Czapek-Dox culture, three distinct metabolites were purified: ascochlorin (**1**), ascofuranol (**2**), and (*R*)-mevalonolactone (**3**). Figure 3 illustrates their respective structures By comparing their spectroscopic properties to the existing literature data, compounds **1–3** were successfully identified and dereplicated. Ascochlorin (**1**) was determined to have a molecular formula of $C_{23}H_{29}ClO_4$ based on its HR-ESIMS, revealing two identifiable mass adducts: $[M+H]^+$ and $[M+Na]^+$. The structural assignment was further confirmed by ^{1}H-NMR spectra, which exhibited diagnostic peaks such as the aldehyde proton at δ

10.14, chelated OH at δ 12.72, one aromatic methyl group signal at δ 2.57, and the other four methyl group signals at δ 1.92, 0.83, 0.81, and 0.70. Similarly, ascofuranol (**2**) was found to possess a molecular formula of $C_{23}H_{31}ClO_5$ based on HR-ESIMS, with two identifiable mass adducts: $[M+H]^+$ and $[M+Na]^+$. The structural assignment was supported by ^{1}H-NMR spectra, highlighting diagnostic peaks such as the aldehyde proton at δ 10.14, chelated OH at δ 12.70, one aromatic methyl signal at δ 2.60, geminal dimethyl groups at δ 1.28 and 1.21, and olefinic protons resonating at δ 5.49 and δ 5.15. (*R*)-Mevalonolactone (**3**) had a molecular formula of $C_6H_{10}O_3$ as deduced from its HR-ESIMS from the $[M+K]^+$ adduct and the dimer $[2M+Na]^+$. ^{1}H-NMR spectra confirm the structural assignment for the presence of diagnostic peaks: a singlet methyl group at δ 1.28 and the two diastereotopic protons at δ 4.62 and δ 4.41. All the spectra are reported in Supplementary Figures S1–S6.

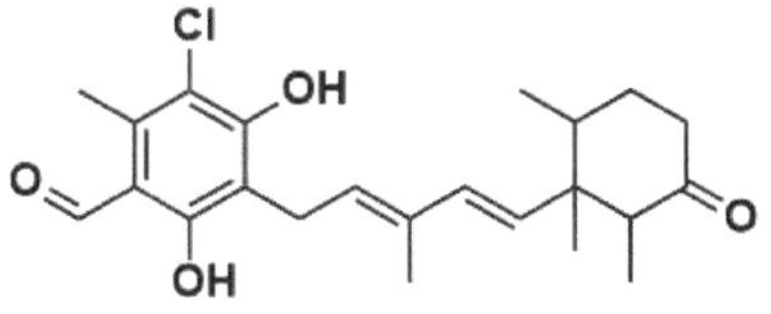

Ascochlorin **1**

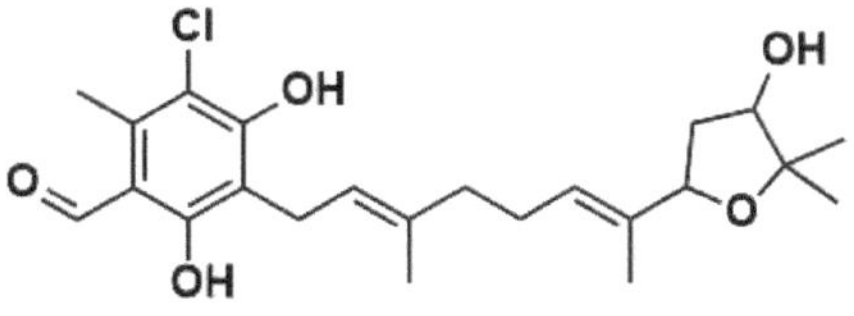

Ascofuranol **2**

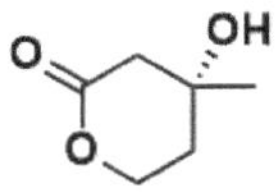

(*R*)-Mevalonolactone **3**

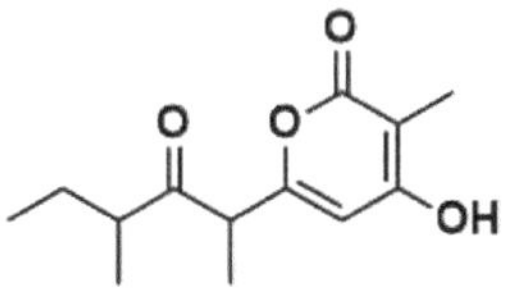

Ascosalipyrone **4**

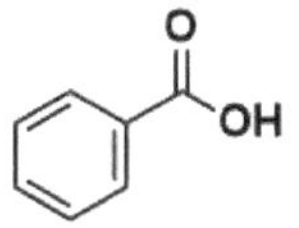

Benzoic acid **5**

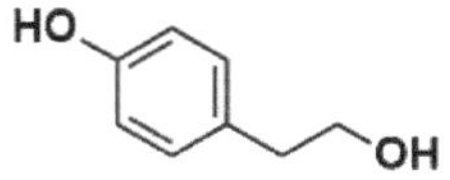

Tyrosol **6**

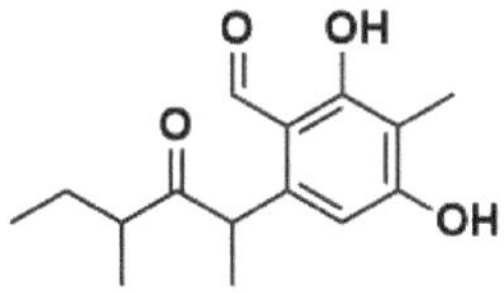

Ascosalitoxin **7**

Figure 3. Structure of ascochlorin (**1**), ascofuranol (**2**), (*R*)-mevalonolactone (**3**), ascosalipyrone (**4**), benzoic acid (**5**), tyrosol (**6**), ascosalitoxin (**7**).

The PDB culture yielded three unique metabolites: ascosalipyrone (**4**), benzoic acid (**5**), and tyrosol (**6**), that were dereplicated according to their spectroscopic properties reported in the literature (illustrated in Supplementary Figures S7–S12 provide the ^{1}H-NMR and ESI/MS spectra). Ascosalipyrone (**4**) was determined to have a molecular formula of $C_{13}H_{18}O_4$ based on its HR-ESIMS, revealing two identifiable mass adducts: $[M+H]^+$ and the dimer $[2M+Na]^+$. The structural assignment was further confirmed by ^{1}H-NMR spectra, which exhibited diagnostic peaks such as the deshielded olefinic proton at δ 5.95, two multiplets at δ 2.69 and δ 1.68, and the four signals of methyl groups at δ 1.94, 1.38, 1.05, and 0.82.

The two simple aromatic compounds benzoic acid (**5**) and tyrosol (**6**) were determined to have molecular formulas $C_7H_6O_2$ and $C_8H_{10}O_2$, respectively. The HR-ESIMS of compound **5** revealed two adducts $[M-H_2O+H]^+$ and $[M+H]^+$, while for compound **6**, the adduct $[M-H_2O+H]^+$ and the dimer $[2M+H]^+$ were again detected (Supplementary Figures S10 and S12). The structural assignment of benzoic acid (**5**) was further confirmed by ^{1}H-NMR spectra, which reveal the typical pattern of monosubstituted benzene with one doublet at δ 8.10 of the two *ortho*-equivalent protons and two triplets at δ 7.62 and δ 7.48. The ^{1}H-NMR spectrum of tyrosol (**6**) showed the typical signal pattern of a para-disubstituted benzene with two doublets, each for two equivalent protons, at δ 7.10 and 6.79, and the two triplets of the two methylene of the 2-hydroxy ethyl residue at δ 3.82 and 2.8.

Lastly, the rice culture produced two distinct metabolites: ascosalipyrone (**4**) and ascosalitoxin (**7**) (illustrated in Figure 3). Also, compound **7** was dereplicated by comparing the spectroscopic properties with those reported in the previous study. Supplementary Figures S13 and S14 display its ^{1}H-NMR and ESI/MS spectra. Ascosalitoxin (**7**) was determined to have a molecular formula of $C_{13}H_{18}O_4$ based on its HR-ESIMS, revealed by the identifiable mass adduct $[M+H]^+$. The structural assignment was further confirmed by ^{1}H-NMR spectra, which exhibited diagnostic peaks such as the aldehyde proton at δ 10.23, chelated OH at δ 12.68, one aromatic proton signal at δ 6.23, and the four methyl group signals at δ 2.11, 1.43, 1.08, and 0.72, respectively.

All the dereplicated metabolites have been previously reported as fungal metabolites Nevertheless, their presence in *A. fabae* in vitro cultures is being reported here for the first time.

2.3. Bioassay of Pure Compounds

The degree of phytotoxicity caused by pure metabolites from *A. fabae* grown on Czapek-Dox, PDB, and rice substrates varied according to the host species and the applied concentration. In general terms, faba bean and narbon vetch were the most susceptible hosts to all the metabolites applied and at any concentrations, followed by common vetch (Figure 4, Supplementary Table S2, Supplementary Figure S15). By contrast, low or no phytotoxicity was induced in both lentil and pea leaves, not significantly different from the negative controls (Supplementary Table S2, Supplementary Figure S15).

Observed by the legume host, species belonging to the genus *Vicia* were the most susceptible (faba bean, narbon vetch, and common vetch), while in pea and lentil hosts, poor or no phytotoxicity was observed. As expected, faba bean was susceptible to all metabolites, at least at the highest concentration tested. In particular, ascosalitoxin (**7**) and benzoic acid (**5**) cause damaged areas of 29.8 and 30.8 mm^2 and 15 and 16 mm^2 at applied concentrations of 10 and 100 μM, respectively. Tyrosol (**6**) was phytotoxic at any concentration tested, with damaged areas higher than 17 mm^2. The other metabolites tested were also phytotoxic, especially at 100 μM. From our results, narbon vetch was the most susceptible legume species tested here, susceptible to all the pure metabolites but with resulting necrotic lesions bigger than those measured in faba bean (Figure 4; Supplementary Table S2; Supplementary Figure S15). Phytotoxicity from ascochlorin (**1**), ascofuranol (**2**), benzoic acid (**5**), tyrosol (**6**), and ascosalitoxin (**7**) was not dose dependent, showing activity at any concentration tested. By contrast, (*R*)-mevalonolactone (**3**) and ascosalipyrone (**4**) showed phytotoxicity only at the higher concentration tested (values higher than 30 and 46 mm^2, respectively). Common vetch was less affected by the metabolite's application, showing significant necrotic areas only with ascofuranol (**2**), benzoic acid (**5**), and ascosalitoxin (**7**) at the highest concentration rate.

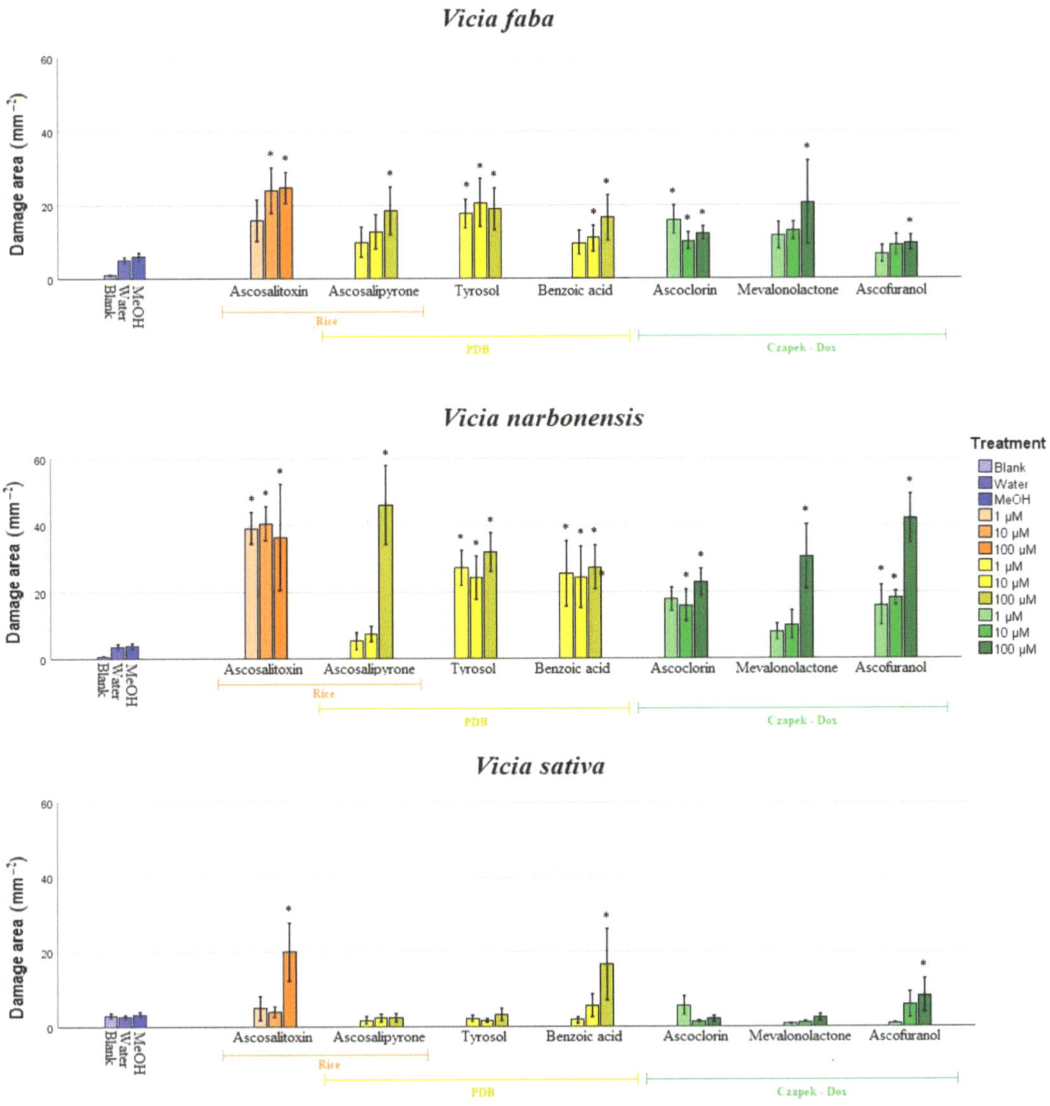

Figure 4. Necrotic area (mm^2) incited by metabolites **1–7** at different concentrations (1, 10, and 100 µM showed as increased color intensity) on leaves of *Vicia faba*, *V. narbonensis*, *V. sativa* (LSD test, $p < 0.01$). In orange metabolites isolated from rice substrate, in yellow, metabolites isolated from PDB culture; in green, metabolites isolated from Czapek-dox; in blue, negative control: blank uninoculated, water and MeOH 5% controls. Asterisk (*) indicates values significantly different from control MeOH 5%.

3. Discussion

Among the diseases affecting legumes, Ascochyta blight, incited from the fungal pathogen *Ascochyta fabae*, is one of the most critical necrotic diseases globally present in all legume cultivation areas [17]. Numerous studies suggest that symptoms associated with Ascochyta blight disease seem to be triggered when there is a shift in host physiology, particularly during periods of plant tissue stress [19]. In fact, various chemical and physical factors, whether directly or indirectly, play a role in activating metabolic pathways, which may include the phytotoxic secondary metabolites generated by the fungus. The legume-associated *Ascochyta* spp. produce different metabolites with pathogenesis-determining cytotoxic capacity, many of which display significant toxicity to plants [19,22]. To shed light on the interaction between *A. fabae* and its host plants and to obtain new insights into the role of secondary metabolites involved in pathogenicity, we conducted a comprehensive study to isolate and characterize the most abundant phytotoxic secondary metabolites produced by this pathogen under in vitro conditions. Due to the difference found in the bibliography concerning the culture media described for isolation of phytotoxins produced by *Ascochyta* spp. [19,22–24], our study was conducted growing *A. fabae* on three commonly used growth media: PDB, Czapek-Dox, and rice substrate. Despite variations in culture media and substrates employed, the mycelial growth and spore production performed well. The mycelium initially displayed a pale cream color, transitioning into shades of greyish white, dark greenish, and creamy white, aligning with expectations. However, the subsequent investigation into the metabolic profile revealed the significant impact of cultural conditions on the production of secondary metabolites. This outcome is consistent with prior research involving the One Strain Many Compounds Strategy (OSMAC) applied to other fungal and bacteria species [25]. Still, this is the first time that this strategy has been applied to an isolate of *A. fabae*. Exploring diverse cultural conditions is essential for comprehensively exploring the selected microorganism's chemical space and biosynthetic pathways, effectively simulating *in vivo* conditions. This is particularly relevant in chemical ecology studies aimed at elucidating the role of specialized metabolites in host–pathogen interactions and identifying chemical biomarkers for early disease detection [25,26].

After filtration of the mycelium and extraction of the cultures, the phytotoxicity of each resulting fungal extracts was tested on the host plant and related legumes. The bioassays revealed differences among the extracts, with that obtained from the Czapek-Dox medium being the most active, followed by that from PDB, and finally, from rice substrate Regarding the host susceptibility, species belonging to the genus *Vicia* spp. were the most susceptible to all the extracts, with faba bean showing the most damage, as expected, since it is the primary host, followed by narbon vetch and common vetch. Lentils and peas, on the other hand, displayed lower susceptibility to the phytotoxic activity of the extracts. These results align with previous findings from cross-inoculation studies with different *Ascochyta* spp. isolates on a panel of legume hosts [11]. The authors found that *A. fabae* principally infected beans (common bean, faba bean, and soybean) and common vetch, while negligible damages were observed in both peas and lentils. These results suggested that the specificity observed might be attributed to bioactive secondary metabolites in the extracts, which could play a role in specific host interactions.

Indeed, when chemical investigation was carried out on the three organic extracts, differences in metabolic composition were appreciated. The prevalent metabolic constituents produced during the in vitro growth by the Ascochyta blight pathogen were isolated by chromatographic methods and dereplicated by extensive spectroscopic studies. As a result, the main compounds identified were ascochlorin, ascofuranol, (*R*)-mevalonolactone, ascosalipyron, benzoic acid, tyrosol, and ascosalitoxin. This was the first time where these metabolites had been purified and dereplicated from an *A. fabae* isolate. Still, their isolation and amount highly depended on the selected cultural condition. In detail, we isolated and dereplicated ascochlorin and ascofuranol together with (*R*)-mevalonolactone in the Czapek-Dox medium. In contrast, ascosalipyron, benzoic acid and tyrosol were isolated and dereplicated in the PDB medium. Finally, when *A. fabae* was grown on rice substrate the main constituents of the extract were ascosalipyron and ascosalitoxin.

Ascochlorin and ascofuranol are the class natural compounds of meroterpenoids of polyketide–terpene hybrid origin. Ascochlorin was originally isolated from a culture extract of *A. viciae* [27] and later from the entomopathogenic fungus *Verticillium hemipterigenum* [28] This compound bears a structural resemblance to ubiquinol, an integral component of the respiratory chain for ATP synthesis, exerting inhibitory effects on protozoan alternate oxidase at the ubiquinol-binding site [29]. Notably, ascochlorin has demonstrated diverse biological activities, including antiviral and antibiotic properties, as evident in studies targeting *Candida albicans* [27]. Additionally, it hinders the respiratory chain of ascomycetes yeast *Pichia anomala* by affecting the coenzyme Q [30]. Furthermore, it functions as a non-toxic anticancer agent by inducing G1 cell cycle arrest through p21 induction in a c-Myc-dependent manner rather than p53-dependent [31]. Ascofuranol, a derivative of ascofuranone, was initially isolated from *A. viciae* [32] and was later identified in *A. rabiei* extracts [33]. Ascofuranol exerts its inhibitory action on the alternative oxidase of Trypanosoma by targeting the ubiquinol-binding domain [32]. Ascosalitoxin is a trisubstituted salicylic aldehyde derivative and a biosynthetic precursor of the ascochitine [21]. While this compound was initially isolated from *Ascochyta pisi* [23], it has also been discovered from an endophytic fungus isolated from the medicinal plant *Hintonia latiflora* [34]. Ascosalitoxin has demonstrated cytotoxic activity against human tumor cell lines, manifesting inhibitory effects on the HL-60 cell line [35]. Ascosalipyrone, a polyketide, was first isolated from *A. salicorniae* [36]. It displays potential biological activity as an inhibitor of protein phosphatases [37]. Additionally, it shows antiplasmodial activity against the K1 and NF 54 strains of *Plasmodium falciparum* in conjunction with antimicrobial activity and inhibition of the tyrosine kinase p56lck [36]. In our study, ascosalipyrone was dereplicated from PDB and rice substrate extracts. Notably, the former exhibited higher phytotoxic activity, possibly attributable to the lower production of ascosalipyrone on the rice substrate. In the PDB fungal extracts, two other metabolites were also found: tyrosol and benzoic acid, two simple phenolic metabolites synthesized via the shikimate and phenylpropanoid pathways. They could contribute to infection and phytotoxicity. Nevertheless, it is essential to acknowledge that these metabolites might also fulfill other roles in disease progression or fungal development. Tyrosol is a derivative of phenethyl alcohol. While it has previously been isolated from *A. lentis* and *A. lentis* var. *lathyri* [22], this study marks its first isolation from *A. fabae*. Tyrosol is recognized as a phytotoxic metabolite isolated from both plants and fungi [38]. It frequently appears in cultures of botryosphaeraceous fungi [38] and has been associated with "quorum sensing" in the human pathogenic fungus *Candida albicans* [39]. Tyrosol exhibits antioxidant and anti-inflammatory properties [40] and protects against oxidative stress in renal cells alongside hydroxytyrosol [41]. Furthermore, studies have linked the cytotoxicity of tyrosol and its derivatives with the inhibition of DNA replication initiation [42]. Its potential suitability for stroke therapy in rats has also been explored [43]. On the other hand, benzoic acid has been identified in *Streptomyces lavandulae* [44,45], as well as in *Lactobacillus plantarum*, where it exhibited antimicrobial activity against Gram-negative bacteria such as *Pantoea agglomerans* (*Enterobacter agglomerans*) and *Fusarium avenaceum* (*Gibberella panacea*). In faba beans infected with Fusarium wilt, benzoic acid has been observed to reduce tissue and cell structure resistance, decrease photosynthesis, and increase cell wall degrading enzyme activity [46]. Additionally, it has been shown to inhibit primary root elongation in *Arabidopsis* seedlings, resulting in reduced sizes [47]. (*R*)-Mevalonolactone, a lactone belonging to the δ-valerolactone class, plays a pivotal role as an essential intermediate in the mevalonate biosynthetic pathway. This biosynthetic route is crucial for synthesizing isoprenoids, versatile compounds with diverse functions in various cellular processes [48,49]. Notably, (*R*)-mevalonolactone has been isolated from different pathogenic and non-pathogenic fungi cultivated in vitro, including *Colletotrichum lupini*, *Diaporthaceae* sp. PSU-SP2/4, *Alternaria euphorbicola*, *Pseudallescheria boydii*, and *Phomopsis archeri* [50–53]. (*R*)-Mevalonolactone was found to enhance chlorophyll content in Leman fronds and inhibit root elongation in cress. Additionally, it led to a considerable reduction in seed germination of *Pelipanche ramosa* [50]. Nevertheless, no phytotoxic effects have been reported for this metabolite.

All these metabolites underwent a phytotoxicity bioassay on the same panel of legume crops of the crude extracts. Notably, prior to this study, there was a lack of information available in the literature regarding the phytotoxic activity of some of the dereplicated metabolites. They all showed different degrees of phytotoxicity regarding legumes and concentration, with the phytotoxic effect more evident in *Vicia* species. In detail, ascochlorin displays intense phytotoxic activity as necrosis on leaves in both faba bean and narbon vetch. Surprisingly, it does not induce significant damage in common vetch despite being first isolated from *A. viciae*. Ascofuranol has a dose-dependent effect in faba beans and peas while in narbon vetch, necrotic damages are high at all concentrations tested. Ascosalitoxin was the most active metabolite isolated, inducing necrosis in all legume crops tested except lentils. This agrees with previous studies where phytotoxic activity from ascosalitoxin on pea leaves and pods and on tomato seedlings was described [23]. Ascosalitoxin was extracted from rice extract. Although the fungal rice extract had the lowest activity in *Vicia* spp., the pure compound caused the most damage. The difference in activity between the fungal extract and the pure compound may be due to its concentration in the organic extract. For ascosalipyrone this is the first evidence regarding its phytotoxic activity, as no previously available information was described. It was active on faba bean, narbon vetch and pea leaves, but only at the highest concentration tested (100 μM). Similar behavior was observed for (*R*)-mevalonolactone being the most phytotoxin on faba bean and narbon vetch, showing a dose-dependent effect. Tyrosol displayed no dose-dependent effect against faba bean and narbon vetch, causing significant damage even at the lowest concentration of 1 μM. Nevertheless, contrary to previous results [19], lentil is only slightly susceptible while no significantly diseased leaves were observed in treated vetch or pea. Since tyrosol is a ubiquitous metabolite in plants, this might exceed the plant's usual levels, leading to necrosis at even lower compound concentrations. Interestingly, benzoic acid is the only compound that exhibits activity in all leguminous plants, but its behavior varies. In narbon vetch, its activity does not depend on concentration. In contrast, in all others, it does, with faba beans showing activity from 10 μM and lentils, peas, and beans only at their highest concentration applied.

The observed variations in bioassay results between crude extracts and pure metabolites may be ascribed to differences in the tested concentrations and production disparities within the various culture media and the potential synergistic or antagonistic effects that may exist among the metabolites generated in each medium. When dealing with complex mixtures of natural products, the dereplication and identification of the specific components responsible for their activities and comprehending the mechanisms involved in their interactions remains a tricky challenge. Such mechanisms can be multifaceted and vary depending on the cultivation methods, preparation, and processing of these compounds, as observed in previous research [54,55]. Modern analytical chemistry techniques, chemoinformatic tools, and metabolomics play a pivotal role in the dereplication of intricate organic extracts by identifying and cataloguing known metabolites and promoting the search for novel compounds. Additionally, it offers a powerful tool for quantifying minor components within these extracts, aiding in accurately assessing their abundance [56–60]. Furthermore, it is essential to highlight that the low amount and the high number of chiral carbons in ascochlorin ascofuranol, ascosalipyrone, and ascosalitoxin did not allow their complete stereochemical characterization using the spectroscopic method. Existing information on the stereochemistry of these metabolites is limited [23,61]. Future research should prioritize the assignment of chiral carbon configurations to fully elucidate their role in the Ascochyta-legume interaction. The absolute assignment of fungal secondary metabolite configurations through advanced spectroscopic methods, including NMR and optical techniques, is indispensable for comprehensively understanding their biological relevance [62–64]. Accurate molecular structure determination provides insights into the compound's bioactivity and potential ecological roles.

Finally, it is essential to highlight that high-molecular-weight phytotoxins were not studied under the conditions of this research. In previous studies involving other fungal species, hydrophilic high-molecular-weight metabolites, such as polysaccharide peptides with phototoxic properties that could have a role as elicitors, have been detected and studied in vitro [65–67].

In conclusion, our research has provided insights into the phytotoxic secondary metabolites produced by *A. fabae* under varying in vitro conditions, unveiling a rich diversity of compounds with differential phytotoxic effects. Notably, prior to this study, only ascochitine was known to be produced by *A. fabae*. We have dereplicated a panel of seven metabolites belonging to different classes of natural compounds that could be used for targeted in-depth investigations. Nevertheless, the observed variations in bioassay results between crude extracts and pure metabolites underline the intricate nature of these interactions, influenced by synergistic or antagonistic effects among the metabolites and further studies using more sensitive techniques are also needed to identify the minor constituents of the fungal exudate. These findings pave the way for further research to elucidate these seven metabolites' underlying mechanisms and ecological implications in legume–plant interactions. Understanding these complex relationships is essential for advancing our knowledge of host–pathogen interactions and developing more specific strategies for Ascochyta blight management and early detection.

4. Materials and Methods

4.1. Fungal Strain, Culture Medium and Growth Conditions

A previously well-characterized monoconidial strain of *Ascochyta fabae* (Af-CO99-01) [68], isolated from a diseased faba bean (*Vicia faba*) crop and belonging to the fungal collection maintained at the Institute for Sustainable Agriculture (IAS-CSIC, Córdoba, Spain), was selected for these experiments. The pathogen was preserved in sterile cellulose filter papers. Before the experiment, inoculum was prepared by multiplying spores of the isolate on potato dextrose agar (PDA) (Sigma Aldrich, Saint-Quentin Fallavier, France) medium under controlled conditions as previously described [11]. Then, the isolate was differentially growth in two artificial media and one solid substrate as follows: (i) 10 flasks containing 1 L of Czapek-Dox medium [69]. Each flask was inoculated with a 1-week-old mycelial plate of the isolate on PDA. The cultures were incubated at 24 °C (stirring conditions, 150 rpm), in absence of light for 21 days. The fungal mycelium was then removed by filtration through four layers of filter paper, centrifuged and kept at −20 °C until the next analysis; (ii) 10 flasks containing 1 L of potato dextrose broth (PDB) (BD Difco®, Crystal Lake, NJ, USA) medium. Each flask was inoculated with a 1-week-old mycelial plate of the isolate on PDA and kept at similar conditions to those mentioned in point (i); (iii) 1 L flask containing 400 g of common rice. Water was added to the flask (45%, vol/vol) and allowed 24 h to be absorbed. Then, the material was sterilized at 121 °C for 30 min. Inoculation was carried out with a 1-week-old mycelial plate of the isolate on PDA. The culture was then incubated in conditions described by Reveglia et al. [70].

4.2. General Experimental Procedure for Chemical Analysis

Analytical and preparative TLCs were carried out on silica gel (Merck, Kieselgel 60, F254, 0.25, and 0.5 mm) and reverse phase (Merck, Kieselgel 60 RP-18, F254, 0.20 mm) plates. The spots were visualized by exposure to UV radiation (254 and/or 312 nm) or by spraying first with 10% H_2SO_4 in MeOH, and then with 5% phosphomolybdic acid in EtOH, followed by heating at 110 °C for 10 min on a hot plate. Column chromatography was performed using silica gel (Merck, Kieselgel 60, 0.063–0.200 mm). Solvents *n*-hexane MeOH, *i*-PrOH, $CHCl_3$, and CH_2Cl_2 were purchased from Panreac AppliChem (Barcelona, Spain). Unless otherwise noted, optical rotation was measured in MeOH on a Jasco (Tokyo, Japan) polarimeter, whereas the CD spectrum was recorded on a JASCO J-815 CD in MeOH. ^{1}H and ^{13}C NMR and 2D NMR spectra were recorded at 400 or 500, and 100 or 125 MHz in $CDCl_3$ on Bruker and Varian instruments. The same solvent was used as an internal standard. HR-ESIMS analyses were performed using the LC/MS TOF system (AGILENT 6230B, HPLC 1260 Infinity) column Phenomenex LUNA (C18 (2) 5 μm 150 × 4.6 mm). ^{1}H-NMR and ESI/MS (+) spectra of the identified compounds are reported in the Supplementary Figures S1–S14.

4.3. Extraction and Purification of Secondary Metabolites Produced in Czapek-Dox Culture

The culture filtrates (10 L) of *A. fabae* were lyophilized and dissolved in 1/10 distilled water of the original volume. The solution was exhaustively extracted with EtOAc

(3×300 mL). The organic extracts were combined, dried (Na_2SO_4), and evaporated under reduced pressure. The corresponding residue (439 mg) was purified by silica gel column, eluted with $CHCl_3$-*i*-PrOH (95:5), yielding six homogeneous fraction groups. The residue of the first fraction (80 mg) was purified by TLC, eluted with $CHCl_3$ affording two white amorphous solids identified as ascochlorin (**1**, 1.7 mg) and ascofuranol (**2**, 2 mg). The residue of the fourth fraction (80 mg) was purified by TLC, eluted with $CHCl_3$-*i*-PrOH (97:3), affording a white amorphous solid identified as (*R*)-mevalonolactone (**3**, 1.9 mg).

Ascochlorin (**1**): ^{1}H-NMR and ESI/MS (+) data agree with those previously reported [27,71].

Ascofuranol (**2**): ^{1}H-NMR and ESI/MS (+) data agree with those previously reported [32].

(*R*)-Mevalonolactone (**3**): ^{1}H-NMR and ESI/MS (+) data agree with those previously reported [50].

4.4. Extraction and Purification of Secondary Metabolites Produced in PDB Culture

The culture filtrates (10 L) of *A. fabae* were lyophilized and dissolved in 1/10 distilled water of original volume. The solution was exhaustively extracted with EtOAc (3×300 mL). The organic extracts were combined, dried (Na_2SO_4), and evaporated under reduced pressure. The corresponding residue (441 mg) was purified by silica gel column, eluted with $CHCl_3$-*i*-PrOH (95:5), yielding seven homogeneous fraction groups. The residue of the second fraction (34 mg) was purified by TLC, eluted with $CHCl_3$-*i*-PrOH (97:3), affording two white amorphous solids identified as ascosalipyrone (**4**, 10 mg), and as benzoic acid (**5**, 8 mg). The residue of the third fraction (60 mg) was purified by TLC and eluted with $CHCl_3$-*i*-PrOH (95:5), affording a white amorphous solid identified as tyrosol (**6**, 1.6 mg).

Ascosalipyrone (**4**): ^{1}H-NMR and ESI/MS (+) data agree with those previously reported [36].

Benzoic acid (**5**): ^{1}H-NMR and ESI/MS (+) data agree with those previously reported. [44].

Tyrosol (**6**): ^{1}H-NMR and ESI/MS (+) data agree with those previously reported [72].

4.5. Extraction and Purification of Secondary Metabolites Produced in Rice Culture

The solid culture of *A. fabae* (440 g) was subjected to air-drying at 27 °C for a minimum of two weeks before the extraction process. Subsequently, the dried material was finely ground using a laboratory mill and then subjected to extraction with a mixture of 500 mL of MeOH–H_2O (1% NaCl) in a 1:1 ratio. Afterward, the mixture underwent centrifugation at 10,000 rpm for 1 h. The resulting pellet was subjected to a second round of extraction using the same solvent mixture under identical conditions. The two supernatants obtained were combined, treated with *n*-hexane (2×500 mL) for defatting, and further extracted with CH_2Cl_2 (3×500 mL). The organic extracts in CH_2Cl_2 were pooled, desiccated using Na_2SO_4, and subsequently concentrated under reduced pressure to produce a brown solid residue weighing 226 mg. The corresponding residue was purified by silica gel column, eluted with $CHCl_3$-*i*-PrOH (95:5), yielding six homogeneous fraction groups. The residue of the second fraction (4.7 mg) was purified by TLC eluted with $CHCl_3$-*i*-PrOH (97:3). This afforded a white amorphous solid identified as ascosalitoxin (**7**, 0.8 mg). The residue of fraction six (18 mg) was purified by TLC, eluted with $CHCl_3$-*i*-PrOH (95:5), yielding another amorphous solid identified as ascosalipyrone (**4**, 1 mg).

Ascosalitoxin (**7**): ^{1}H-NMR and ESI/MS (+) data agree with those previously reported [23,34].

4.6. Bioassays

The phytotoxic effects of all the *A. fabae* organic extracts and those of pure compounds **1**–**7** were evaluated using a detached leaf method [73]. Several legume crops (listed in Table 2) were selected and grown in chamber as follows: seeds were sown in pots

(6 × 6 × 10 cm) filled with a potting mixture (sand/peat, 1:3 vol/vol), then were grown in a growth chamber at 20 ± 2 °C and 65% relative humidity under a photoperiod with 14 h light/10 h dark at a light intensity of 200 μmol m^{-2} s^{-1} photon flux density supplied by high-output white fluorescent tubes until the fifth leaf stage was achieved [70]. Leaves from each legume specie were excised and placed, adaxial side up, on 4% technical agar in Petri dishes. The three organic fungal extracts were dissolved in MeOH (5%) and then added to the assay concentration with distilled water of 0.5, 1, and 2 mg/mL. Similarly, bioassays performed with pure compounds **1–7** and were arranged in Petri dishes as described above and assayed at 1, 10, and 100 μM concentrations. For each legume specie, fungal extract, compound, and concentration assayed, cut leaves were arranged in a randomized design with three replicates per treatment, each replicate having four leaves.

Table 2. Legume species and genotypes grow under controlled conditions and are used in detached leaves assays.

Legume	Plant Specie	Genotype
Faba bean	*Vicia faba*	Baraca
Narbon vetch	*V. narbonensis*	VN01
Common vetch	*V. sativa*	Buzza
Lentil	*Lens culinaris*	Pardina
Pea	*Pisum sativum*	Messire

4.7. Data Analysis

A completely randomized design was used in all detached leaves essays. The presence of symptoms through the appearance of dark spots or discoloration of the plant tissue was monitored, introducing a method of image acquisition by an android smartphone. The smartphone was equipped with CMOS image sensor and SMD LED background light illumination to provide a constant brightness for all the images captured and reduce the effect of ambient lighting condition. Samsung galaxy J2 smartphone (Samsung Engineering Co., Ltd., Seoul, Republic of Korea) was used to acquire 2 images per detached leaves and per plate to be analyzed. All the images collected were in an RGB color space. The damage area (mm^2) was measured on the smartphone-captured images, with the help of ImageJ (1.46 r) program (free license). The significance of the differences in leaf damage between plant species, treatments, and concentrations was estimated by one-way analysis of variance (ANOVA). All statistical analyses were performed using the Statistix 9.0 package (Analytical Software, Tallahase, FL, USA). Significance of differences between means was determined by calculating least significant difference (LSD).

One-dimensional and two-dimensional NRM data were analyzed and interpreted by MNova software v. 14 (MestreLab Research S.L, Santiago de Compostela, Spain).

Supplementary Materials: The following supporting information can be downloaded at: https://www.mdpi.com/article/10.3390/toxins15120693/s1. Supplementary Figure S1. ^{1}H-NMR spectrum of ascochlorin (**1**) ($CDCl_3$, 400 MHz); Supplementary Figure S2. ESI/MS (+) spectrum of ascochlorin (**1**); Supplementary Figure S3. ^{1}H-NMR spectrum of ascofuranol (**2**) ($CDCl_3$, 400 MHz); Supplementary Figure S4. ESI/MS (+) spectrum of ascofuranol (**2**); Supplementary Figure S5. ^{1}H-NMR spectrum of (*R*)-mevalonolactone (**3**) ($CDCl_3$, 400 MHz); Supplementary Figure S6. ESI/MS (+) spectrum of (*R*)-mevalonolactone (**3**); Supplementary Figure S7. ^{1}H-NMR spectrum of ascosalipyrone (**4**) ($CDCl_3$, 400 MHz); Supplementary Figure S8. ESI/MS (+) spectrum of ascosalipyrone (**4**); Supplementary Figure S9. ^{1}H-NMR spectrum of benzoic acid (**5**) ($CDCl_3$, 400 MHz); Supplementary Figure S10. ESI/MS (+) spectrum of benzoic acid (**5**); Supplementary Figure S11. ^{1}H-NMR spectrum of tyrosol (**6**) ($CDCl_3$, 400 MHz); Supplementary Figure S12. ESI/MS (+) spectrum of tyrosol (**6**); Supplementary Figure S13. ^{1}H-NMR spectrum of ascosalitoxin (**7**) ($CDCl_3$, 400 MHz); Supplementary Figure S14. ESI/MS (+) spectrum of ascosalitoxin (**7**); Supplementary Figure S15. Images of the symptoms of each of the compounds. Supplementary Table S1. Diseased area (mm^2) measured on detached leaves of several legume crops with exudates from the fungus *A. fabae* growth in vitro on

3 different culture media (Czapek-Dox = CD, potato dextrose broth = PDB, and rice) at concentrations of 0.5, 1, and 2 mg/mL. Negative (blank untreated, water and MeOH 5%) controls were also included. The experiment was repeated four times. Supplementary Table S2. Diseased area (mm^2) measured in leaves detached from various legume crops with metabolites produced by the exudate of the *A. fabae* fungus from the three-growth media at concentrations of 1, 10, and 100 μM. Negative controls (untreated blank, water, and MeOH 5%) were also included. *p*-value compared with value from MeOH 5% control.

Author Contributions: Conceptualization, E.B., P.R. and D.R.; methodology, P.R. and E.B.; validation, D.R., A.E. and A.C.; investigation, E.B., P.R., F.J.A.-J. and V.C.G.; data curation, P.R., E.B., V.C.G. and F.J.A.-J.; writing—original draft preparation, E.B. and P.R.; writing—review and editing, F.J.A.-J., A.E., A.C. and D.R.; visualization, P.R. and F.J.A.-J.; supervision, E.B. and D.R.; funding acquisition, D.R. All authors have read and agreed to the published version of the manuscript.

Funding: This research was funded by projects PCI2020-111974 (PRIMA-DiVicia) and PID2020-114668RB-I00 (MCIN/AEI/10.13039/501100011033).

Institutional Review Board Statement: Not applicable.

Informed Consent Statement: Not applicable.

Data Availability Statement: All the data that arose from this research are included in the manuscript and in the supplementary material.

Conflicts of Interest: The authors declare no conflict of interest.

References

1. Rubiales, D.; Annicchiarico, P.; Vaz Patto, M.C.; Julier, B. Legume breeding for the agroecological transition of global agri-food systems: A European perspective. *Front. Plant Sci.* **2021**, *12*, 782574. [CrossRef] [PubMed]
2. Ferreira, H.; Pinto, E.; Vasconcelos, M.W. Legumes as a cornerstone of the transition toward more sustainable agri-food systems and diets in Europe. *Front. Sustain. Food Syst.* **2021**, *5*, 694121. [CrossRef]
3. Rubiales, D.; Duc, G.; Stoddard, F. Faba beans in sustainable agriculture. *Field Crops Res.* **2010**, *115*, 201–233. [CrossRef]
4. Gharzeddin, K.; Maalouf, F.; Khoury, B.; Abou Khater, L.; Christmann, S.; Jamal El Dine, N.A. Efficiency of different breeding strategies in improving the faba bean productivity for sustainable agriculture. *Euphytica* **2019**, *215*, 203. [CrossRef]
5. Yitayih, G.; Fininsa, C.; Terefe, H.; Shibabaw, A. Integrated management approaches reduced yield loss, and increased productivity in faba bean, due to gall disease in northwestern Ethiopia. *Arch. Phytopathol. Plant Prot.* **2022**, *55*, 1592–1610. [CrossRef]
6. Karkanis, A.; Ntatsi, G.; Lepse, L.; Fernández, J.A.; Vågen, I.M.; Rewald, B.; Alsina, I.; Kronberga, A.; Balliu, A.; Olle, M.; et al. Faba bean cultivation-revealing novel managing practices for more sustainable and competitive European cropping systems. *Front. Plant Sci.* **2018**, *9*, 1115. [CrossRef]
7. Tivoli, B.; Banniza, S. *Comparison of the Epidemiology of Ascochyta Blights on Grain Legumes*; Springer: Berlin/Heidelberg, Germany, 2007.
8. Hernandez-Bello, M.; Chilvers, M.; Akamatsu, H.; Peever, T. Host specificity of *Ascochyta* spp. infecting legumes of the *Viciae* and *Cicerae* tribes and pathogenicity of an interspecific hybrid. *Phytopathology* **2006**, *96*, 1148–1156. [CrossRef] [PubMed]
9. Zhang, C.; Chen, W.; Sankaran, S. High-throughput field phenotyping of Ascochyta blight disease severity in chickpea. *Crop Prot.* **2019**, *125*, 104885. [CrossRef]
10. Bretag, T.W.; Keane, P.J.; Price, T.V. The epidemiology and control of ascochyta blight in field peas: A review. *Aust. J. Agric. Res.* **2006**, *57*, 883–902. [CrossRef]
11. Barilli, E.; Cobos, M.J.; Rubiales, D. Clarification on host range of *Didymella pinodes* the causal agent of pea Ascochyta blight. *Front. Plant Sci.* **2016**, *7*, 592. [CrossRef]
12. Ahmed, S.; Abang, M.; Maalouf, F. Integrated management of Ascochyta blight (*Didymella fabae*) on faba bean under Mediterranean conditions. *Crop Prot.* **2016**, *81*, 65–69. [CrossRef]
13. Koder, S.B.; Nawale, R.; Katyayani, K.K.S.; Rana, M.; Srivastava, S. Symptoms, biology and management of ascochyta blight (Phoma exigua) of French beans: A review. *Agric. Sci. Dig. Res. J.* **2022**, *42*, 657–664. [CrossRef]
14. Trapero-Casas, A.; Kaiser, W.J. Influence of temperature, wetness period, plant age, and inoculum concentration on infection and development of Ascochyta blight of chickpea. *Phytopathology* **1992**, *82*, 589–596. [CrossRef]
15. Rubiales, D.; Fondevilla, S.; Chen, W.; Gentzbittel, L.; Higgins, T.J.; Castillejo, M.A.; Singh, K.B.; Rispail, N. Achievements and challenges in legume breeding for pest and disease resistance. *Crit. Rev. Plant Sci.* **2015**, *34*, 195–236. [CrossRef]
16. Pratap, A.; Douglas, C.; Prajapati, U.; Kumari, G.; War, A.R.; Tomar, R.; Pandey, A.K.; Dubey, S. Breeding progress and future challenges: Biotic stresses. In *The Mungbean Genome. Compendium of Plant Genomes*; Springer: Cham, Switzerland, 2020; pp. 55–80.
17. Rubiales, D.; Ávila, C.M.; Sillero, J.C.; Hybl, M.; Narits, L.; Sass, O.; Flores, F. Identification and multi-environment validation of resistance to *Ascochyta fabae* in faba bean (*Vicia faba*). *Field Crops Res.* **2012**, *126*, 165–170. [CrossRef]

18. Mengiste, T. Plant immunity to necrotrophs. *Annu. Rev. Phytopathol.* **2012**, *50*, 267–294. [CrossRef] [PubMed]
19. Kim, W.; Chen, W. Phytotoxic metabolites produced by legume-associated *Ascochyta* and its related genera in the Dothideomycetes. *Toxins* **2019**, *11*, 627. [CrossRef] [PubMed]
20. Oku, H.; Nakanishi, T. A toxic metabolite from *Ascochyta fabae* having antibiotic activity. *Phytopathology* **1963**, *53*, 1321–1325.
21. Kim, W.; Lichtenzveig, J.; Syme, R.A.; Williams, A.H.; Peever, T.L.; Chen, W. Identification of a polyketide synthase gene responsible for Ascochitine biosynthesis in *Ascochyta fabae* and its abrogation in sister taxa. *Msphere* **2019**, *4*, e00622-19. [CrossRef]
22. Agudo-Jurado, F.J.; Reveglia, P.; Rubiales, D.; Evidente, A.; Barilli, E. Status of Phytotoxins Isolated from Necrotrophic Fungi Causing Diseases on Grain Legumes. *Int. J. Mol. Sci.* **2023**, *24*, 5116. [CrossRef]
23. Evidente, A.; Capasso, R.; Vurro, M.; Bottalico, A. Ascosalitoxin, a phytotoxic trisubstituted salicylic aldehyde from *Ascochyta pisi*. *Phytochemistry* **1993**, *34*, 995–998. [CrossRef]
24. Beed, F.; Strange, R.; Onfroy, C.; Tivoli, B. Virulence for faba bean and production of ascochitine by *Ascochyta fabae*. *Plant Pathol.* **1994**, *43*, 987–997. [CrossRef]
25. Pan, R.; Bai, X.; Chen, J.; Zhang, H.; Wang, H. Exploring structural diversity of microbe secondary metabolites using OSMAC strategy: A literature review. *Front. Microbiol.* **2019**, *10*, 294. [CrossRef] [PubMed]
26. Farinella, V.F.; Kawafune, E.S.; Tangerina, M.M.; Domingos, H.V.; Costa-Lotufo, L.V.; Ferreira, M.J. OSMAC strategy integrated with molecular networking for accessing griseofulvin derivatives from endophytic fungi of *Moquiniastrum polymorphum* (Asteraceae). *Molecules* **2021**, *26*, 7316. [CrossRef] [PubMed]
27. Tamura, G.; Suzuki, S.; Takatsuki, A.; Ando, K.; Arima, K. Ascochlorin, a new antibiotic, found by paper-disc agar-diffusion method. I isolation, biological and chemical properties of ascochlorin (studies on antiviral and antitumor antibiotics. I). *J. Antibiot.* **1968**, *21*, 539–544. [CrossRef] [PubMed]
28. Seephonkai, P.; Isaka, M.; Kittakoop, P.; Boonudomlap, U.; Thebtaranonth, Y. A novel ascochlorin glycoside from the insect pathogenic fungus *Verticillium hemipterigenum* BCC 2370. *J. Antibiot.* **2004**, *57*, 10–16. [CrossRef] [PubMed]
29. Mogi, T.; Miyoshi, H. Properties of cytochrome bd plastoquinol oxidase from the cyanobacterium *Synechocystis* sp. PCC 6803. *J. Biochem.* **2009**, *145*, 395–401. [CrossRef]
30. Berry, E.A.; Huang, L.S.; Lee, D.W.; Daldal, F.; Nagai, K.; Minagawa, N. Ascochlorin is a novel, specific inhibitor of the mitochondrial cytochrome bc1 complex. *Biochim. Biophys. Acta BBA Bioenerg.* **2010**, *1797*, 360–370. [CrossRef]
31. Jeong, J.H.; Jeong, Y.J.; Cho, H.J.; Shin, J.M.; Kang, J.H.; Park, K.K.; Park, Y.Y.; Chung, I.K.; Chang, H.W.; Magae, J. Ascochlorin inhibits growth factor-induced HIF-1α activation and tumor-angiogenesis through the suppression of EGFR/ERK/p70S6K signaling pathway in human cervical carcinoma cells. *J. Cell. Biochem.* **2012**, *113*, 1302–1313. [CrossRef]
32. Sasaki, H.; Hosokawa, T.; Sawada, M.; Ando, K. Isolation and structure of ascofuranone and ascofranol, antibiotics with hypolipidemic activity. *J. Antibiot.* **1973**, *26*, 676–680. [CrossRef]
33. Hamid, K. *Separation and Phytotoxicity of Solanapyrone Compounds Produced by Ascochyta rabiei (Pass.) Labr. and Their Metabolism by Chickpea (Cicer arietinum L.)*; University of London, University College London (United Kingdom): London, UK, 1999.
34. Leyte-Lugo, M.; González-Andrade, M.; González, M.d.C.; Glenn, A.E.; Cerda-García-Rojas, C.M.; Mata, R. (+)-Ascosalitoxin and vermelhotin, a calmodulin inhibitor, from an endophytic fungus isolated from *Hintonia latiflora*. *J. Nat. Prod.* **2012**, *75*, 1571–1577. [CrossRef] [PubMed]
35. Yu, C.; Nian, Y.; Chen, H.; Liang, S.; Sun, M.; Pei, Y.; Wang, H. Pyranone Derivatives with antitumor activities, from the endophytic fungus *Phoma* sp. YN02-P-3. *Front. Chem.* **2022**, *10*, 950726. [CrossRef] [PubMed]
36. Osterhage, C.; Kaminsky, R.; König, G.M.; Wright, A.D. Ascosalipyrrolidinone a, an antimicrobial alkaloid, from the obligate marine fungus *Ascochyta salicorniae*. *J. Org. Chem.* **2000**, *65*, 6412–6417. [CrossRef] [PubMed]
37. Seibert, S.F.; Eguereva, E.; Krick, A.; Kehraus, S.; Voloshina, E.; Raabe, G.; Fleischhauer, J.; Leistner, E.; Wiese, M.; Prinz, H. Polyketides from the marine-derived fungus *Ascochyta salicorniae* and their potential to inhibit protein phosphatases. *Org. Biomol. Chem.* **2006**, *4*, 2233–2240. [CrossRef] [PubMed]
38. Salvatore, M.M.; Alves, A.; Andolfi, A. Secondary metabolites of *Lasiodiplodia theobromae*: Distribution, chemical diversity, bioactivity, and implications of their occurrence. *Toxins* **2020**, *12*, 457. [CrossRef] [PubMed]
39. Chen, H.; Fujita, M.; Feng, Q.; Clardy, J.; Fink, G.R. Tyrosol is a quorum-sensing molecule in *Candida albicans*. *Proc. Natl. Acad. Sci. USA* **2004**, *101*, 5048–5052. [CrossRef] [PubMed]
40. Muriana, F.J.; Montserrat-de la Paz, S.; Lucas, R.; Bermudez, B.; Jaramillo, S.; Morales, J.C.; Abia, R.; Lopez, S. Tyrosol and its metabolites as antioxidative and anti-inflammatory molecules in human endothelial cells. *Food Funct.* **2017**, *8*, 2905–2914. [CrossRef]
41. Loru, D.; Incani, A.; Deiana, M.; Corona, G.; Atzeri, A.; Melis, M.; Rosa, A.; Dessì, M. Protective effect of hydroxytyrosol and tyrosol against oxidative stress in kidney cells. *Toxicol. Ind. Health* **2009**, *25*, 301–310. [CrossRef]
42. Karković Marković, A.; Torić, J.; Barbarić, M.; Jakobušić Brala, C. Hydroxytyrosol, tyrosol and derivatives and their potential effects on human health. *Molecules* **2019**, *24*, 2001. [CrossRef]
43. Bu, Y.; Rho, S.; Kim, J.; Kim, M.Y.; Lee, D.H.; Kim, S.Y.; Choi, H.; Kim, H. Neuroprotective effect of tyrosol on transient focal cerebral ischemia in rats. *Neurosci. Lett.* **2007**, *414*, 218–221. [CrossRef]
44. Ohtsuki, T.; Sato, K.; Sugimoto, N.; Akiyama, H.; Kawamura, Y. Absolute quantification for benzoic acid in processed foods using quantitative proton nuclear magnetic resonance spectroscopy. *Talanta* **2012**, *99*, 342–348. [CrossRef] [PubMed]

45. Shibata, M.; Uyeda, M.; Kido, Y.; Toya, N.; Nakashima, R.; Terazumi, R. A new antibiotic K-82 A and minor components, produced by *Streptomyces lavendulae*, strain no. K-82. *J. Antibiot.* **1980**, *33*, 1231–1235. [CrossRef] [PubMed]
46. Yang, W.; Guo, Y.; Li, Y.; Lv, J.; Dong, K.; Dong, Y. Benzoic Acid Phytotoxicity the Structural Resistance and Photosynthetic Physiology of Faba Bean and Promotes Fusarium Wilt Incidence. *SSRN Electron. J.* **2022**. [CrossRef]
47. Zhang, K.; Sun, P.; Khan, A.; Zhang, Y. Photochemistry of biochar during ageing process: Reactive oxygen species generation and benzoic acid degradation. *Sci. Total Environ.* **2021**, *765*, 144630. [CrossRef] [PubMed]
48. Buhaescu, I.; Izzedine, H. Mevalonate pathway: A review of clinical and therapeutical implications. *Clin. Biochem.* **2007**, *40*, 575–584. [CrossRef] [PubMed]
49. Lasunción, M.A.; Martinez-Botas, J.; Martin-Sanchez, C.; Busto, R.; Gómez-Coronado, D. Cell cycle dependence on the mevalonate pathway: Role of cholesterol and non-sterol isoprenoids. *Biochem. Pharm.* **2022**, *196*, 114623. [CrossRef] [PubMed]
50. Masi, M.; Nocera, P.; Boari, A.; Zonno, M.C.; Pescitelli, G.; Sarrocco, S.; Baroncelli, R.; Vannacci, G.; Vurro, M.; Evidente, A. Secondary metabolites produced by *Colletotrichum lupini*, the causal agent of anthachnose of lupin (*Lupinus* spp.). *Mycologia* **2020**, *112*, 533–542. [CrossRef] [PubMed]
51. Khamthong, N.; Rukachaisirikul, V.; Phongpaichit, S.; Preedanon, S.; Sakayaroj, J. An antibacterial cytochalasin derivative from the marine-derived fungus *Diaporthaceae* sp. PSU-SP2/4. *Phytochem. Lett.* **2014**, *10*, 5–9. [CrossRef]
52. Hemtasin, C.; Kanokmedhakul, S.; Kanokmedhakul, K.; Hahnvajanawong, C.; Soytong, K.; Prabpai, S.; Kongsaeree, P. Cytotoxic pentacyclic and tetracyclic aromatic sesquiterpenes from *Phomopsis archeri*. *J. Nat. Prod.* **2011**, *74*, 609–613. [CrossRef]
53. Varejão, E.V.V.; Demuner, A.J.; Barbosa, L.C.d.A.; Barreto, R.W. Phytotoxic effects of metabolites from *Alternaria euphorbiicola* against its host plant *Euphorbia heterophylla*. *Quím. Nova* **2013**, *36*, 1004–1007. [CrossRef]
54. Junio, H.A.; Sy-Cordero, A.A.; Ettefagh, K.A.; Burns, J.T.; Micko, K.T.; Graf, T.N.; Richter, S.J.; Cannon, R.E.; Oberlies, N.H.; Cech, N.B. Synergy-directed fractionation of botanical medicines: A case study with goldenseal (*Hydrastis canadensis*). *J. Nat. Prod.* **2011**, *74*, 1621–1629. [CrossRef]
55. Caesar, L.K.; Cech, N.B. Synergy and antagonism in natural product extracts: When 1 + 1 does not equal 2. *Nat. Prod. Rep.* **2019**, *36*, 869–888. [CrossRef] [PubMed]
56. Gauglitz, J.M.; West, K.A.; Bittremieux, W.; Williams, C.L.; Weldon, K.C.; Panitchpakdi, M.; Di Ottavio, F.; Aceves, C.M.; Brown, E.; Sikora, N.C. Enhancing untargeted metabolomics using metadata-based source annotation. *Nat. Biotechnol.* **2022**, *40*, 1774–1779. [CrossRef] [PubMed]
57. Li, Y.; Fiehn, O. Flash entropy search to query all mass spectral libraries in real time. *Nat. Methods* **2023**, *20*, 1475–1478. [CrossRef]
58. Burns, D.C.; Mazzola, E.P.; Reynolds, W.F. The role of computer-assisted structure elucidation (CASE) programs in the structure elucidation of complex natural products. *Nat. Prod. Rep.* **2019**, *36*, 919–933. [CrossRef] [PubMed]
59. Marcarino, M.O.; Zanardi, M.M.; Cicetti, S.; Sarotti, A.M. NMR calculations with quantum methods: Development of new tools for structural elucidation and beyond. *Acc. Chem. Res.* **2020**, *53*, 1922–1932. [CrossRef]
60. Beniddir, M.A.; Kang, K.B.; Genta-Jouve, G.; Huber, F.; Rogers, S.; Van Der Hooft, J.J. Advances in decomposing complex metabolite mixtures using substructure-and network-based computational metabolomics approaches. *Nat. Prod. Rep.* **2021**, *38*, 1967–1993. [CrossRef]
61. Mori, K.; Takechi, S. Synthesis of the natural enantiomers of ascochlorin, ascofuranone and ascofuranol. *Tetrahedron* **1985**, *41*, 3049–3062. [CrossRef]
62. Menna, M.; Imperatore, C.; Mangoni, A.; Della Sala, G.; Taglialatela-Scafati, O. Challenges in the configuration assignment of natural products. A case-selective perspective. *Nat. Prod. Rep.* **2019**, *36*, 476–489. [CrossRef]
63. Bitchagno, G.T.M.; Nchiozem-Ngnitedem, V.-A.; Melchert, D.; Fobofou, S.A. Demystifying racemic natural products in the homochiral world. *Nat. Rev. Chem.* **2022**, *6*, 806–822. [CrossRef]
64. Pereda-Miranda, R.; Bautista, E.; Martínez-Fructuoso, L.; Fragoso-Serrano, M. From Relative to Absolute Stereochemistry of Secondary Metabolites: Applications in Plant Chemistry. *Rev. Bras. Farmacogn.* **2023**, *33*, 1–48. [CrossRef]
65. Lo Presti, L.; Lanver, D.; Schweizer, G.; Tanaka, S.; Liang, L.; Tollot, M.; Zuccaro, A.; Reissmann, S.; Kahmann, R. Fungal effectors and plant susceptibility. *Annu. Rev. Plant Biol.* **2015**, *66*, 513–545. [CrossRef] [PubMed]
66. Chen, H.; Singh, H.; Bhardwaj, N.; Bhardwaj, S.K.; Khatri, M.; Kim, K.H.; Peng, W. An exploration on the toxicity mechanisms of phytotoxins and their potential utilities. *Crit. Rev. Environ. Sci. Technol.* **2022**, *52*, 395–435. [CrossRef]
67. Guo, J.; Cheng, Y. Advances in fungal elicitor-triggered plant immunity. *Int. J. Mol. Sci.* **2022**, *23*, 12003. [CrossRef] [PubMed]
68. Sillero, J.C.; Rojas-Molina, M.M.; Ávila, C.M.; Rubiales, D. Induction of systemic acquired resistance against rust, ascochyta blight and broomrape in faba bean by exogenous application of salicylic acid and benzothiadiazole. *Crop Prot.* **2012**, *34*, 65–69. [CrossRef]
69. Gulder, T.A.; Hong, H.; Correa, J.; Egereva, E.; Wiese, J.; Imhoff, J.F.; Gross, H. Isolation, structure elucidation and total synthesis of lajollamide A from the marine fungus *Asteromyces cruciatus*. *Mar. Drugs.* **2012**, *10*, 2912–2935. [CrossRef] [PubMed]
70. Reveglia, P.; Agudo-Jurado, F.J.; Barilli, E.; Masi, M.; Evidente, A.; Rubiales, D. Uncovering phytotoxic compounds produced by *Colletotrichum* spp. involved in legume diseases using an OSMAC–metabolomics approach. *J. Fungi* **2023**, *9*, 610. [CrossRef] [PubMed]
71. Sasaki, H.; Hosokawa, T.; Nawata, Y.; Ando, K. Isolation and structure of ascochlorin and its analogs. *Agric. Biol. Chem.* **1974**, *38*, 1463–1466. [CrossRef]

72. Kimura, Y.; Tamura, S. Isolation of L-β-phenyllactic acid and tyrosol as plant growth regulators from *Gloeosporium laeticolor*. *Agric. Biol. Chem.* **1973**, *37*, 2925. [CrossRef]
73. Sillero, J.; Fondevilla, S.; Davidson, J.; Patto, M.V.; Warkentin, T.; Thomas, J.; Rubiales, D. Screening techniques and sources of resistance to rusts and mildews in grain legumes. *Euphytica* **2006**, *147*, 255–272. [CrossRef]

toxins

MDPI

Article

Alkaline pH, Low Iron Availability, Poor Nitrogen Sources and CWI MAPK Signaling Are Associated with Increased Fusaric Acid Production in *Fusarium oxysporum*

Davide Palmieri [1,*], David Segorbe [2,†], Manuel S. López-Berges [2], Filippo De Curtis [1], Giuseppe Lima [1], Antonio Di Pietro [2] and David Turrà [3,4,*]

1 Department of Agricultural, Environmental and Food Sciences, University of Molise, 86100 Campobasso, Italy
2 Departamento de Genética, Campus de Excelencia Internacional Agroalimentario ceiA3, Universidad de Córdoba, 14014 Córdoba, Spain
3 Department of Agricultural Sciences, Università di Napoli Federico II, 80055 Portici, Italy
4 Center for Studies on Bioinspired Agro-Enviromental Technology, Università di Napoli Federico II, 80055 Portici, Italy
* Correspondence: davide.palmieri@unimol.it (D.P.); davturra@unina.it (D.T.)
† Current address: Instituto Maimonides de Investigación Biomédica de Cordoba (IMIBIC), Universitdad de Córdoba, 14014 Córdoba, Spain.

Abstract: Fusaric acid (FA) is one of the first secondary metabolites isolated from phytopathogenic fungi belonging to the genus *Fusarium*. This molecule exerts a toxic effect on plants, rhizobacteria, fungi and animals, and it plays a crucial role in both plant and animal pathogenesis. In plants, metal chelation by FA is considered one of the possible mechanisms of action. Here, we evaluated the effect of different nitrogen sources, iron content, extracellular pH and cellular signalling pathways on the production of FA siderophores by the pathogen *Fusarium oxysporum* (*Fol*). Our results show that the nitrogen source affects iron chelating activity and FA production. Moreover, alkaline pH and iron limitation boost FA production, while acidic pH and iron sufficiency repress it independent of the nitrogen source. FA production is also positively regulated by the cell wall integrity (CWI) mitogen-activated protein kinase (MAPK) pathway and inhibited by the iron homeostasis transcriptional regulator HapX. Collectively, this study demonstrates that factors promoting virulence (i.e., alkaline pH, low iron availability, poor nitrogen sources and CWI MAPK signalling) are also associated with increased FA production in *Fol*. The obtained new insights on FA biosynthesis regulation can be used to prevent both *Fol* infection potential and toxin contamination.

Keywords: *Fusarium oxysporum*; fusaric acid; pH; iron limitation; chelating activity; signaling

Key Contribution: Production of fusaric acid in *Fusarium oxysporum* is associated with virulence-promoting conditions: alkaline pH, low iron availability, poor nitrogen sources and CWI MAPK signalling.

Citation: Palmieri, D.; Segorbe, D.; López-Berges, M.S.; De Curtis, F.; Lima, G.; Di Pietro, A.; Turrà, D. Alkaline pH, Low Iron Availability, Poor Nitrogen Sources and CWI MAPK Signaling Are Associated with Increased Fusaric Acid Production in *Fusarium oxysporum*. *Toxins* **2023**, *15*, 50. https://doi.org/10.3390/toxins15010050

Received: 22 November 2022
Revised: 18 December 2022
Accepted: 29 December 2022
Published: 6 January 2023

1. Introduction

Fusarium oxysporum comprises a cosmopolitan complex of fungal species [1] including both non-pathogenic and pathogenic forms [2], which can infect plants, animals and humans [3]. Plant pathogenic strains cause tracheomycosis or foot and root rots (Fusarium wilt) in a large number of plant species and are grouped into over 150 pathogenic forms (formae speciales) [4]. *F. oxysporum* f. sp. *lycopersici* (*Fol*) is the pathogenic form that causes wilting of tomato plants. *Fusarium* species are known to synthesize several biologically active compounds with different roles in plant pathogenesis and microbial competition [5]. Fusaric acid (5-butylpyridine-2-carboxylic acid) (FA), the first fungal metabolite discovered to be implicated in tomato pathogenesis [6], is one of the most widely distributed mycotoxins in the genus *Fusarium* and has been used as an efficient indicator of *Fusarium* contamination in food and feed grains [7]. Plant treatment with FA causes the rapid development of disease symptoms such as internerval necrosis and foliar desiccation even in the absence of the pathogen [8]. FA toxicity in plants has been attributed to different mechanisms of action, including direct membrane damage, electrolyte loss, decrease in cellular ATP levels, metallo-enzyme inhibition, oxidative burst and metal chelation [6,9–11]. In addition to its phytotoxic effect, FA also shows varying degrees of inhibitory activity on rhizobacterial populations. For instance, species of the genera *Bacillus* and *Paenibacillus* are susceptible, while those belonging to *Pseudomonas* are highly resistant [12]. Intriguingly, FA resistance in these species has been shown to rely on the expression of two major siderophores, pyoverdine and enantio-pyochelin, suggesting that the inhibitory effect of FA toxicity on bacteria, similar to plants, depends on its chelating activity [13].

In *Fusarium fujikuroi* the expression of FA biosynthesis genes has been shown to be regulated by the nitrogen-responsive GATA transcription factor AreB and the pH-responsive transcription factor PacC [14]. Similarly, FA levels in *Fol* are controlled via PacC-mediated modulation of chromatin condensation at the *fub1* locus, which encodes a major FA biosynthetic gene [15]. Additionally, in a banana pathogenic isolate of *F. oxysporum* f. sp. *cubense*, several components of the CWI MAPK cascade have been shown to act as positive regulators of FA biosynthetic genes and FA production [16].

In *Fol*, three different MAPKs (Fmk1, Mpk1 and Hog1) regulating distinct virulence functions have been described. While Fmk1 is essential for invasive growth and plant infection, the other two MAPKs, Mpk1 and Hog1, contribute to plant infection both via Fmk1-shared and -independent functions, albeit to a lesser extent [17–19]. This work aimed at evaluating the role of different environmental factors such as nitrogen source, extracellular pH and iron content in the regulation of FA production in *Fol*. Furthermore, we tested the contribution of the three MAPK pathways as well as the iron and pH response regulators HapX and PacC, respectively, on FA biosynthesis.

2. Results

2.1. Nitrogen Source Affects Extracellular pH in F. oxysporum f. sp. lycopersici

We tested the effect of different nitrogen sources on extracellular pH modification, iron chelating activity and FA production by *Fol*. Microconidia were inoculated in minimal medium (pH 4.5) supplemented with either urea, sodium nitrate, ammonium sulphate or ammonium nitrate as the sole nitrogen source. While urea and sodium nitrate elicited an increase in extracellular pH, ammonium sulphate and ammonium nitrate induced extracellular acidification (Table 1; Figure 1). To investigate the role of MAPK pathways in pH modulation, we measured extracellular pH changes in *fmk1*Δ, *hog1*Δ and *mpk1*Δ knockout mutants. Interestingly, deletion of the cell wall integrity (CWI) MAPK Mpk1 resulted in increased extracellular alkalinisation on urea and sodium nitrate but did not affect ammonium-dependent acidification. Similarly, mutations in the seven-transmembrane α-pheromone receptor Ste2 or the conserved components of the CWI pathway Bck1 and Mkk2 also led to an increase in pH (Table 1), suggesting for a role of the sex pheromone perception machinery and the CWI pathway in the regulation of this process.

2.2. Siderophore Production Is pH- and Iron-Sensing Dependent

To detect siderophore production by *Fol*, a CAS assay was performed after 5 days of incubation in the different test conditions. We found that the chelating activity in fungal supernatants was more than 40% higher in media containing urea or sodium nitrate showing high pH, compared to those supplemented with ammonium sulphate or ammonium nitrate which had low pH (Table 1). Furthermore, chelating activity was significantly higher ($p \leq 0.05$) in isogenic mutants lacking Ste2 or conserved components of the CWI MAPK pathway, but not in *fmk1*Δ and *hog1*Δ mutants, compared with the wild-type strain (Table 1). The correlation between pH signalling and siderophore production was further supported by the finding that deletion the of alkaline pH-responsive factor PacC (*pacC*Δ) resulted in decreased chelating activity in urea and nitrate media, whereas expression of a dominant activating PacC allele ($pacC^c$), which represses acidic-regulated functions [20,21], resulted in increased chelating activity in ammonium-containing media (Table 1).

Table 1. Effect of different nitrogen sources on extracellular pH modification, chelating ability and fusaric acid content in the culture supernatants of the indicated *F. oxysporum* f. sp. *lycopersici* (*Fol*) strains. For each fungal strain, values marked by common letters are not different according to Tukey's test ($p \leq 0.05$). For each nitrogen source values marked with the * symbol are statistically different ($p \leq 0.05$; according to Tukey's test) from wild-type values. The values in the table are averages of three independent experiments with three replicates each.

Fol Strain	Nitrogen Source	pH			Chelating Activity			Fusaric Acid [1]		
Wild type	Urea	7.02	a		78.00	a		37	a	
	Sodium nitrate	7.81	b		68.40	b		82	b	
	Ammonium sulphate	3.07	c		27.55	c		n.d.	c	
	Ammonium nitrate	3.64	d		25.55	c		n.d.	c	
fmk1Δ	Urea	6.94	a		75.78	a		41	a	
	Sodium nitrate	7.85	b		69.46	b		75	b	
	Ammonium sulphate	2.88	c		22.98	c		n.d.	c	
	Ammonium nitrate	4.16	d		23.90	c		n.d.	c	
hog1Δ	Urea	6.81	a		75.75	a		36	a	
	Sodium nitrate	7.12	b		65.37	b		85	b	
	Ammonium sulphate	2.93	c		25.55	c		n.d.	c	
	Ammonium nitrate	3.60	d		25.16	c		n.d.	c	
mpk1Δ	Urea	8.95	a	*	89.05	a	*	12	a	*
	Sodium nitrate	8.22	b	*	95.16	a	*	42	b	*
	Ammonium sulphate	3.01	c		21.09	b		n.d.	c	
	Ammonium nitrate	4.16	d		23.51	b		n.d.	c	
ste2Δ	Urea	8.40	a	*	92.05	a	*	9	a	*
	Sodium nitrate	8.33	a	*	91.16	a	*	39	b	*
	Ammonium sulphate	3.07	b		28.09	b		n.d.	c	
	Ammonium nitrate	3.92	c		27.51	b		n.d.	c	
bck1Δ	Urea	8.80	a	*	90.59	a	*	11	a	*
	Sodium nitrate	8.52	a	*	92.13	a	*	45	b	*
	Ammonium sulphate	2.94	b		21.09	b		n.d.	c	
	Ammonium nitrate	3.91	c		24.76	b		n.d.	c	
mkk2Δ	Urea	8.71	a	*	93.93	a	*	8	a	*
	Sodium nitrate	8.35	a	*	93.02	a	*	62	b	*
	Ammonium sulphate	3.12	b		28.43	b		n.d.	c	
	Ammonium nitrate	4.00	c		23.46	b		n.d.	c	
hapXΔ	Urea	7.05	a		84.80	a	*	63	a	*
	Sodium nitrate	7.89	b		86.41	a	*	70	a	
	Ammonium sulphate	3.02	c		60.56	b	*	27	b	*
	Ammonium nitrate	3.98	d		66.75	b	*	0.22	b	*
$pacC^c$	Urea	7.18	a		77.89	a		37	a	
	Sodium nitrate	7.77	b		67.77	b		50	b	*
	Ammonium sulphate	3.12	c		58.28	c	*	22	c	*
	Ammonium nitrate	4.06	d		56.28	c	*	12	d	*
pacCΔ	Urea	7.08	a		35.55	a	*	n.d.	a	
	Sodium nitrate	7.58	b		32.25	a	*	n.d.	a	
	Ammonium sulphate	3.05	c		28.35	b		n.d.	a	*
	Ammonium nitrate	4.18	d		29.25	b		n.d.	a	*

[1] Fusaric acid concentration is expressed in μg of the compound per mg of dry fungal biomass. n.d.= not detectable.

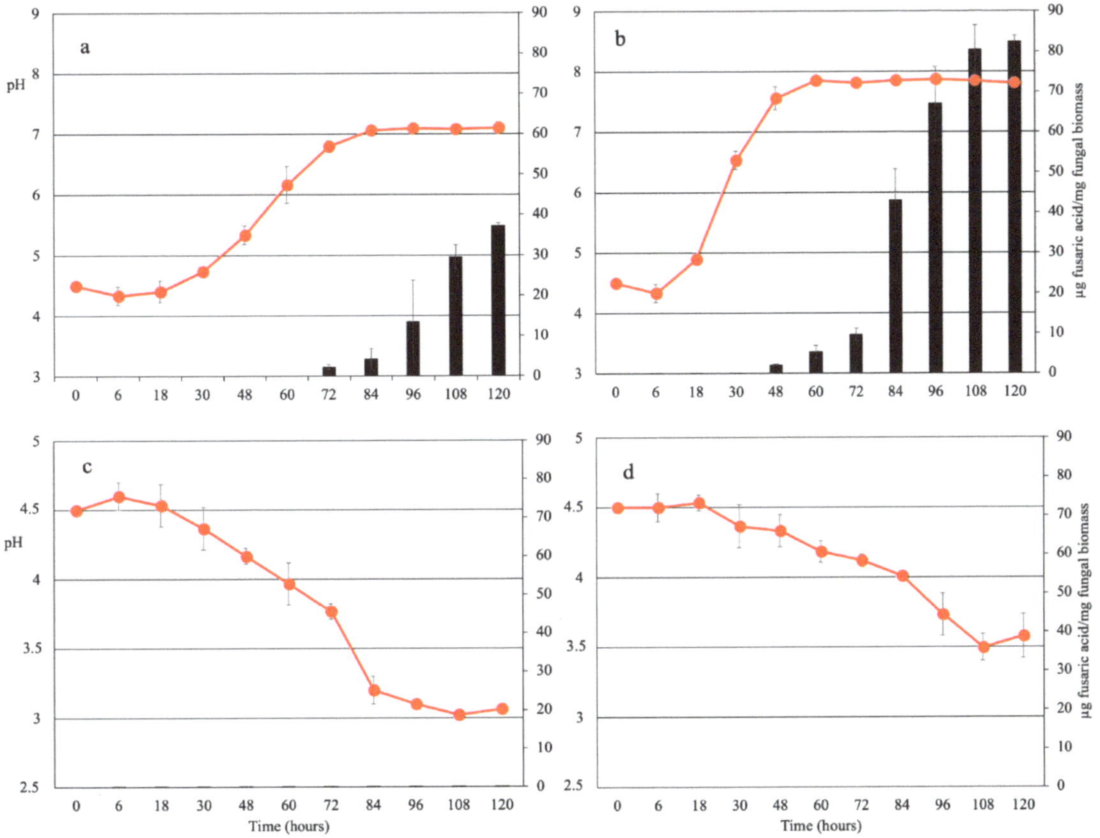

Figure 1. Trend of pH (red line) and fusaric acid concentration (black bars) in the culture supernatants of *Fusarium oxysporum* f. sp. *lycopersici* grown in minimal medium supplemented with urea (**a**), sodium nitrate (**b**), ammonium sulphate (**c**) or ammonium nitrate (**d**) as sole nitrogen sources. Bars represent standard deviations from three independent replicates. Experiments were performed three times, with similar results.

Previous studies revealed that deletion of the iron homeostasis regulator HapX induces a slight increase in extracellular chelating activity under iron-limiting conditions when using glutamine (Gln) as the nitrogen source [22]. Here, we detected a significant increase in extracellular chelating activity in *hapX*Δ as compared to the wild type, which was even more dramatic when ammonium was used as a nitrogen source.

2.3. Fusaric Acid Production Is Regulated by Environmental pH and Iron Availability

Fusaric acid (FA) has been suggested to function in metal cation chelation [13,15]. Here, we found that FA concentrations increased steadily in supernatants of the wild-type strain grown on urea or sodium nitrate, whereas no FA was detected in cultures supplemented with ammonium even after prolonged incubation (Figures 1 and 2; Table 1). These findings suggest that either the nitrogen source or environmental pH regulates FA production. In line with the second hypothesis, buffering the pH to 4.5 completely abolished FA production on urea- or sodium nitrate-containing media, while increasing the pH to 7.0 activated FA production on ammonium-supplemented media (Figure 3). Further corroborating the finding of a pH-dependent FA regulation mechanism in *Fol*, inappropriate pH sensing in the *pacC*Δ and *pacC^c* mutants resulted in altered FA levels at alkaline or acidic pH, respectively.

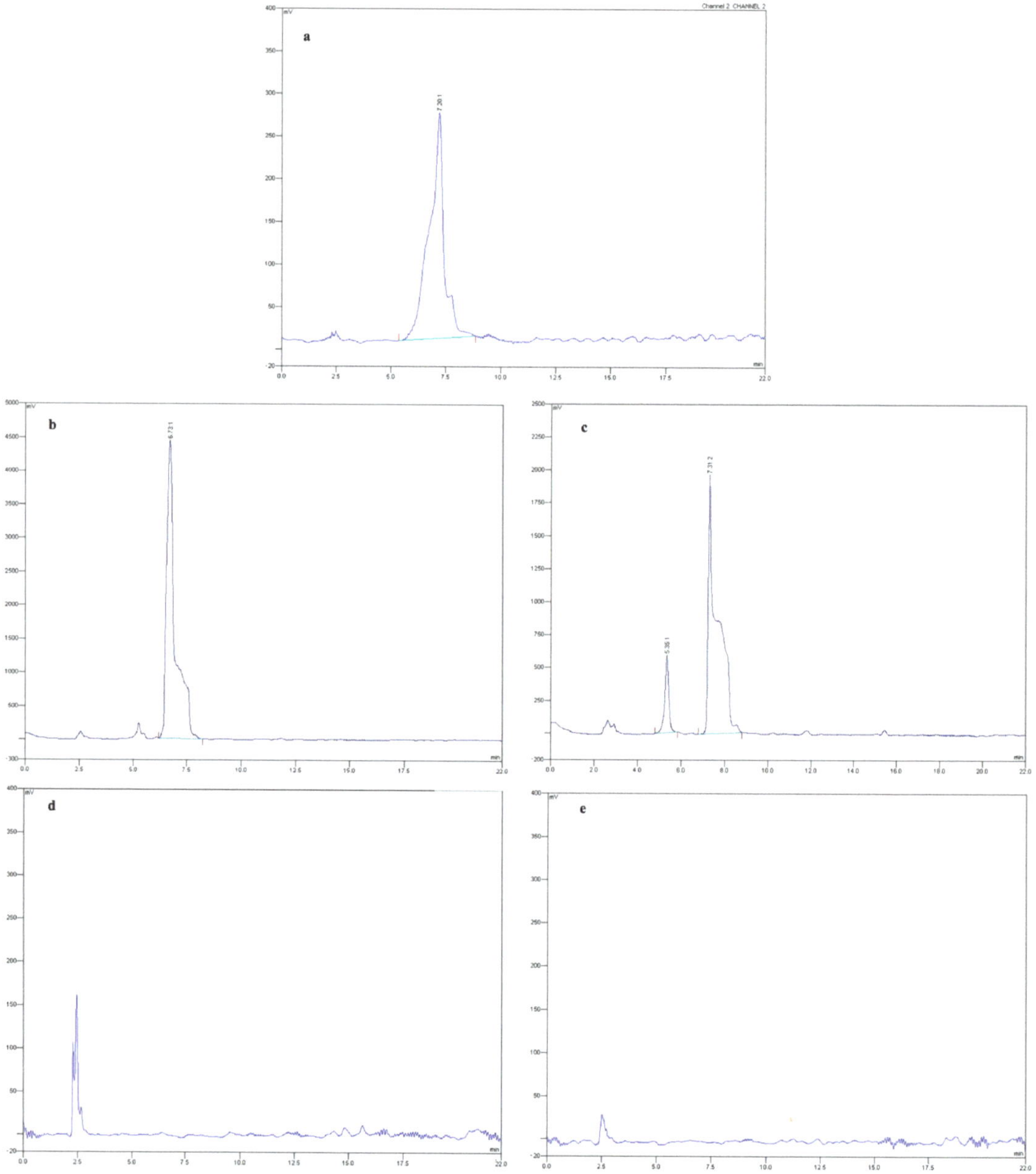

Figure 2. HPLC chromatograms obtained by injecting 20 μg mL^{-1} of a fusaric acid standard (**a**) or an ethyl acetate fraction obtained from *Fusarium oxysporum* f. sp. *lycopersici* cultures grown in the presence of urea (**b**), sodium nitrate (**c**), ammonium sulphate (**d**) or ammonium nitrate (**e**) as sole nitrogen sources. The red vertical lines in the graph mark the start and end of each peak.

In general, FA production appeared to correlate with chelating activity in fungal supernatants, particularly in sodium nitrate-supplemented cultures, which contained high levels of chelating activity and FA (Table 1). Interestingly, the addition of the general ion chelator EDTA or the specific iron-chelating bacterial siderophore pyoverdine resulted in increased FA concentrations regardless of the nitrogen source used, even though pyoverdine stimulation was most effective on sodium nitrate (Figure 3). By contrast, iron addition dramatically decreased FA production in all tested conditions (Figure 3), suggesting that iron sensing plays an important role in the regulation of FA biosynthesis. Indeed, the deletion of the iron-response transcriptional regulator HapX led to increased FA production in all tested media except for that containing sodium nitrate (Table 1).

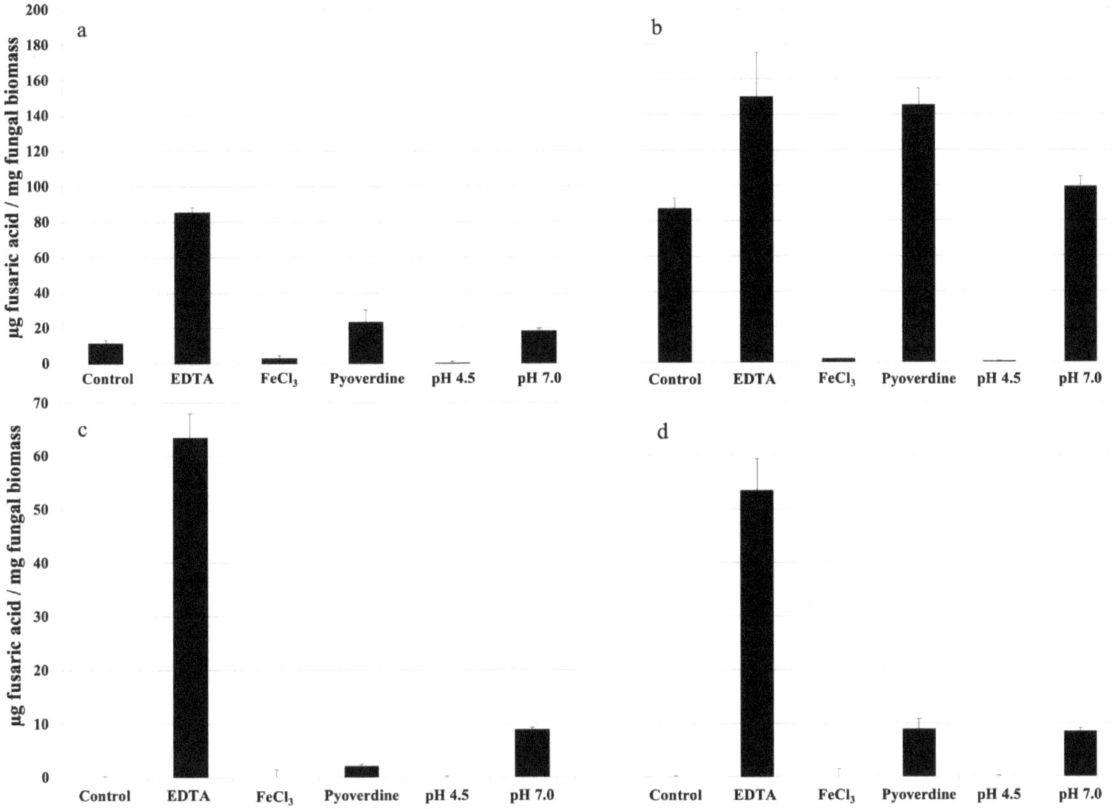

Figure 3. Fusaric acid content in the culture filtrates of *F. oxysporum* f. sp. *lycopersici* grown in minimal medium containing urea (**a**), sodium nitrate (**b**), ammonium sulphate (**c**) or ammonium nitrate (**d**) as sole nitrogen sources and supplemented with 0.2 mM EDTA, 100 µM $FeCl_3$ or 0.2 mM pyoverdine, or pH buffered with 100 mM MES to pH 4.5 or 7. Bars represent standard deviations from three independent replicates. Experiments were performed three times, with similar results.

Unexpectedly, the *ste2*Δ, *bck1*Δ, *mkk2*Δ and *mpk1*Δ mutants showed lower levels of FA production in both urea- and sodium nitrate-supplemented media, despite the higher chelating activity detected in these conditions (Table 1).

3. Discussion

Since its discovery more than 70 years ago, fusaric acid (FA) has been among the most studied fungal secondary metabolites produced by *Fusarium* phytopathogenic species [7,23]. Its wide spectrum toxicity towards plants, animals, bacteria and fungi has attracted the attention of many scientists with the aim of identifying its biosynthetic gene cluster, the environmental conditions eliciting its production/secretion and its mode of action. Recently, different genes (*fub1*, *fub2*, *fub3*, *fub4* and *fub5*) have been described as being responsible for FA biosynthesis in plant pathogenic *Fusarium* species, and their transcription has been found to be regulated by several environmental factors, including ambient pH, nitrogen source, nutrient availability and presence of a plant host [24]. Although the toxicity mechanism of FA is not fully understood, an increasing body of evidence suggests that metal chelation represents a major mechanism for the toxic effect of FA on plants, mammals and competing rhizobacteria [13,15]. In this work, we investigated the effect of environmental conditions on FA production by *Fol*. Previous work by Lopez-Berges and co-workers [25] showed that *Fol* is able to use a large variety of nitrogen sources. While a readily metabolized source ammonium inhibited virulence-related functions, a non-preferred source nitrate promoted such functions [25]. Moreover, it was shown that the ability of fungal pathogens to invade and kill plants depends upon cellular iron homeostasis, environmental iron availability and rhizosphere pH [22,26–29]. High iron availability and acidic pH inhibit virulence, while low iron availability and alkaline pH promote infection [29].

Here, we found that *Fol* cultures grown in the presence of ammonium show acidic pH values, while those supplemented with nitrate or urea show high pH values. It is important to note that iron availability in soils depends largely on redox potential and pH, where iron solubility decreases as soil pH increases [30]. To overcome reduced iron availability, soil-inhabiting microbes have evolved a battery of high-affinity, low-molecular-weight iron chelators known as siderophores, which are secreted into the environment for efficient acquisition of limited iron pools [31]. In line with this, *Fol* cultures grown on nitrogen sources leading to alkaline pH values showed higher chelating activity than those grown in acidic conditions. Interestingly, a similar pattern was observed for FA accumulation in culture supernatants, suggesting a possible role in FA production under iron-limiting conditions. In support of this idea, external addition of the chelating agent EDTA or the bacterial siderophore pyoverdine, as well as buffering the medium to pH 7.0, induced an increase in FA levels, while exogenous addition of iron or buffering to pH 4.5 resulted in reduced FA production. Thus, FA biosynthesis in *Fol* appears to be regulated by environmental pH and, consequently, iron availability. In line with this, *Fol* mutants in PacC, which are affected in external pH sensing, were altered in FA production and chelating activity. This is in agreement with previous reports indicating the requirement of PacC for efficient expression of *fub* genes in *F. fujikuroi* and siderophore production in *Aspergillus nidulans* at alkaline pH [14,32]. It is noteworthy that, similarly to siderophore biosynthesis, FA production also appears to depend on iron homeostasis in *Fol* because deletion of the iron homeostasis regulator HapX [22], a repressor of siderophore biosynthesis [33], led to an overall increase in FA levels and chelating activity. Thus, FA production in *Fol* might be regulated via two independent mechanisms based on pH and iron sensing.

In the banana pathogen *F. oxysporum* f. sp. *cubense*, Bck1, Mkk2 and Mpk1, three conserved elements of the CWI MAPK signalling cascade, were shown to positively regulate the expression of FA biosynthetic genes and FA production [16]. Here, we found that *Fol* mutants lacking Mpk1, which is required for host sensing and virulence [18], produced less FA, suggesting that FA production in *F. oxysporum* is regulated by the CWI MAPK pathway. Surprisingly, the α-pheromone specific receptor Ste2, which was recently shown to signal via the CWI MAPK pathway to regulate chemotropism and conidial germination in *Fol* [18,34,35], also showed lower FA accumulation, suggesting a new role of pheromone autocrine signalling in FA production. Importantly, this effect was independent of extracellular pH and chelating activity, indicating that pheromone signalling-mediated FA production functions downstream of pH and Fe sensing in *Fol*.

Collectively, our results show that virulence-promoting conditions such as alkaline pH, low iron availability, poor nitrogen sources and CWI MAPK signalling are associated with an increase in FA production, suggesting that *Fol* has evolved both independent and overlapping strategies to fine-tune the production of this important mycotoxin.

4. Materials and Methods

4.1. Fungal Isolates and Culture Condition

Fungal strains derived from *Fusarium oxysporum* f. sp. *lycopersici* (*Fol*) isolate 4287 (FGSC 9935) and used in this study are reported in Table 2. For microconidia production, fungal strains were grown in Potato Dextrose Broth (PDB; Difco; Fisher Scientific; Rodano, MI, Italy) at 28 °C with shaking at 180 rpm for 5 days. For in vitro fusaric acid (FA) detection, Puhalla minimal medium ($MgSO_4 \cdot 7 H_2O$ 2 mM, KH_2PO_4 7 mM, KCl 6 mM, Sucrose 90 mM) adjusted to pH 5.0 and supplemented with 25 mM of different nitrogen sources ($NaNO_3$; $(NH_4)_2SO_4$; NH_4NO_3; CH_4N_2O) was used [36]. Where indicated, the medium was pH buffered to 7.0 or 5.0 with 100 mM 4-morpholineethanesulfonic acid monohydrate (MES) or supplemented with 100 µM $FeCl_3$, 0.2 mM EDTA or 0.2 mM pyoverdine. Fungal strains were inoculated in the growth medium at a final concentration of 5×10^5 conidia mL^{-1} and incubated for 7 days at 28 °C on a rotary shaker regulated at 180 rpm. The dry weight of the fungal biomass and pH of the culture broth were evaluated periodically.

Table 2. *Fusarium oxysporum* f. sp. *lycopersici* (*Fol*) wild-type and mutant strains used in the experiments.

Fol Strain	Genotype	Gene Function	Reference
FGSC 4287	Wild type		[19]
fmk1Δ	*fmk1::PHLEO*	MAPK	[19]
mpk1Δ	*mpk1::HYG*	MAPK	[18]
hog1Δ	*hog1::HYG*	MAPK	[17]
ste2Δ	*ste2::HYG*	GPCR	[18]
mkk2Δ	*mkk2::HYG*	MAPKK	[18]
bck1Δ	*bck1::HYG*	MAPKKK	[18]
hapXΔ	*hapX::HYG*	Transcription factor	[22]
pacCΔ	*pacC::HYG*	Transcription factor	[21]
$pacC^C$	$pacC^C$*::HYG*	Transcription factor	[21]

4.2. Chrome Azurol S Assay

Siderophore quantification in fungal supernatants was carried out by using the liquid chrome azurol S assay (CAS) (as previously described [37]. The percentage of chelating activity (CA%) was indirectly quantified by measuring the OD_{655} of the culture supernatant (ODs) and the uninoculated medium (ODc), used as a control, 60 min after the start of the reaction, with the following formula: CA% = [(ODc − ODs)/ODc] × 100.

4.3. Fusaric Acid Extraction and Quantification

For FA extraction from fungal cultures, supernatants were collected and filtered through Whatman no. 4 filter paper (Whatman Ltd., Maidstone, UK), adjusted to pH 2.0 with HCl (37% v/v) and extracted with ethyl acetate (1:1 v/v). Ethyl acetate phases were separately collected, dried by rotary evaporation under reduced pressure and resuspended in methanol. FA content was quantified through high-performance liquid chromatography (HPLC-UV; Varian Analytical Instruments; Model 9010; Palo Alto, CA, USA) by using previously reported methods and experimental conditions [38,39] and expressed in µg of FA per mg of dry fungal biomass. To obtain an FA calibration curve, methanol-dissolved FA standard solution (Merck Life Science; Milano, MI, Italy) was injected at concentrations ranging from 0.02 to 2.0 mg mL^{-1}. A linear relationship between peak areas and the investigated FA concentrations was obtained ($Y = 0.001x + 0.0105$; R^2 value of 0.997). Method validation was performed by spiking MM blanks with known concentrations of FA. The average recovery rate was 96% and always exceeded 95%.

4.4. Statistical Analyses

Data were submitted to variance analysis (ANOVA) using the SPSS software v. 16.0 (SPSS Inc., Chicago, IL, USA) and means compared with Tukey's test. Before analyses, percentages of chelating activity were converted into Bliss angular values (arcsine square root of the percentage value). All experiments were repeated at least three times, with similar results. Homogeneity of variance for independent repetitions of each experiment was tested, and data from separate experiments having homogeneous variances were pooled.

Author Contributions: Conceptualization, D.P. and D.T.; methodology, D.S.; validation, D.P., F.D.C., G.L., A.D.P. and D.T.; resources, M.S.L.-B.; writing—original draft preparation, D.P.; writing—review and editing, A.D.P. and D.T.; supervision, D.T., F.D.C. and G.L.; funding acquisition, D.T., A.D.P. and G.L. All authors have read and agreed to the published version of the manuscript.

Funding: This work was supported by grants from the Spanish Ministry of Science and Innovation (MICINN, grant PID2019-108045RB-I00) and Junta de Andalucía (P20_00179) to A.D.P.; grants by the Italian Ministry of Education, University and Research (PRIN-BiPP grant 2020T58TA3) and the Università degli Studi di Napoli Federico II (FRA-Line B-2020-TOPOPATH grant PG/2021/0034842) to D.T.; and grants by the Italian Ministry of Education (PRIN 20089LSZ2A_003) to G.L. This study was carried out within the Agritech National Research Center and received funding from the European Union Next-GenerationEU (PIANO NAZIONALE DI RIPRESA E RESILIENZA (PNRR)—MISSIONE 4 COMPONENTE 2, INVESTIMENTO 1.4–D.D. 1032 17/06/2022, CN00000022). This manuscript reflects only the authors' views and opinions, neither the European Union nor the European Commission can be considered responsible for them.

Institutional Review Board Statement: Not applicable.

Informed Consent Statement: Not applicable.

Data Availability Statement: Not applicable.

Conflicts of Interest: The authors declare no conflict of interest.

References

1. Gordon, T.R.; Martyn, R.D. The evolutionary biology of *Fusarium oxysporum*. *Annu. Rev. Phytopathol.* **1997**, *35*, 111–128. [CrossRef] [PubMed]
2. Fuchs, J.G.; Moënne-Loccoz, Y.; Défago, G. Nonpathogenic *Fusarium oxysporum* strain fo47 induces resistance to Fusarium wilt in tomato. *Plant Dis.* **1997**, *81*, 492–496. [CrossRef] [PubMed]
3. Kang, S.; Demers, J.; del Mar Jimenez-Gasco, M.; Rep, M. Fusarium oxysporum. In *Genomics of Plant-Associated Fungi and Oomycetes: Dicot Pathogens*; Dean, R.A., Lichens-Park, A., Kole, C., Eds.; Springer: Berlin/Heidelberg, Germany, 2014; pp. 99–119.
4. Michielse, C.B.; Rep, M. Pathogen profile update: *Fusarium oxysporum*. *Mol. Plant Pathol.* **2009**, *10*, 311–324. [CrossRef] [PubMed]
5. Keller, N.P.; Turner, G.; Bennett, J.W. Fungal secondary metabolism [mdash] from biochemistry to genomics. *Nat. Rev. Microbiol.* **2005**, *3*, 937–947. [CrossRef]
6. Gaumann, E. Fusaric acid as a wilt toxin. *Phytopathology* **1957**, *47*, 342–357.
7. Bacon, C.W.; Porter, J.K.; Norred, W.P.; Leslie, J.F. Production of fusaric acid by *Fusarium* species. *Appl. Environ. Microbiol.* **1996**, *62*, 4039–4043. [CrossRef]
8. Dong, X.; Ling, N.; Wang, M.; Shen, Q.; Guo, S. Fusaric acid is a crucial factor in the disturbance of leaf water imbalance in fusarium-infected banana plants. *Plant. Physiol. Biochem.* **2012**, *60*, 171–179. [CrossRef]
9. Bouizgarne, B.; El-Maarouf-Bouteau, H.; Frankart, C.; Reboutier, D.; Madiona, K.; Pennarun, A.M.; Monestiez, M.; Trouverie, J.; Amiar, Z.; Briand, J.; et al. Early physiological responses of *Arabidopsis thaliana* cells to fusaric acid: Toxic and signalling effects. *New Phytol.* **2006**, *169*, 209–218. [CrossRef]
10. Stipanovic, R.D.; Puckhaber, L.S.; Liu, J.; Bell, A.A. Phytotoxicity of fusaric acid and analogs to cotton. *Toxicon* **2011**, *57*, 176–178. [CrossRef]
11. Singh, V.K.; Upadhyay, R.S. Fusaric acid induced cell death and changes in oxidative metabolism of *Solanum lycopersicum*. *Bot. Stud.* **2014**, *55*, 66. [CrossRef]
12. Landa, B.B.; Cachinero-Díaz, J.M.; Lemanceau, P.; Jiménez-Díaz, R.M.; Alabouvette, C. Effect of fusaric acid and phytoanticipins on growth of rhizobacteria and *Fusarium oxysporum*. *Can. J. Microbiol.* **2002**, *48*, 971–985. [CrossRef] [PubMed]
13. Ruiz, J.A.; Bernar, E.M.; Jung, K. Production of siderophores increases resistance to fusaric acid in *Pseudomonas protegens* pf-5. *PLoS ONE* **2015**, *10*, e0117040. [CrossRef] [PubMed]
14. Niehaus, E.M.; von Bargen, K.W.; Espino, J.J.; Pfannmuller, A.; Humpf, H.U.; Tudzynski, B. Characterization of the fusaric acid gene cluster in *Fusarium fujikuroi*. *Appl. Microbiol. Biotechnol.* **2014**, *98*, 1749–1762. [CrossRef] [PubMed]
15. López-Díaz, C.; Rahjoo, V.; Sulyok, M.; Ghionna, V.; Martín-Vicente, A.; Capilla, J.; Di Pietro, A.; López-Berges, M.S. Fusaric acid contributes to virulence of *Fusarium oxysporum* on plant and mammalian hosts. *Mol. Plant Pathol.* **2018**, *19*, 440–453. [CrossRef]
16. Ding, Z.; Li, M.; Sun, F.; Xi, P.; Sun, L.; Zhang, L.; Jiang, Z. Mitogen-activated protein kinases are associated with the regulation of physiological traits and virulence in *Fusarium oxysporum* f. sp. *cubense*. *PLoS ONE* **2015**, *10*, e0122634. [CrossRef]
17. Segorbe, D.; Di Pietro, A.; Pérez-Nadales, E.; Turrà, D. Three *Fusarium oxysporum* mitogen-activated protein kinases (mapks) have distinct and complementary roles in stress adaptation and cross-kingdom pathogenicity. *Mol. Plant Pathol.* **2016**, *18*, 912–924. [CrossRef]
18. Turrà, D.; El Ghalid, M.; Rossi, F.; Di Pietro, A. Fungal pathogen uses sex pheromone receptor for chemotropic sensing of host plant signals. *Nature* **2015**, *527*, 521–524. [CrossRef]

19. Di Pietro, A.; García-Maceira, F.I.; Méglecz, E.; Roncero, M.I.G. A map kinase of the vascular wilt fungus *Fusarium oxysporum* is essential for root penetration and pathogenesis. *Mol. Microbiol.* **2001**, *39*, 1140–1152. [CrossRef]
20. Prusky, D.; McEvoy, J.L.; Saftner, R.; Conway, W.S.; Jones, R. Relationship between host acidification and virulence of *Penicillium* spp. on apple and citrus fruit. *Phytopathology* **2004**, *94*, 44–51. [CrossRef]
21. Caracuel, Z.; Roncero, M.I.; Espeso, E.A.; Gonzalez-Verdejo, C.I.; Garcia-Maceira, F.I.; Di Pietro, A. The ph signalling transcription factor pacc controls virulence in the plant pathogen *Fusarium oxysporum*. *Mol. Microbiol.* **2003**, *48*, 765–779. [CrossRef]
22. López-Berges, M.S.; Capilla, J.; Turrà, D.; Schafferer, L.; Matthijs, S.; Jöchl, C.; Cornelis, P.; Guarro, J.; Haas, H.; Di Pietro, A. Hapx-mediated iron homeostasis is essential for rhizosphere competence and virulence of the soilborne pathogen *Fusarium oxysporum*. *Plant Cell* **2012**, *24*, 3805–3822. [CrossRef] [PubMed]
23. Yabuta, T.; Kambe, K.; Hayashi, T. Biochemistry of the bakanae-fungus. I. Fusarinic acid, a new product of the bakanae fungus. *Agric. Chem. Soc. Jpn* **1937**, *10*, 1059–1068.
24. Brown, D.W.; Butchko, R.A.; Busman, M.; Proctor, R.H. Identification of gene clusters associated with fusaric acid, fusarin, and perithecial pigment production in *Fusarium verticillioides*. *Fungal Genet. Biol.* **2012**, *49*, 521–532. [CrossRef]
25. López-Berges, M.S.; Rispail, N.; Prados-Rosales, R.C.; Di Pietro, A. A nitrogen response pathway regulates virulence functions in *Fusarium oxysporum* via the protein kinase tor and the bzip protein meab. *Plant Cell* **2010**, *22*, 2459–2475. [CrossRef] [PubMed]
26. Masachis, S.; Segorbe, D.; Turra, D.; Leon-Ruiz, M.; Furst, U.; El Ghalid, M.; Leonard, G.; Lopez-Berges, M.S.; Richards, T.A.; Felix, G. A fungal pathogen secretes plant alkalinizing peptides to increase infection. *Nat. Microbiol.* **2016**, *1*, 16043. [CrossRef]
27. Lopez-Berges, M.S.; Turra, D.; Capilla, J.; Schafferer, L.; Matthijs, S.; Jochl, C.; Cornelis, P.; Guarro, J.; Haas, H.; Di Pietro, A. Iron competition in fungus-plant interactions: The battle takes place in the rhizosphere. *Plant Signal. Behav.* **2013**, *8*, e23012. [CrossRef]
28. Fernandes, T.R.; Segorbe, D. How alkalinization drives fungal pathogenicity. *PLoS Pathog.* **2017**, *13*, e1006621. [CrossRef]
29. Dong, X.; Wang, M.; Ling, N.; Shen, Q.; Guo, S. Effects of iron and boron combinations on the suppression of Fusarium wilt in banana. *Sci. Rep.* **2016**, *6*, 38944. [CrossRef]
30. Colombo, C.; Palumbo, G.; He, J.Z.; Pinton, R.; Cesco, S. Review on iron availability in soil: Interaction of fe minerals, plants, and microbes. *J. Soils Sedim.* **2014**, *14*, 538–548. [CrossRef]
31. Lemanceau, P.; Bauer, P.; Kraemer, S.; Briat, J.-F. Iron dynamics in the rhizosphere as a case study for analyzing interactions between soils, plants and microbes. *Plant Soil* **2009**, *321*, 513–535. [CrossRef]
32. Eisendle, M.; Oberegger, H.; Buttinger, R.; Illmer, P.; Haas, H. Biosynthesis and uptake of siderophores is controlled by the pacc-mediated ambient-ph regulatory system in *Aspergillus nidulans*. *Eukaryot. Cell* **2004**, *3*, 561–563. [CrossRef] [PubMed]
33. Hsu, P.-C.; Yang, C.-Y.; Lan, C.-Y. *Candida albicans* hap43 is a repressor induced under low-iron conditions and is essential for iron-responsive transcriptional regulation and virulence. *Eukaryot. Cell* **2011**, *10*, 207–225. [CrossRef]
34. Vitale, S.; Partida-Hanon, A.; Serrano, S.; Martinez-Del-Pozo, A.; Di Pietro, A.; Turra, D.; Bruix, M. Structure-activity relationship of alpha mating pheromone from the fungal pathogen *Fusarium oxysporum*. *J. Biol. Chem.* **2017**, *292*, 3591–3602. [CrossRef]
35. Vitale, S.; Di Pietro, A.; Turra, D. Autocrine pheromone signalling regulates community behaviour in the fungal pathogen *Fusarium oxysporum*. *Nat. Microbiol.* **2019**, *4*, 1443–1449. [CrossRef] [PubMed]
36. Puhalla, J.E. Compatibility reactions on solid medium and interstrain inhibition in *Ustilago maydis*. *Genetics* **1968**, *60*, 461–474. [CrossRef] [PubMed]
37. Pérez-Miranda, S.; Cabirol, N.; George-Téllez, R.; Zamudio-Rivera, L.S.; Fernández, F.J. O-cas, a fast and universal method for siderophore detection. *J. Microbiol. Meth.* **2007**, *70*, 127–131. [CrossRef] [PubMed]
38. Amalfitano, C.; Pengue, R.; Andolfi, A.; Vurro, M.; Zonno, M.C.; Evidente, A. Hplc analysis of fusaric acid, 9,10-dehydrofusaric acid and their methyl esters, toxic metabolites from weed pathogenic *Fusarium* species. *Phytochem. Anal.* **2002**, *13*, 277–282. [CrossRef]
39. Marzano, M.; Gallo, A.; Altomare, C. Improvement of biocontrol efficacy of *Trichoderma harzianum vs. Fusarium oxysporum* f. sp. *lycopersici* through uv-induced tolerance to fusaric acid. *Biol. Control.* **2013**, *67*, 397–408. [CrossRef]

toxins

MDPI

Article

In Silico Evaluation of Sesquiterpenes and Benzoxazinoids Phytotoxins against M^pro^, RNA Replicase and Spike Protein of SARS-CoV-2 by Molecular Dynamics. Inspired by Nature

Francisco J. R. Mejías [1,2], Alexandra G. Durán [1], Nuria Chinchilla [1], Rosa M. Varela [1], José A. Álvarez [3], José M. G. Molinillo [1], Francisco García-Cozar [4] and Francisco A. Macías [1,*]

[1] Allelopathy Group, Department of Organic Chemistry, Institute of Biomolecules (INBIO), Campus CEIA3, School of Science, University of Cádiz, C/República Saharaui, 7, 11510 Puerto Real, Spain
[2] Center for Molecular Biosciences (CMBI), Institute of Pharmacy/Pharmacognosy, University of Innsbruck, 6020 Innsbruck, Austria
[3] Department of Physical Chemistry, Faculty of Sciences, INBIO, University of Cádiz, 11510 Puerto Real, Spain
[4] Department of Biomedicine, Biotechnology and Public Health, University of Cádiz and Institute of Biomedical Research Cádiz (INIBICA), 11009 Cádiz, Spain
* Correspondence: famacias@gm.uca.es

Abstract: In the work described here, a number of sesquiterpenes and benzoxazinoids from natural sources, along with their easily accessible derivatives, were evaluated against the main protease, RNA replicase and spike glycoprotein of SARS-CoV-2 by molecular docking. These natural products and their derivatives have previously shown remarkable antiviral activities. The most relevant compounds were the 4-fluoro derivatives of santamarine, reynosin and 2-amino-3*H*-phenoxazin-3-one in terms of the docking score. Those compounds fulfill the Lipinski's rule, so they were selected for the analysis by molecular dynamics, and the kinetic stabilities of the complexes were assessed. The addition of the 4-fluorobenzoate fragment to the natural products enhances their potential against all of the proteins tested, and the complex stability after 50 ns validates the inhibition calculated. The derivatives prepared from reynosin and 2-amino-3*H*-phenoxazin-3-one are able to generate more hydrogen bonds with the M^pro^, thus enhancing the stability of the protein–ligand and generating a long-term complex for inhibition. The 4-fluoro derivate of santamarine and reynosin shows to be really active against the spike protein, with the RMSD site fluctuation lower than 1.5 Å. Stabilization is mainly achieved by the hydrogen-bond interactions, and the stabilization is improved by the 4-fluorobenzoate fragment being added. Those compounds tested in silico reach as candidates from natural sources to fight this virus, and the results concluded that the addition of the 4-fluorobenzoate fragment to the natural products enhances their inhibition potential against the main protease, RNA replicase and spike protein of SARS-CoV-2.

Keywords: molecular dynamics; docking; SARS-CoV-2; COVID-19; sesquiterpene; benzoxazinoid

Key Contribution: Molecular dynamic studies demonstrated that natural and derivative sesquiterpenoids and benzoxazinoids represent an interesting possibility in the fight against SARS-CoV-2.

Citation: Mejías, F.J.R.; Durán, A.G.; Chinchilla, N.; Varela, R.M.; Álvarez, J.A.; Molinillo, J.M.G.; García-Cozar, F.; Macías, F.A. In Silico Evaluation of Sesquiterpenes and Benzoxazinoids Phytotoxins against M^pro^, RNA Replicase and Spike Protein of SARS-CoV-2 by Molecular Dynamics. Inspired by Nature. *Toxins* **2022**, *14*, 599. https://doi.org/10.3390/toxins14090599

Received: 5 August 2022
Accepted: 26 August 2022
Published: 29 August 2022

Publisher's Note: MDPI stays neutral with regard to jurisdictional claims in published maps and institutional affiliations.

1. Introduction

Coronaviruses (CoVs) are large positive-strand, enveloped non-segmented RNA viruses that generally cause enteric and respiratory illnesses in animals and humans [1]. Although most CoVs that affect humans produce only mild respiratory diseases, with little or no mortality, the previous epidemics of two pathogenic CoVs, namely severe acute respiratory syndrome coronavirus (SARS-CoV) and Middle East respiratory syndrome coronavirus (MERS-CoV), led to major health alerts.

Traditional medicine based on plants has been used for preventive treatments for COVID-19 in countries all over the world. Furthermore, some nutrient supplements obtained from herbal sources have also proven effective in reducing virus transmission and decreasing infection [2]. Among the families of compounds that are potential drugs in traditional medicine, sesquiterpenes are relevant due to their broad-spectrum drug nature, e.g., artemisinin, and this family of compounds is found in *A. annua*. The in vitro efficacy of artemisinin-based treatments in combating SARS-CoV-2 has shown that treatment with artesunate, artemether, *A. annua* extracts and artemisinin hindered viral infections of human lung cancer A549-hACE2 cells, VeroE6 cells and human hepatoma Huh7.5 cells. Among these four treatments, artesunate showed the strongest anti-SARS-CoV-2 activity (7–12 μg/mL) [3,4]. Given the promising results obtained with terpenoids, in silico evaluation seems to be a promising tool to select leads for future bioassays against SARS-CoV-2.

Previous in silico studies have demonstrated the efficacy of natural products fighting against SARS-CoV-2. A plant-derived alkaloid, such as cryptoquindoline and 6-oxoisoiguesterin isolated from *Cryptolepis sanguinolenta* and *Salacia madagascariensis*, displayed inhibition against the M^{pro} [5]. Forrestall et al. also evaluated the activity against the M^{pro} by molecular docking of different natural products with 2-pyridone scaffolds, mainly based on diterpene skeletons [6]. On the other hand, Narkhede et al. did not use a skeleton criterion and selected different kinds of natural products with previous antiviral activity [7]. In the same case, compared to the other, neither sesquiterpene nor benzoxazinoids have been studied in depth by molecular dynamics and docking.

The work described here concerned the evaluation of inhibitors for the three main targets of SARS-CoV-2 (M^{pro} [8,9], spike glycoprotein [10,11] and RNA replicase [12,13]) by molecular docking and molecular dynamics simulation studies on bioactive natural products and derivatives obtained from natural sources. These compounds can be obtained on a multigram scale or can be synthesized in a single step, and they are readily available and are relatively inexpensive.

2. Results and Discussion

2.1. Molecular Docking Studies

A total of 12 sesquiterpene lactones and 14 benzoxazinoids (Figure 1A,B) were selected from the natural products and derivatives with notable bioactivity and structural similarity to the reference standards (Figure 1C). The results for these compounds were compared with those obtained for the standards. All of the compounds have previously shown anticancer activity (mostly anti-leukemia) or some other cytotoxicity [14–16]. Antiviral activity is also displayed, as in the case of costunolide, DHC and alantolactone, against the Hepatitis C virus [17]. Inhibition of this virus has been also observed after the application of artichoke extracts containing cynaropicrin [18]. APO and different benzoxazinoids present activity against human cytomegalovirus and herpes simplex virus type 1 [19,20]. Favipiravir and hydroxychloroquine contain two fused rings with at least one heteroatom in the structure, as do the benzoxazinoids **DIBOA**, **DIMBOA**, **DDIBOA** and **APO**. In addition, the presence of a halogen in the structures of the standards inspired us to include 4-fluorobenzoate derivatives in the study. Methyl 4-fluorobenzoate (**Met-4F-Benzo**) was included in the test in order to ascertain whether the activity can be attributed to this fragment alone. In contrast, artemisinin is an antimalarial compound isolated from Artemisia annua, and this is already being tested [21,22]. Artemisinin has a lactone sesquiterpene skeleton (C-15 and cyclic ester in the main structure), as do the costunolide, dehydrocostuslactone (DHC), cynaropicrin and alantolactone (alanto) derivatives. Azithromycin was included in the study as a negative standard due to its different backbone and its reported lack of efficacy against COVID-19 disease [23].

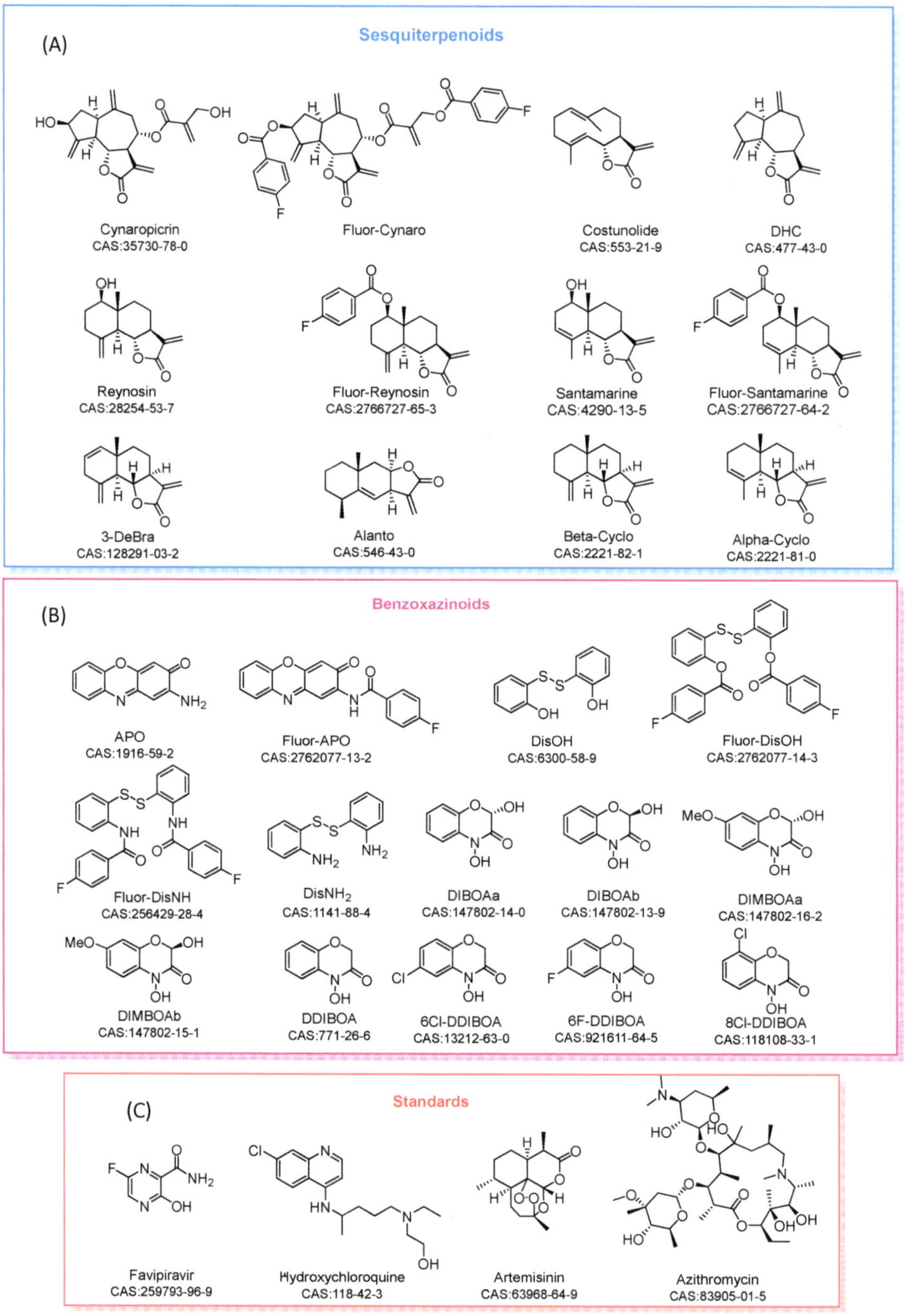

Figure 1. (**A**) Sesquiterpenoids tested in the molecular docking analysis. (**B**) Benzoxazinoids tested and (**C**) standards employed.

The binding energies of the sesquiterpenoids toward the M^{pro}, RNA replicase and the spike protein of SARS-CoV-2 in comparison with the standards are provided in Table 1.

Table 1. Binding energy values of sesquiterpenoids selected in the study on Mpro, RNA replicase and spike protein of SARS-CoV-2.

Compounds	ΔG (Kcal/mol)		
	Main Protease	**RNA Replicase**	**Spike Protein**
Azithromycin	−1.20 ± 0.47	−0.76 ± 0.88	−4.64 ± 0.78
Hydroxychloroquine	−3.45 ± 0.16	−2.67 ± 0.81	−4.29 ± 0.76
Favipiravir	−3.21 ± 0.16	−3.58 ± 0.24	−3.93 ± 0.42
Artemisinin	−6.25 ± 0.23	−6.07 ± 0.07	−5.96 ± 0.19
Cynaropicrin	−3.49 ± 0.07	−4.02 ± 0.25	−4.19 ± 0.28
Met-4F-Benzo	−5.32 ± 0.64	−5.71 ± 0.93	−5.81 ± 0.48
Fluor-Cynaro	−3.97 ± 1.01	−5.56 ± 0.73	−8.13 ± 1.08
Costunolide	−6.11 ± 0.41	−5.77 ± 0.20	−6.15 ± 0.20
DHC	−6.08 ± 0.30	−5.57 ± 0.34	−6.00 ± 0.28
Reynosin	−5.54 ± 0.48	−5.92 ± 0.41	−6.11 ± 0.18
Santamarine	−5.81 ± 0.59	−5.97 ± 0.48	−6.12 ± 0.31
Fluor-Reynosin	−7.37 ± 0.50	−7.10 ± 0.93	−7.89 ± 0.77
Fluor-Santamarine	−7.77 ± 0.77	−6.35 ± 0.54	−7.68 ± 0.74
Alanto	−5.82 ± 0.22	−6.57 ± 0.26	−6.46 ± 0.17
Alpha-Cyclo	−5.99 ± 0.37	−5.95 ± 0.36	−6.20 ± 0.25
Beta-Cyclo	−5.98 ± 0.49	−6.02 ± 0.52	−6.20 ± 0.29
3-DeBra	−6.36 ± 0.37	−6.04 ± 0.37	−6.19 ± 0.25

The binding energy values show the remarkable activity of artemisinin, which has not been tested previously, on all of the proteins tested. Furthermore, artemisinin has similar binding energies to costunolide and **DHC**, two compounds isolated on a multigram scale from *Saussurea Lappa* (Decne.) Sch.Bip [24]. Nevertheless, the highest activities were obtained for the 4-fluorobenzoate derivatives of reynosin and santamarine (**Fluor-Reynosin** and **Fluor-Santamarine**). In terms of the M^{pro} and RNA replicase inhibition values (Table 1), artemisinin gave values in the range 25–35 μM, while **Fluor-Reynosin** and **Fluor-Santamarine** were in the range 1–20 μM. The results of the studies on the spike protein are consistent with the recognition function that this receptor protein has. In this case (Table 1), the bis (4-fluorobenzoate) derivative of cynaropicrin (**Fluor-Cynaro**) was the most active, with an inhibition constant of 1.10 μM on the spike protein.

Small changes in the skeleton did not result in significant changes in the binding energy. A comparison of the results for reynosin, santamarine, alantolactone (**alanto**), β-cyclocostunolide (**beta-cyclo**), α-cyclocostunolide (**alpha-cyclo**) and 3-deoxybrachylaenolide (**3-DeBra**) clearly shows that the arrangement of the skeleton does not lead to changes in the inhibition in computational studies and even the presence of a hydroxyl group or double bond in the first ring of the structure did not alter the energy markedly. An analysis of the ligand binding site and the intermolecular forces (Figures S1–S3 and Table 1) indicated that the lactone group appears to be the main component required for activity. Nevertheless, **alanto** displayed a significant binding value, which was better than those for similar lactones, against the RNA replicase. **Alanto** differs from the other sesquiterpenes in the lactone arrangement, and this indicates that the remaining carbon skeleton must play a relevant role.

As far as the benzoxazinoids (Table 2) are concerned, the results are similar to those described for the sesquiterpenoids. These compounds all showed a binding energy toward the M^{pro} that was lower than that of the standard artemisinin, but they are more active than the standards with similar skeletons (hydroxychloroquine and favipiravir). In addition, the

4-fluorobenzoate derivative of APO (**Fluor-APO**) has values similar to artemisinin. The RNA replicase shows different profiles, with APO and the 4-fluorobenzoate derivative of 2,2′-disulfanediyldianiline (**Fluor-DisNH**) being more active than they were against the M^{pro}. The spike protein did not seem to recognize this kind of skeleton easily, but the presence of halogen atoms (Figure S5) linked at the edge of the fluorobenzoate fragment does appear to be relevant.

Table 2. Binding energy values of benzoxazinoids selected in the study on M^{pro}, RNA replicase and the spike protein of SARS-CoV-2.

Compounds	ΔG (Kcal/mol)		
	Main Protease	**RNA Replicase**	**Spike Protein**
Azithromycin	-1.20 ± 0.47	-0.76 ± 0.88	-4.64 ± 0.78
Hydroxychloroquine	-3.45 ± 0.16	-2.67 ± 0.81	-4.29 ± 0.76
Favipiravir	-3.21 ± 0.16	-3.58 ± 0.24	-3.93 ± 0.42
Artemisinin	-6.25 ± 0.23	-6.07 ± 0.07	-5.96 ± 0.19
Met-4F-Benzo	-3.49 ± 0.08	-4.02 ± 0.25	-4.19 ± 0.28
APO	-5.13 ± 0.31	-5.93 ± 0.66	-5.52 ± 0.24
DisOH	-4.84 ± 0.69	-4.74 ± 0.84	-4.66 ± 0.59
$DisNH_2$	-4.48 ± 0.22	-4.68 ± 0.44	-4.88 ± 0.38
Fluor-APO	-6.01 ± 0.53	-6.08 ± 0.41	-7.79 ± 0.88
Fluor-DisOH	-5.71 ± 1.36	-4.67 ± 0.69	-5.01 ± 0.86
Fluor-DisNH	-4.45 ± 1.31	-5.77 ± 0.55	-5.91 ± 0.93
DIBOAa	-4.05 ± 0.28	-4.05 ± 0.34	-4.94 ± 0.33
DIBOAb	-3.90 ± 0.17	-4.50 ± 0.49	-4.33 ± 0.28
DIMBOAa	-3.93 ± 0.17	-4.03 ± 0.38	-4.61 ± 0.30
DIMBOAb	-3.91 ± 0.13	-3.71 ± 0.47	-4.53 ± 0.36
DDIBOA	-4.12 ± 0.17	-4.19 ± 0.19	-4.41 ± 0.27
6Cl-DDIBOA	-4.42 ± 0.11	-4.28 ± 0.24	-4.77 ± 0.21
6F-DDIBOA	-4.07 ± 0.28	-4.30 ± 0.36	-4.28 ± 0.19
6F-DDIBOA	-4.46 ± 0.22	-4.57 ± 0.38	-4.57 ± 0.18

Previous studies regarding similar proteins have highlighted the efficacy of this kind of compound. Xue et al. showed that Michael acceptors groups in molecules, with the same function as sesquiterpenes lactones with an exocyclic double bond, are really important to inhibit the main protease of coronaviruses [25]. This is in concordance with the data displayed in Tables 1 and 2, where the sesquiterpenes present higher inhibition values than the benzoxazinoids in general terms. The studies on similar proteins to the RNA replicase and spike protein of coronaviruses is really limited, and there are no small molecules with reported inhibition. However, interesting studies on the M^{pro} of COVID-03 displayed the ability of dibenzyl sulphides (structurally similar to DisOH and $DisNH_2$) to link cysteine and histidine [26]. This interaction is observed in the M^{pro} with mimics of the benzoxazinoids tested (DisOH and $DisNH_2$) whose main interaction in the binding site involves histide and cysteine. In the last case, Lu et al. remarked the relevance of the sulfur–sulfur interaction [26].

On comparing the standards employed against the SARS-CoV main protease (Figure 2A), it is clear that small differences between the SARS-CoV-2 and SARS-CoV viruses are sufficient to cause differences in ligand binding. According to Xu et al., these two viruses share 96% sequence similarity [27]. The most remarkable example is hydroxychloroquine, which has an inhibition constant in the mM range against SARS-CoV-2 and an inhibition constant of 60 μM against SARS-CoV. Even the site of action of the compound is radically different. The arrangement between the ligand and the target protein is shown in Figure 2B,C, and the different spatial positions in SARS-CoV-2 and SARS-CoV is clear. In the former case, threonine is the main interaction site and this is linked by a hydrogen bond with the terminal hydroxyl group of hydroxychloroquine. In contrast, the SARS-CoV protein binds to the terminal hydroxyl group through a glutamic acid residue and a nitrogen in the structure shows a secondary union with the protein, in this case by a leucine residue. This is a relevant finding according to the experimental results previously published by Liu et al., who reported IC50 values of hydroxychloroquine [28] against SARS-CoV-2 that were ~500 times higher than the IC50 values previously reported against SARS-CoV by Vincent et al. in 2005 [29]. Accordingly, in our computational studies, the IC50 value for hydroxychloroquine against SARS-CoV-2 was only ~200 times higher than for SARS-CoV. On the other hand, azithromycin does not show any activity against the main protease, as one would expect due to the similarities in the previous peptidic inhibitors [30].

In the evaluation of sesquiterpenes and benzoxazinoids, the compounds **Fluor-Reynosin** and **Fluor-Santamarine** are the most promising for the bioassay evaluation. The sites of action for these compounds, i.e., in the main protease and RNA replicase, are the same as for artemisinin. Notwithstanding, the results of an in-depth study on the mode of action of this standard showed that its inhibitory activity is due to a 'desolvation effect' caused by a physical impediment toward the protein to be stabilized with solvent in the cytosol. In contrast, **Fluor-Reynosin** and **Fluor-Santamarine**, despite sharing the same action site with artemisinin, are able to establish stronger intermolecular forces. The binding of two histidines instead of one in the case of M^{pro} and one unit of arginine and one valine in the RNA replicase are observed due to the presence of the 4-fluorobenzoate group. Furthermore, this group links with leucine141 and cisteine145, two principal targets in the protease for sesquiterpenoids and benzoxazinoids. Both structures explore new sites of action (Figures S1–S3) that are overlooked by azithromycin, favipiravir and hydroxychloroquine. This situation is exemplified in Figure S4 for the main protease.

Fluor-Cynaro offers an interesting result in the case of the spike protein due to its long-branched edges, which leads to the establishment of more interactions with the protein than for other ligands. The presence of fluoro-substituents, a high number of carbonyl groups and double-bonded carbons allows more secondary forces to participate in the interaction. The site of action of this compound preferentially enables intermolecular forces with asparagine and glutamic acid, as shown in Figure S5. **Fluor-APO** also presents a remarkable profile along the whole viral protein, and it is more effective than all of the standards in the case of the RNA protease but is best in the case of the spike protein. In addition, it is important to highlight that both compounds can be synthesized in one step in 99% yield by the reaction of the precursor with 4-fluorobenzoyl chloride. Furthermore, both of the precursor natural products (cynaropicrin and **APO**) can be obtained on a multigram scale. [31,32] On considering the results for **DIBOA**, **DIMBOA**, **DDIBOA** and the halogenated derivatives of **DDIBOA**, it is clear that the functionalization of the aromatic ring is not the key aspect. Nevertheless, amide formation, as in the case of **APO**, with the addition of a fluorinated fragment seems to be important. Thus, an extra ring in the structure contributes to a higher binding energy. Furthermore, **Met-4F-Benzo**, the corresponding added fragment, did not show relevant activity when it was not linked to the natural product.

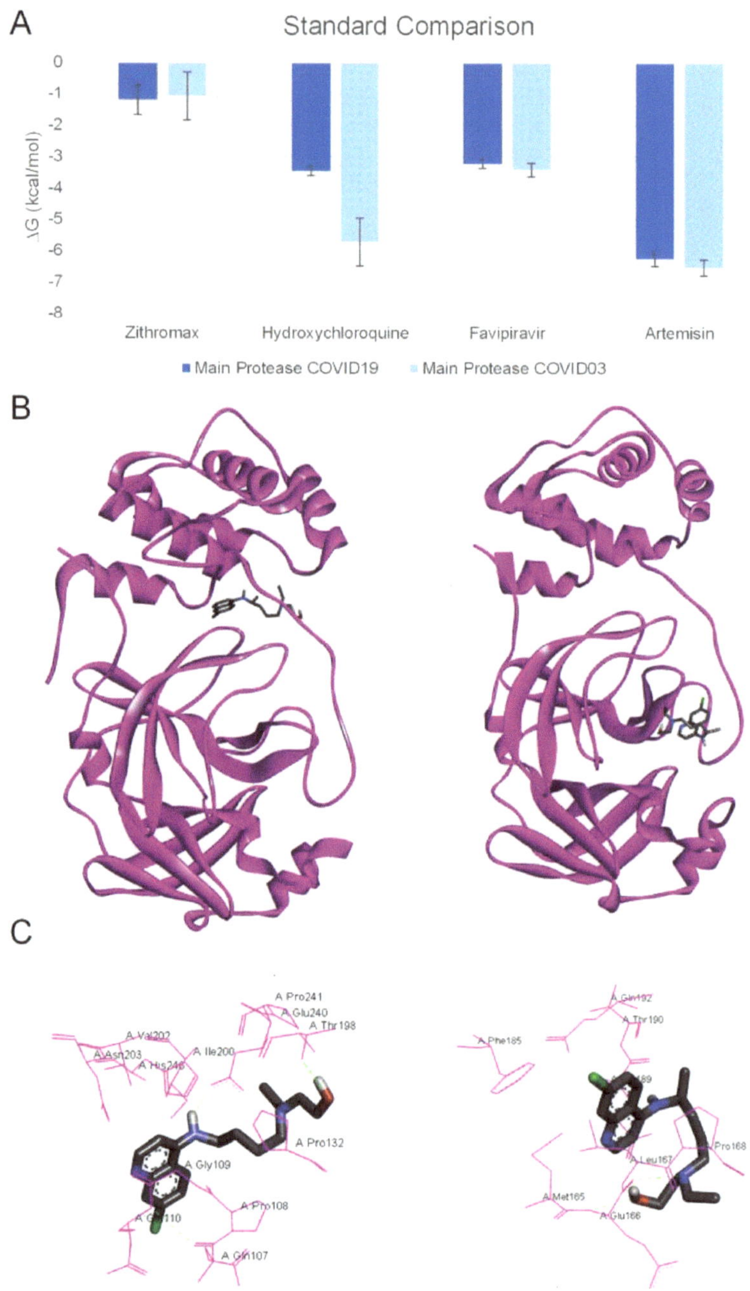

Figure 2. (**A**) Comparison between binding energy values of standard compounds against M^{pro} of SARS-CoV and M^{pro} SARS-CoV-2. (**B Left**) Site of action of hydroxychloroquine on M^{pro} SARS-CoV-2. (**B Right**) Site of action of hydroxychloroquine on M^{pro} SARS-CoV. (**C Left**) Amino acid residues that establish intermolecular forces with hydroxychloroquine on M^{pro} SARS-CoV-2. (**C Right**) Amino acid residues that establish intermolecular forces with hydroxychloroquine on M^{pro} SARS-CoV.

The most promising compounds were considered in the context of Lipinski's rule in order to evaluate their pharmacological potential in terms of oral bioavailability. The rules and standards are shown in Table 3A. This rule offers a first approach to understand the ADME (absorption, distribution, metabolism and elimination) properties for the compounds selected. The Lipinski 'rule-of-five' has had a major impact on the daily practice of medicinal chemistry across the pharmaceutical industry and served as a very useful guideline for orally bioavailable small-molecule drug discovery [33,34]. It can be seen how azithromycin is limited by its high molecular weight and hydrogen-bond acceptors, which could prevent the correct orientation toward protein targets. Nevertheless, all of the sesquiterpenoids and benzoxazinoids shown in Tables 1 and 2, except for **Fluor-Cynaro**, fulfill the requirements and could be important options in the future development of SARS-CoV-2 inhibitors. This model is dealing only with transport by passive diffusion (a major route for drug molecules permeating thorugh cell membranes). However, diffusion mechanims and complexation with ions also help in the transport. This may present some of the drugs in Table 3B,C as potential drugs with good ADME properties although it is not fulfilling the oral bioavailability Lipinski's rule. Further analysis may be required in the future to analyze **Fluor-DisNH, Fluor-DisOH** and **Fluor-Cynaro** in more details.

Table 3. Lipinski's rules evaluation of compounds evaluated in molecular docking.

(A). Lipinski's rules for standard compounds tested.				
No	**Standard**	**Molecular Formula**	**Lipinski's Rule of 5**	
			Properties	**Value**
1	6-fluoropyrazine-2-carboxamide (Favipiravir)	$C_5H_4FN_3O$	M.W. (≤500 amu)	141.11
			cLog *P* (≤5)	–0.50873
			H-bond donors (≤5)	1
			H-bond acceptors (≤10)	5
			Violations	0
2	Hydroxychloroquine	$C_{18}H_{26}ClN_3O$	M.W. (≤500 amu)	335.88
			cLog *P* (≤5)	4.11588
			H-bond donors (≤5)	2
			H-bond acceptors (≤10)	4
			Violations	0
3	Artemisinin	$C_{15}H_{22}O_5$	M.W. (≤500 amu)	282.34
			cLog *P* (≤5)	2.71630
			H-bond donors (≤5)	0
			H-bond acceptors (≤10)	5
			Violations	0
4	Azithromycin	$C_{38}H_{72}N_2O_{12}$	M.W. (≤500 amu)	749.00
			cLog *P* (≤5)	2.63825
			H-bond donors (≤5)	5
			H-bond acceptors (≤10)	14
			Violations	2

Table 3. *Cont.*

(B). Lipinski's rules for the most relevant sesquiterpenoid compounds tested.				
No	**Sesquiterpenoids**	**Molecular Formula**	**Lipinski's Rule of 5**	
			Properties	**Value**
1	Cynaropicrin	$C_{19}H_{22}O_6$	M.W. (≤500 amu)	346.38
			cLog *P* (≤5)	0.045825
			H-bond donors (≤5)	2
			H-bond acceptors (≤10)	6
			Violations	0
2	3,3′-di(4′-fluorobenzoyloxy) cynaropicrin (Fluor-Cynaro)	$C_{33}H_{28}F_2O_8$	M.W. (≤500 amu)	590.58
			cLog *P* (≤5)	5.82662
			H-bond donors (≤5)	0
			H-bond acceptors (≤10)	10
			Violations	2
3	Costunolide	$C_{15}H_{20}O_2$	M.W. (≤500 amu)	232.32
			cLog *P* (≤5)	3.79
			H-bond donors (≤5)	0
			H-bond acceptors (≤10)	2
			Violations	0
4	Dehydrocostuslactone (DHC)	$C_{15}H_{18}O_2$	M.W. (≤500 amu)	230.31
			cLog *P* (≤5)	2.786
			H-bond donors (≤5)	0
			H-bond acceptors (≤10)	2
			Violations	0
5	Reynosin	$C_{15}H_{20}O_3$	M.W. (≤500 amu)	248.32
			cLog *P* (≤5)	1.183
			H-bond donors (≤5)	1
			H-bond acceptors (≤10)	3
			Violations	0
6	1-(4′-fluorobenzoyloxy) reynosin (Fluor-Reynosin)	$C_{22}H_{23}FO_4$	M.W. (≤500 amu)	370.42
			cLog *P* (≤5)	4.201
			H-bond donors (≤5)	0
			H-bond acceptors (≤10)	5
			Violations	0

Table 3. *Cont.*

(B). Lipinski's rules for the most relevant sesquiterpenoid compounds tested.				
No	**Sesquiterpenoids**	**Molecular Formula**	**Lipinski's Rule of 5**	
			Properties	**Value**
7	Santamarine	$C_{15}H_{20}O_3$	M.W. (≤500 amu)	248.32
			cLog *P* (≤5)	1.183
			H-bond donors (≤5)	1
			H-bond acceptors (≤10)	3
			Violations	0
8	1-(4-fluorobenzoyloxy) santamarine (Fluor-Santamarine)	$C_{22}H_{23}FO_4$	M.W. (≤500 amu)	370.42
			cLog *P* (≤5)	4.201
			H-bond donors (≤5)	0
			H-bond acceptors (≤10)	5
			Violations	0
9	Alantolactone (Alanto)	$C_{15}H_{20}O_2$	M.W. (≤500 amu)	232.32
			cLog *P* (≤5)	3.27
			H-bond donors (≤5)	0
			H-bond acceptors (≤10)	2
			Violations	0
10	β-cyclocostunolide (Beta-Cyclo)	$C_{15}H_{20}O_2$	M.W. (≤500 amu)	232.32
			cLog *P* (≤5)	3.27
			H-bond donors (≤5)	0
			H-bond acceptors (≤10)	2
			Violations	0
11	α-cyclocostunolide (Alpha-Cyclo)	$C_{15}H_{20}O_2$	M.W. (≤500 amu)	232.32
			cLog *P* (≤5)	3.27
			H-bond donors (≤5)	0
			H-bond acceptors (≤10)	2
			Violations	0
12	3-deoxybrachylaenolide (3-DeBra)	$C_{15}H_{16}O_3$	M.W. (≤500 amu)	244.29
			cLog *P* (≤5)	1.024
			H-bond donors (≤5)	0
			H-bond acceptors (≤10)	3
			Violations	0

Table 3. *Cont.*

(C). Lipinski's rules for the most relevant aminophenoxazinoids tested.				
No	**Benzoxazinoids**	**Molecular Formula**	**Lipinski's Rule of 5**	
			Properties	**Value**
13	2-amino-3*H*-phenoxazin-3-one (APO)	$C_{12}H_8N_2O_2$	M.W. (≤500 amu)	212.21
			cLog *P* (≤5)	1.13575
			H-bond donors (≤5)	1
			H-bond acceptors (≤10)	4
			Violations	0
14	4-fluoro-*N*-(3-oxo-3*H*-phenoxazin-2-yl)benzamide (Fluor-APO)	$C_{19}H_{11}FN_2O_3$	M.W. (≤500 amu)	334.31
			cLog *P* (≤5)	2.97045
			H-bond donors (≤5)	1
			H-bond acceptors (≤10)	6
			Violations	0
15	2,2′-disulfanediyldiphenol (DisOH)	$C_{12}H_{10}O_2S_2$	M.W. (≤500 amu)	250.33
			cLog *P* (≤5)	3.0194
			H-bond donors (≤5)	2
			H-bond acceptors (≤10)	2
			Violations	0
16	disulfanediylbis(2,1-phenylene) bis(4-fluorobenzoate) (Fluor-DisOH)	$C_{26}H_{16}F_2O_4S_2$	M.W. (≤500 amu)	494.53
			cLog *P* (≤5)	7.2229
			H-bond donors (≤5)	0
			H-bond acceptors (≤10)	6
			Violations	1
17	2,2′-dithiodianiline ($DisNH_2$)	$C_{12}H_{12}N_2S_2$	M.W. (≤500 amu)	248.36
			cLog *P* (≤5)	2.736
			H-bond donors (≤5)	2
			H-bond acceptors (≤10)	2
			Violations	0
18	*N*,*N*′-(disulfanediylbis(2,1-phenylene))bis(4-fluorobenzamide) (Fluor-DisNH)	$C_{26}H_{18}F_2N_2O_2S_2$	M.W. (≤500 amu)	492.56
			cLog *P* (≤5)	5.06192
			H-bond donors (≤5)	2
			H-bond acceptors (≤10)	4
			Violations	1

2.2. Molecular Dynamics Simulations

The MD simulations were run after obtaining the docked positions of the most relevant ligands (**Fluor-Reynosin**, **Fluor-Santamarine** and **Fluor-APO**) (Figures S6–S15). On considering 6LU7, it can be seen from Figure 3 that the RMSD fluctuated by less than 1–1.5 Å for **Fluor-APO** and **Fluor-Reynosin,** and this is consistent with the stable complexes during the whole simulation (50 ns). This finding is also in agreement with the snapshots shown in Figures S8–S10. It is clear from these results that the docked position was fully predicted by molecular docking with these two promising compounds. However, **Fluor-Santamarine** did not give a stable complex in any of the three replicates carried out. According to the score obtained in the docking, both compounds show a similar activity profile, but the different location of the double bond (i.e., exocyclic or endocyclic) seems to determine the stability of the complex at the site of action. The addition of the 4-fluoro benzoate fragment allows to enhance the inhibition of the protein according to the docking score, but isomerism in the double bond allows to generate a long-term complex ligand–protein that shows permanent inhibition. This stability is also observed in the protein–ligand interaction energies in Table 4, which also contains the low Lennard–Jones energy of **Fluor-Santamarine** with the M^{pro} in comparison with the other stable complexes. Furthermore, this stability seems to be directly related to the total and average number of hydrogen bonds per ns. **Fluor-Reynosin** and **Fluor-APO** are able to generate more hydrogen bonds with the protein, thus enhancing the stability of the protein–ligand complex. A structural change in the RMSD is observed during the first 20 ns for **Fluor-Reynosin** and **Fluor-APO,** and these, according to the snapshots shown in Figures S8 and S9, are just rotations of the molecule that do not affect the active site.

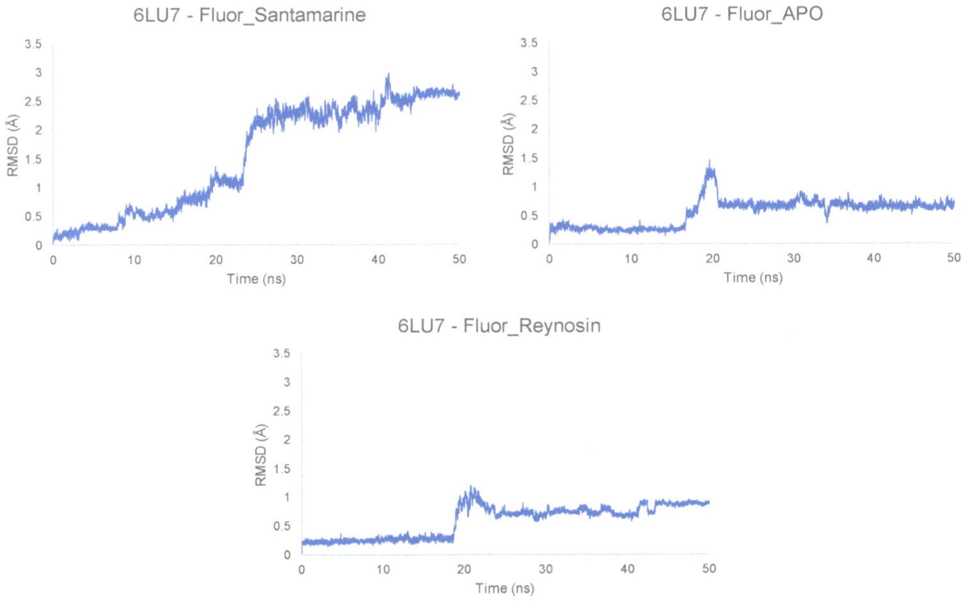

Figure 3. Root mean square deviation (RMSD) of the different ligands in the protein–ligand complex with the main protease (6LU7) of SARS-CoV-2.

Table 4. Relevant energy values and intermolecular interactions of every protein with a ligand, surrounded by ions and water molecules.

Protein–LIG Energy (kJ/mol) Lennard–Jones								
	6M0J			**6LU7**			**6W4B**	
Fluor-APO	Fluor-Santamarine	Fluor-Reynosin	Fluor-APO	Fluor-Santamarine	Fluor-Reynosin	Fluor-APO	Fluor-Santamarine	Fluor-Reynosin
−8.846 ± 4.279	−123.866 ± 3.611	−113.915 ± 2.960	−105.696 ± 2.446	−68.819 ± 3.583	−126.618 ± 2.007	−54.026 ± 2.800	−118.928 ± 1.982	−125.207 ± 10.865
Protein–LIG Total Number of H-Bonds along 50 ns								
	6M0J			**6LU7**			**6W4B**	
Fluor-APO	Fluor-Santamarine	Fluor-Reynosin	Fluor-APO	Fluor-Santamarine	Fluor-Reynosin	Fluor-APO	Fluor-Santamarine	Fluor-Reynosin
355	1267	1674	3600	2490	3708	1293	3571	2385
Protein–LIG Average Number of H-Bonds per ns								
	6M0J			**6LU7**			**6W4B**	
Fluor-APO	Fluor-Santamarine	Fluor-Reynosin	Fluor-APO	Fluor-Santamarine	Fluor-Reynosin	Fluor-APO	Fluor-Santamarine	Fluor-Reynosin
0.07	0.25	0.33	0.72	0.50	0.74	0.26	0.91	0.48
Protein–LIG Average Distance of H-Bonds (nm)								
	6M0J			**6LU7**			**6W4B**	
Fluor-APO	Fluor-Santamarine	Fluor-Reynosin	Fluor-APO	Fluor-Santamarine	Fluor-Reynosin	Fluor-APO	Fluor-Santamarine	Fluor-Reynosin
0.2925	0.3075	0.2825	0.2875	0.2975	0.3125	0.3275	0.2875	0.2825
Protein–LIG Lifetime of H-Bonds (ps)								
	6M0J			**6LU7**			**6W4B**	
Fluor-APO	Fluor-Santamarine	Fluor-Reynosin	Fluor-APO	Fluor-Santamarine	Fluor-Reynosin	Fluor-APO	Fluor-Santamarine	Fluor-Reynosin
19.63	18.08	14.03	65.95	24.34	19.81	27.57	74.94	75.55

In the case of the RNA replicase (6W4B), the RMSD fluctuations for the eudesmanolide derivatives (**Fluor-Reynosin** and **Fluor-Santamarine**) and **Fluor-APO** show stabilization throughout the simulation, with values that do not exceed 1.5 Å (Figures 4 and S7). None of the steps exceed 0.5 Å, and this confirms the stability of the complexes. Nevertheless, **Fluor-APO** experiences a significant continuous variation in geometry throughout the simulation. According to the snapshots (Figure S14), this is not only due to the rotation or rocking of the fluorobenzoate fragment but movement of the whole compound out from the site of action of the protein, thus indicating a kinetically unstable complex. This situation was confirmed by the lower protein–ligand average interaction energy of **Fluor-APO** with the 6W4B protein (RNA replicase) when compared to the other compounds (Table 4). Once again, hydrogen bonding seems to be the main contribution to complex stability. According to the number of hydrogen bonds and their average lifetime, **Fluor-APO** is the worst ligand in terms of inhibiting the action of the RNA replicase in comparison with the other fluorobenzoate derivatives. This finding is consistent with the results shown in Tables 1 and 2, where it can be seen that the docking energy value for **Fluor-APO** with the RNA replicase is markedly lower than those for the other two compounds analyzed. In addition, **Fluor-APO** also has the lowest average number of hydrogen bonds per nanosecond, which is consistent with the continuous increase in the RMSD value as the ligand moves away.

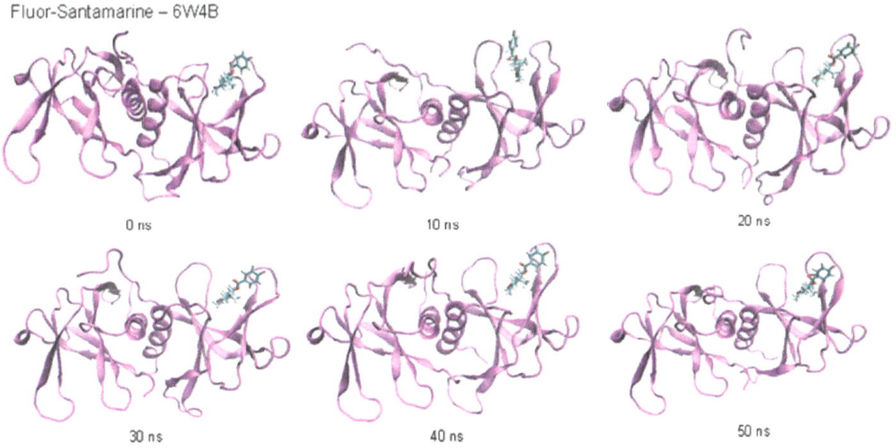

Figure 4. Root mean square deviation (RMSD) of Fluor-Santamatine in the protein–ligand complex with the RNA replicase (6W4B) of SARS-CoV-2.

The spike (6M0J) receptor-binding protein–ligand complexes were also analyzed. It can be seen from Figure S6 that the **Fluor-Santamarine** and **Fluor-Reynosin** complexes are stable after 50 ns, while **Fluor-APO** is relatively unstable with an RMSD fluctuation above 9 Å, which means that the ligand position is not stable at that docking point. The score values from the docking studies show that **Fluor-APO** is a promising compound, but the MD simulations show a kinetically unstable complex. This is graphically represented in the snapshots, where **Fluor-APO** changes its position markedly with respect to the spike protein (Figure S11). This situation is consistent with the energy values of the ligands, where the protein–ligand energy differs between **Fluor-APO** and the other two ligands by a factor of greater than fifteen. The number of hydrogen bonds is a relevant parameter in terms of the energy and stability of the complex and, in this case, complexes with the 6M0J protein seem to generate structures with lower stability in comparison to other proteins (Table 4. The number of hydrogen bonds is reduced dramatically, with **Fluor-Reynosin** showing only 1674 H-bonds. This value is extremely small in comparison with the numbers of hydrogen bonds generated in the cases of the other proteins, although the protein–ligand interaction energies have comparable values. It appears that other intermolecular forces that have more profound energetic implications must be involved in the interaction with the protein to contribute to the stability of the **Fluor-Reynosin** and **Fluor-Santamarine** complexes.

3. Conclusions

In silico studies such as molecular docking and dynamic methods represent a relevant and rapid advance in the search for new drugs from derivatives of natural compounds against SARS-CoV-2. The results reported here highlight the potential use of sesquiterpenoids and benzoxazinoids to fight this virus. The molecules evaluated in this study have a different site of action when compared with compounds from the same families that have previously shown activity against the virus in preliminary studies. Furthermore, the results of the molecular dynamics studies corroborated the docking results, thus showing the stability of the protein–ligand complex by the RMSD fluctuations—especially the complexes with the M^{pro} and RNA replicase. Our team is currently analyzing and selecting possible candidates based on the docking scores and physicochemical properties in an effort to identify the best candidates for molecular dynamics studies. The results reported here indicate that the addition of the 4-fluorobenzoate fragment to the natural products enhances their potential against all of the proteins tested. This option would allow the production of a large number of drug leads, and it would be possible to synthesize the most remarkable compounds (**Fluor-Reynosin, Fluor-Santamarine** and **Fluor-APO**) in just one step.

4. Materials and Methods

4.1. Molecular Docking Studies

The 2D structures of the assayed compounds were generated with ChemBioDraw 20.0 and were converted to 3D structures with GaussView 6.0.16 software (Wallingford, CT, USA). Proteins were obtained from the Protein Data Bank (www.rcsb.org, accessed on 1 April 2020). The proteins selected were 2GTB (main protease of SARS-CoV), 6LU7 (main protease of SARS-CoV-2), 6W4B (RNA replicase of SARS-CoV-2) and 6M0J (spike receptor binding of SARS-CoV-2). A grid box (120 × 120 × 120 Å) was generated and centered on the proteins. Kollman charges were applied to each protein to simulate the electrostatic potential of amino acids. AutoDockTools (v. 1.5.6) was employed to define the previous steps. DFT B3LYP/6-311G(d,p) minimization was employed prior to carrying out the docking. Autodock 4.2 and the Lamarckian GA algorithm with 20 GA runs were employed to develop the local docking, with a value of 1.0 used as the variance of the Cauchy distribution for gene mutations. All calculations correspond to the most populated cluster, with at least three members that fulfill an RMSD tolerance below 2.000 Å (Tables S1–S4). Discovery Studio Visualizer 19.0 was used for the refinement of the docking results. Chemical Identifier Resolver [35] was employed for the calculation of properties related to Lipinski's rule.

4.2. Molecular Dynamics Simulation

The studies were carried out starting from the minimum energy protein–ligand conformation obtained from the previous molecular docking studies. GROMACS (2019.6 version) was employed in conjunction with CHARMM36 force-field (march-2019) and SPCE water model. The ligand topologies and parameters were obtained using the SwissParam server (www.swissparam.ch, accessed on 5 June 2021) [36]. A dodecahedral box was generated and the protein–ligand complexes (6LU7, 6W4 and 6M0J) were at least 1 nm from the edges of the box, with a distance of at least 2 nm between periodic images of the protein in order to fulfill the minimum image convention. A 0.1 M NaCl concentration was simulated in the system to mimic physiological conditions. An energy minimization was applied until the maximum force was less than 10 kJ/mol. The system was then equilibrated for 0.1 ns with 2 fs per step at 300 K using canonical equilibration. Equilibration of the pressure was then carried out by the isothermal–isobaric method using the Parrinello–Rahman barostat. The system was equilibrated for 0.1 ns, also with 2 fs per step, at 300 K. The full equilibrated system was submitted to a molecular dynamics simulation for 50 ns with 2 fs per step. Correction of the trajectory was carried out by protein recentering within the dodecahedral box. Snapshots of the trajectory were collected every 10 ns. The average number of hydrogen bonds and average distance of these bonds were calculated using a 0.35 nm cut-off distance.

Supplementary Materials: The following supporting information can be downloaded at: https://www.mdpi.com/article/10.3390/toxins14090599/s1. Figure S1: Bond mapping of M^{pro} with the most relevant ligand in the study. The image highlights that benzoxazinoids and sesquiterpenes explore a different binding site than the standards. The legend for the compounds is shown in the table below. Figure S2: Bond mapping of the RNA replicase with the most relevant ligand in the study. In this case, the protein shows symmetry, so compounds in the first and fourth grid correspond to the same site. Figure S3: Bond mapping of the spike protein with the most relevant ligand in the study. The image shows that benzoxazinoids and sesquiterpenes explore different binding sites than the standards. Figure S4: Comparative images of M^{pro} site of action of standard (a) azithromycin and (b) favipiravir, with (c) APO and (d) Fluor-Reynosin. (a) and (b) show different sites of action than (c) and (d). In the case of (b), the position is in front of the protein while (c) and (d) are behind. Sesquiterpenoids and benzoxazinoids explore a different kind of site. Figure S5: (a) Binding site of Fluor-Cynaro on the spike protein of SARS-CoV-2. (b) Binding site of Fluor-APO on the spike protein of SARS-CoV-2. (c) Amino acid residues that establish intermolecular forces with Fluor-Cynaro on the spike protein of SARS-CoV-2. (d) Amino acid residues that establish intermolecular forces with Fluor-APO on the spike protein of SARS-CoV-2. Figure S6: Root mean square deviation (RMSD) of the different ligands in protein–ligand complex with spike protein of SARS-CoV-2. Figure S7: Root mean square deviation (RMSD) of the different ligands in protein–ligand complex with RNA replicase of SARS-CoV-2. Figure S8: Snapshot of structural changes at different times of the molecular dynamics of Fluor-APO with main protease of SARS-CoV-2. Figure S9: Snapshot of structural changes at different times of the molecular dynamics of Fluor-Reynosin with main protease of SARS-CoV-2. Figure S10: Snapshot of structural changes at different times of the molecular dynamics of Fluor-Santamarine with main protease of SARS-CoV-2. Figure S11: Snapshot of structural changes at different times of the molecular dynamics of Fluor-APO with spike protein of SARS-CoV-2. Figure S12: Snapshot of structural changes at different times of the molecular dynamics of Fluor-Reynosin with spike protein of SARS-CoV-2. Figure S13: Snapshot of structural changes at different times of the molecular dynamics of Fluor-Santamarine with spike protein of SARS-CoV-2. Figure S14: Snapshot of structural changes at different times of the molecular dynamics of Fluor-APO with RNA replicase of SARS-CoV-2. Figure S15: Snapshot of structural changes at different times of the molecular dynamics of Fluor-Reynosin with RNA replicase of SARS-CoV-2. Table S1: RMSD values of tested compounds against M^{pro} of SARS-CoV-2. Table S2: RMSD values of tested compounds against RNA replicase of SARS-CoV-2. Table S3: RMSD values of tested compounds against spike protein of SARS-CoV-2. Table S4: RMSD values of tested compounds against M^{pro} of SARS-CoV.

Author Contributions: Conceptualization: F.J.R.M., F.A.M. and J.M.G.M.; methodology, F.J.R.M., A.G.D., R.M.V. and N.C.; software: F.J.R.M. and J.A.Á.; validation: F.J.R.M., J.A.Á. and R.M.V.; formal analysis: F.J.R.M., A.G.D., F.G.-C. and R.M.V.; investigation: F.J.R.M. and A.G.D.; resources: J.A.Á., J.M.G.M. and F.A.M.; data curation: F.J.R.M. and R.M.V.; writing—original draft preparation: F.J.R.M. and A.G.D.; writing—review and editing, A.G.D. and F.A.M.; visualization: R.M.V. and F.J.R.M.; supervision: J.M.G.M., F.G.-C., J.A.Á. and F.A.M.; project administration: F.A.M.; funding acquisition: F.A.M. All authors have read and agreed to the published version of the manuscript.

Funding: This research was funded by the Agencia Estatal de Investigación, Ministerio de Ciencia e Innovacion, grant number PID2020-15747RB-I00/AEI/10.13039, Spain. F.J.R.M thanks the Universidad de Cádiz for postdoctoral support with a Margarita-Salas fellowship, funded by the European Union—NextGenerationEU.

Institutional Review Board Statement: Not Applicable.

Informed Consent Statement: Not Applicable.

Acknowledgments: This paper is affectionately dedicated in the memory of Mariola Macías (1984–2020) on her second anniversary. She was an excellent professional, an emergency doctor at Hospital Punta Europa, Algeciras (Cadiz), Spain, a Doctor in Immunology and, above all, a great person. She worked intensively not only in clinical functions but also in research against SARS- CoV-2 and was passionate about Natural Products. Her humanity, kindness, special and unmistakable smile, generosity, dedication and professionalism will never be forgotten. All simulations were performed using computational facilities at the 'Servicio de Supercomputación of Área de Sistemas de Información' of the University of Cádiz. F.J.R.M thanks Iván Carrillo-Berdugo for his MD comments and advice.

Conflicts of Interest: The authors declare no conflict of interest. The funders had no role in the design of the study; in the collection, analyses or interpretation of data; in the writing of the manuscript; or in the decision to publish the results.

References

1. Glass, W.G.; Subbarao, K.; Murphy, B.; Murphy, P.M. Mechanisms of Host Defense Following Severe Acute Respiratory Syndrome-Coronavirus (SARS-CoV) Pulmonary Infection of Mice. *J. Immunol.* **2004**, *173*, 4030–4039. [CrossRef] [PubMed]
2. Yang, Y.; Islam, M.S.; Wang, J.; Li, Y.; Chen, X. Traditional Chinese Medicine in the Treatment of Patients Infected with 2019-New Coronavirus (SARS-CoV-2): A Review and Perspective. *Int. J. Biol. Sci.* **2020**, *16*, 1708–1717. [CrossRef] [PubMed]
3. Farmanpour-Kalalagh, K.; Beyraghdar Kashkooli, A.; Babaei, A.; Rezaei, A.; van der Krol, A.R. Artemisinins in Combating Viral Infections Like SARS-CoV-2, Inflammation and Cancers and Options to Meet Increased Global Demand. *Front. Plant Sci.* **2022**, *13*, 780257. [CrossRef] [PubMed]
4. Nair, M.S.; Huang, Y.; Fidock, D.A.; Polyak, S.J.; Wagoner, J.; Towler, M.J.; Weathers, P.J. Artemisia Annua, L. Extracts Inhibit the in Vitro Replication of SARS-CoV-2 and Two of Its Variants. *J. Ethnopharmacol.* **2021**, *274*, 114016. [CrossRef]
5. Gyebi, G.A.; Ogunro, O.B.; Adegunloye, A.P.; Ogunyemi, O.M.; Afolabi, S.O. Potential Inhibitors of Coronavirus 3-Chymotrypsin-like Protease (3CL ^{pro}): An *in Silico* Screening of Alkaloids and Terpenoids from African Medicinal Plants. *J. Biomol. Struct. Dyn.* **2020**, *39*, 3396–3408. [CrossRef]
6. Forrestall, K.L.; Burley, D.E.; Cash, M.K.; Pottie, I.R.; Darvesh, S. 2-Pyridone Natural Products as Inhibitors of SARS-CoV-2 Main Protease. *Chem. Biol. Interact.* **2021**, *335*, 109348. [CrossRef]
7. Narkhede, R.R.; Pise, A.v.; Cheke, R.S.; Shinde, S.D. Recognition of Natural Products as Potential Inhibitors of COVID-19 Main Protease (Mpro): In-Silico Evidences. *Nat. Prod. Bioprospect* **2020**, *10*, 297–306. [CrossRef]
8. Jin, Z.; Du, X.; Xu, Y.; Deng, Y.; Liu, M.; Zhao, Y.; Zhang, B.; Li, X.; Zhang, L.; Peng, C.; et al. Structure of Mpro from SARS-CoV-2 and Discovery of Its Inhibitors. *Nature* **2020**, *582*, 289–293. [CrossRef]
9. Protein Data Bank. The Crystal Structure of COVID-19 Main Protease in Complex with an Inhibitor N3. Available online: https://www.rcsb.org/structure/6LU7 (accessed on 23 August 2022). [CrossRef]
10. Lan, J.; Ge, J.; Yu, J.; Shan, S.; Zhou, H.; Fan, S.; Zhang, Q.; Shi, X.; Wang, Q.; Zhang, L.; et al. Structure of the SARS-CoV-2 Spike Receptor-Binding Domain Bound to the ACE2 Receptor. *Nature* **2020**, *581*, 215–220. [CrossRef]
11. Protein Data Bank. Crystal Structure of SARS-CoV-2 Spike Receptor-Binding Domain Bound with ACE2. Available online: https://www.rcsb.org/structure/6M0J (accessed on 23 August 2022). [CrossRef]
12. Litter, D.; Gully, B.; Colson, R.; Rossjohn, J. Crystal Structure of the SARS-CoV-2 Non-structural Protein 9, Nsp9. *iScience* **2020**, *23*, 101258–101265. [CrossRef]
13. Protein Data Bank. The Crystal Structure of Nsp9 RNA Binding Protein of SARS CoV-2. Available online: https://www.rcsb.org/structure/6W4B (accessed on 23 August 2022). [CrossRef]
14. Moriya, S.; Miyazawa, K.; Kawaguchi, T.; Che, X.F.; Tomoda, A. Involvement of Endoplasmic Reticulum Stress-Mediated CHOP (GADD153) Induction in the Cytotoxicity of 2-Aminophenoxazine-3-One in Cancer Cells. *Int. J. Oncol.* **2011**, *39*, 981–988. [CrossRef] [PubMed]
15. babaei, G.; Aliarab, A.; Abroon, S.; Rasmi, Y.; Aziz, S.G.G. Application of Sesquiterpene Lactone: A New Promising Way for Cancer Therapy Based on Anticancer Activity. *Biomed. Pharmacother.* **2018**, *106*, 239–246. [CrossRef]
16. Russo, A.; Perri, M.; Cione, E.; di Gioia, M.L.; Nardi, M.; Cristina Caroleo, M. Biochemical and Chemical Characterization of Cynara Cardunculus, L. Extract and Its Potential Use as Co-Adjuvant Therapy of Chronic Myeloid Leukemia. *J. Ethnopharmacol.* **2017**, *202*, 184–191. [CrossRef] [PubMed]
17. Hwang, D.-R.; Wu, Y.-S.; Chang, C.-W.; Lien, T.-W.; Chen, W.-C.; Tan, U.-K.; Hsu, J.T.A.; Hsieh, H.-P. Synthesis and Anti-Viral Activity of a Series of Sesquiterpene Lactones and Analogues in the Subgenomic HCV Replicon System. *Bioorg. Med. Chem.* **2006**, *14*, 83–91. [CrossRef] [PubMed]
18. Elsebai, M.F.; Koutsoudakis, G.; Saludes, V.; Pérez-Vilaró, G.; Turpeinen, A.; Mattila, S.; Pirttilä, A.M.; Fontaine-Vive, F.; Mehiri, M.; Meyerhans, A.; et al. Pan-Genotypic Hepatitis C Virus Inhibition by Natural Products Derived from the Wild Egyptian Artichoke. *J. Virol.* **2016**, *90*, 1918–1930. [CrossRef]
19. Hayashi, K.; Hayashi, T.; Tomoda, A. Phenoxazine Derivatives Inactivate Human Cytomegalovirus, Herpes Simplex Virus-1, and Herpes Simplex Virus-2 In Vitro. *J. Pharmacol. Sci.* **2008**, *106*, 369–375. [CrossRef]

20. Hayashi, K.; Hayashi, T.; Miyazawa, K.; Tomoda, A. Phenoxazine Derivatives Suppress the Infections Caused by Herpes Simplex Virus Type-1 and Herpes Simplex Virus Type-2 Intravaginally Inoculated Into Mice. *J. Pharmacol. Sci.* **2010**, *114*, 85–91. [CrossRef]
21. Touret, F.; de Lamballerie, X. Of Chloroquine and COVID-19. *Antivir. Res.* **2020**, *177*, 104762. [CrossRef]
22. Colson, P.; Rolain, J.M.; Raoult, D. Chloroquine for the 2019 Novel Coronavirus SARS-CoV-2. *Int. J. Antimicrob. Agents* **2020**, *55*, 105923. [CrossRef]
23. Echeverría-Esnal, D.; Martin-Ontiyuelo, C.; Navarrete-Rouco, M.E.; De-Antonio Cuscó, M.; Ferrández, O.; Horcajada, J.P.; Grau, S. Azithromycin in the Treatment of COVID-19: A Review. *Expert Rev. Anti. Infect. Ther.* **2021**, *19*, 147–163. [CrossRef]
24. Cala, A.; Zorrilla, J.G.; Rial, C.; Molinillo, J.M.G.; Varela, R.M.; Macías, F.A. Easy Access to Alkoxy, Amino, Carbamoyl, Hydroxy, and Thiol Derivatives of Sesquiterpene Lactones and Evaluation of Their Bioactivity on Parasitic Weeds. *J. Agric. Food Chem.* **2019**, *67*, 10764–10773. [CrossRef]
25. Xue, X.; Yu, H.; Yang, H.; Xue, F.; Wu, Z.; Shen, W.; Li, J.; Zhou, Z.; Ding, Y.; Zhao, Q.; et al. Structures of Two Coronavirus Main Proteases: Implications for Substrate Binding and Antiviral Drug Design. *J. Virol.* **2008**, *82*, 2515–2527. [CrossRef]
26. Lu, I.-L.; Mahindroo, N.; Liang, P.-H.; Peng, Y.-H.; Kuo, C.-J.; Tsai, K.-C.; Hsieh, H.-P.; Chao, Y.-S.; Wu, S.-Y. Structure-Based Drug Design and Structural Biology Study of Novel Nonpeptide Inhibitors of Severe Acute Respiratory Syndrome Coronavirus Main Protease. *J. Med. Chem.* **2006**, *49*, 5154–5161. [CrossRef]
27. Xu, Z.; Peng, C.; Shi, Y.; Zhu, Z.; Mu, K.; Wang, X.; Zhu, W. Nelfinavir Was Predicted to Be a Potential Inhibitor of 2019-NCov Main Protease by an Integrative Approach Combining Homology Modelling, Molecular Docking and Binding Free Energy Calculation. *BioRxiv* **2020**. [CrossRef]
28. Liu, J.; Cao, R.; Xu, M.; Wang, X.; Zhang, H.; Hu, H.; Li, Y.; Hu, Z.; Zhong, W.; Wang, M. Hydroxychloroquine, a Less Toxic Derivative of Chloroquine, Is Effective in Inhibiting SARS-CoV-2 Infection in Vitro. *Cell Discov.* **2020**, *6*, 16. [CrossRef] [PubMed]
29. Vincent, M.J.; Bergeron, E.; Benjannet, S.; Erickson, B.R.; Rollin, P.E.; Ksiazek, T.G.; Seidah, N.G.; Nichol, S.T. Chloroquine Is a Potent Inhibitor of SARS Coronavirus Infection and Spread. *Virol. J.* **2005**, *2*, 1–10. [CrossRef]
30. Yang, H.; Yang, M.; Ding, Y.; Liu, Y.; Lou, Z.; Zhou, Z.; Sun, L.; Mo, L.; Ye, S.; Pang, H.; et al. The Crystal Structures of Severe Acute Respiratory Syndrome Virus Main Protease and Its Complex with an Inhibitor. *Proc. Natl. Acad. Sci. USA* **2003**, *100*, 13190–13195. [CrossRef]
31. Rial, C.; Novaes, P.; Varela, R.M.; Molinillo, J.M.G.; Macias, F.A. Phytotoxicity of Cardoon (Cynara Cardunculus) Allelochemicals on Standard Target Species and Weeds. *J. Agric. Food Chem.* **2014**, *62*, 6699–6706. [CrossRef]
32. Schulz, M.; Marocco, A.; Tabaglio, V.; Macias, F.A.; Molinillo, J.M.G. Benzoxazinoids in Rye Allelopathy—From Discovery to Application in Sustainable Weed Control and Organic Farming. *J. Chem. Ecol.* **2013**, *39*, 154–174. [CrossRef]
33. Zhang, M.-Q.; Wilkinson, B. Drug Discovery beyond the 'Rule-of-Five'. *Curr. Opin. Biotechnol.* **2007**, *18*, 478–488. [CrossRef]
34. Hou, T.; Wang, J.; Zhang, W.; Xu, X. ADME Evaluation in Drug Discovery. 7. Prediction of Oral Absorption by Correlation and Classification. *J. Chem. Inf. Model.* **2007**, *47*, 208–218. [CrossRef] [PubMed]
35. National Cancer Institute—USA Chemical Indetifier Resolver. Available online: https://cactus.nci.nih.gov/chemical/structure (accessed on 23 August 2022).
36. Zoete, V.; Cuendet, M.A.; Grosdidier, A.; Michielin, O. SwissParam: A Fast Force Field Generation Tool for Small Organic Molecules. *J. Comput. Chem.* **2011**, *32*, 2359–2368. [CrossRef] [PubMed]

toxins

MDPI

Article

Harzianic Acid Activity against *Staphylococcus aureus* and Its Role in Calcium Regulation

Alessia Staropoli [1,2,*,†], Paola Cuomo [2,*,†], Maria Michela Salvatore [1,3], Gaetano De Tommaso [3], Mauro Iuliano [3], Anna Andolfi [3,4], Gian Carlo Tenore [5], Rosanna Capparelli [2] and Francesco Vinale [4,6]

1 Institute for Sustainable Plant Protection, National Research Council, 80055 Portici, Italy; mariamichela.salvatore@unina.it
2 Department of Agricultural Sciences, University of Naples Federico II, 80055 Portici, Italy; rosanna.capparelli@unina.it
3 Department of Chemical Sciences, University of Naples Federico II, 80126 Naples, Italy; gaetano.detommaso@unina.it (G.D.T.); mauro.iuliano@unina.it (M.I.); andolfi@unina.it (A.A.)
4 BAT Center-Interuniversity Center for Studies on Bioinspired Agro-Environmental Technology, University of Naples Federico II, 80055 Portici, Italy; frvinale@unina.it
5 Department of Pharmacy, University of Naples Federico II, 80131 Naples, Italy; giancarlo.tenore@unina.it
6 Department of Veterinary Medicine and Animal Productions, University of Naples Federico II, 80137 Naples, Italy
* Correspondence: alessia.staropoli@ipsp.cnr.it (A.S.); paola.cuomo@unina.it (P.C.)
† These authors contributed equally to this work.

Abstract: *Staphylococcus aureus* is a Gram-positive bacterium, which can be found, as a commensal microorganism, on the skin surface or in the nasal mucosa of the human population. However, *S. aureus* may become pathogenic and cause severe infections, especially in hospitalized patients. As an opportunistic pathogen, in fact, *S. aureus* interferes with the host Ca^{2+} signaling, favoring the spread of the infection and tissue destruction. The identification of novel strategies to restore calcium homeostasis and prevent the associated clinical outcomes is an emerging challenge. Here, we investigate whether harzianic acid, a bioactive metabolite derived from fungi of the genus *Trichoderma*, could control *S. aureus*-induced Ca^{2+} movements. First, we show the capability of harzianic acid to complex calcium divalent cations, using mass spectrometric, potentiometric, spectrophotometric, and nuclear magnetic resonance techniques. Then, we demonstrate that harzianic acid significantly modulates Ca^{2+} increase in HaCaT (human keratinocytes) cells incubated with *S. aureus*. In conclusion, this study suggests harzianic acid as a promising therapeutical alternative against diseases associated with Ca^{2+} homeostasis alteration.

Keywords: calcium; chelation; fungi; secondary metabolites; *Staphylococcus aureus*; *Trichoderma*

Key Contribution: Harzianic acid significantly modulates Ca^{2+} increasing in HaCaT cells incubated with *Staphylococcus aureus*.

Citation: Staropoli, A.; Cuomo, P.; Salvatore, M.M.; De Tommaso, G.; Iuliano, M.; Andolfi, A.; Tenore, G.C.; Capparelli, R.; Vinale, F. Harzianic Acid Activity against *Staphylococcus aureus* and Its Role in Calcium Regulation. *Toxins* **2023**, *15*, 237. https://doi.org/10.3390/toxins15040237

Received: 9 February 2023
Revised: 20 March 2023
Accepted: 21 March 2023
Published: 24 March 2023

1. Introduction

Calcium is a universal intracellular messenger that regulates different cellular activities. It is responsible for controlling cell development and proliferation, as well as fundamental processes such as learning, memories, and muscle contraction [1]. Ca^{2+} signaling and regulation has been widely described in eukaryotic cells due to its involvement in above-mentioned cellular processes [2,3]. Given this scenario, Ca^{2+} signaling is highly regulated and its concentration tightly controlled in various cell compartments [4,5]. For this reason, if slightly exceeding, Ca^{2+} ions may become toxic and stimulate cell death, thus increasing the risk to develop severe pathologies [6]. External stimuli may induce significant changes in cell calcium concentration. It has been reported that bacteria are one of the biotic factors contributing to Ca^{2+} homeostasis alteration, for example, through the release of pore-forming toxins (PFTs) [7].

Staphylococcus aureus is a Gram-positive bacterium that, although commonly considered a commensal, is a major cause of several human infections (e.g., pneumonia, endocarditis, and medical-device-related), including skin and soft tissue infections (SSTIs) [8]. *Staphylococcus aureus* is able to colonize skin and nasal mucosa without causing any symptoms. However, when colonizing immunocompromised individuals, *S. aureus* may build an infection [9,10]. In order to colonize and infect the host cell, *S. aureus* expresses virulence factors such as hemolysin A, a PFT that can form pores and insert into host cell membranes, resulting in a perturbation of calcium levels [7,11]. Alterations of Ca^{2+} concentration, amongst other pathogenesis mechanisms, could mediate bacterial adherence, following its incorporation into the host cells [7,12,13].

Starting from the discovery of penicillin, the interest in natural products has increased, since microbial strains play a key role as major sources of secondary metabolites for drug discovery and application in both medical and agricultural fields [14–16]. These secondary metabolites mediate interactions with plants, microbes, cells, and tissues and are involved in the effects on plants or other organisms [17,18]

Among fungal microbes, *Trichoderma* is the genus recognized as a model to study plant–microbe interactions [19,20]. Therefore, selected strains of *Trichoderma* are broadly commercialized for crop protection and production. [21]. Several strains of *Trichoderma* are also exceptional producers of secondary metabolites with a wide range of biological activities (e.g., antibiosis, plant growth promotion, induction of systemic resistance, transport of metal cations, etc.) [22,23].

Among these bioactive metabolites, there is harzianic acid (HA), a tetramic acid derivative that has demonstrated remarkable biological activities, including antimicrobial activity (e.g., *S. pseudintermedius*, *Rhizoctonia solani*), plant growth promotion (i.e., tomato, olive drupes), and affinity to ferric and other divalent metal ions [24–31].

In this context, harzianic acid may represent a valid therapeutical strategy to prevent detrimental diseases, having shown chelating properties towards bivalent cations [30,31]. The aim of the present study is to demonstrate the affinity of HA for Ca^{2+} ions and its ability to affect calcium mobilization in HaCaT cells upon *S. aureus* infection.

2. Results and Discussion

2.1. Harzianic Acid Inhibits Staphylococcus aureus Growth

To determine whether HA affects *S. aureus* growth, the bacterial growth dynamic was evaluated for 16 h. HA was found to completely inhibit the growth of *S. aureus* at the highest tested concentrations (100 μM to 1000 μM) (Figure 1). Interestingly, bacterial growth suppression did not decrease over time (Figure 1). Of note, HA was also found to exert a modest antimicrobial activity against *S. aureus* at concentrations of 10 and 50 μM. In particular, a gradual and significant decrease in *S. aureus* growth was observed at 16 h of incubation with HA (10 and 50 μM), compared with that of untreated cells ($p < 0.001$) (Figure 1). Attractively, HA showed improved activity against *S. aureus* at 16 h compared with ampicillin, one of the most commonly used broad-spectrum antibiotics. Although the mechanisms underlying the suppression of bacterial growth following HA treatment remain to be determined, as a tetramic acid, HA might exert its antimicrobial activity by impairing the barrier function of the bacterial membrane. High concentrations of HA have been reported to produce pores in the cell membrane of Gram-positive bacteria [32]. However, the mechanism of pore formation is still unclear, but not depending on a direct targeting of the cell membrane. In fact, lacking a highly lipophilic N–substituent, HA seems not to be as effective in penetrating bacterial cell membranes. Generally, tetramic acid molecules possess lipophilic functional groups, exhibiting effective antibacterial activity. This property reflects the capability of these functional groups to (i) dissipate the transmembrane pH of bacteria, (ii) allow proton translocation across the membrane, and (iii) destroy the bacterial cell membrane [33]. In the absence of cell selectivity (prokaryotic cells over eukaryotic cells), it seems evident that tetramic acids also exhibit cytotoxic effects on eukaryotic cells [33]. Many studies, in fact, have focused on synthesizing novel molecules with reduced lipophilicity in order to improve their safety and preserve their antimicrobial effects. Yet, contrary to other tetramic acid derivatives, HA was found to be highly tolerated by eukaryotic cells, specifically HaCaT cells (See Section 2.2). This could find an explanation in its peculiar chemical structure. In such conditions, the capability of HA to chelate Fe^{3+} may represent an effective mechanism hampering bacterial iron availability, thus altering bacterial growth [29].

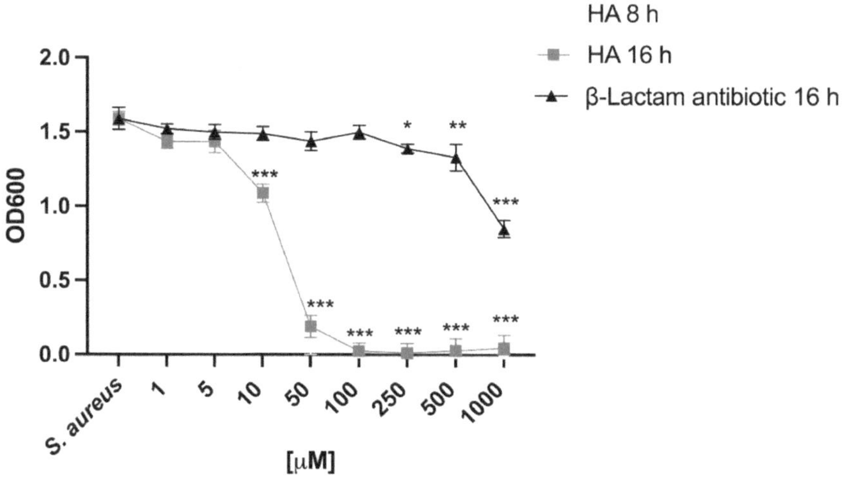

Figure 1. HA impacts *S. aureus* cell growth. *S. aureus* was incubated in the presence of LB medium as general control (*S. aureus*) or a range of HA (from 1000 μM to 1 μM). Growth curves were measured at an optic density of 600 nm (OD600) after 8 and 16 h of incubation. B-lactam antibiotic was used as positive control. Statistical analysis was performed by two-way ANOVA, followed by Bonferroni correction test. Each condition was compared with the untreated control of the corresponding timepoint (*, $p < 0.05$; **, $p < 0.01$; ***, $p < 0.001$).

2.2. Harzianic Acid Does Not Alter HaCaT Cell Viability

To investigate whether HA affects the metabolic activity of human keratinocytes, the cytotoxicity of HA on HaCaT cells was explored. Despite different concentrations of HA were examined (spanning from 0.7 to 500 μM), no cytotoxic effects were detected (Figure 2). However, an unusual bimodal distribution was observed.

Of note, HaCaT cells treated with high concentrations of HA (55 to 500 μM) displayed an increased survival, compared with untreated cells (control; cell without HA treatment) (Figure 2). Yet, this phenomenon was not dependent on the HA dose.

Conversely, concentrations of HA lower than 55 μM decreased cell viability in a dose-dependent manner. However, cell viability was constantly more than 80% compared with the untreated control (Figure 2).

2.3. Harzianic Acid Controls the Cell Host Ca^{2+} Movements

Calcium signalling regulates diverse biological processes. Impairment of cellular calcium levels may alter cell metabolism and cause various diseases. The reasons of such alteration are multiple. It is generally reported that bacterial infections affect Ca^{2+} fluxes in host cells [34].

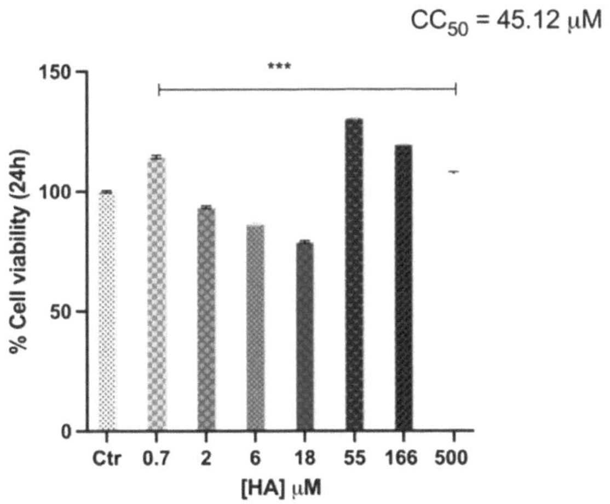

Figure 2. Effect of HA on HaCaT cell viability. HaCaT cells were cultured with different concentrations of HA for 24 h. The bar graph represents means ± SD of three independent experiments, each performed in triplicate. Results are expressed as percentage of untreated control. Statistical significance was determined by one-way ANOVA (***, $p < 0.001$). Statistical analysis was performed by comparing each condition with the untreated control. CC50, indicating cytotoxic concentration 50, was calculated by Graphad software.

Staphylococcus aureus is recognized as the primary cause of skin infections [35]. It is described to invade and survive within the host cells for a long period of time, establishing a persistent infection [36]. Virulence factors, as well as its capability to escape the host immune defence, contribute to the pathogenicity and occurrence of *S. aureus* infection [37].

Staphylococcus aureus produces a variety of virulence factors, which may interfere with the host calcium signalling [13]. To invade the eukaryotic host cells, *S. aureus* produces pore-forming toxins, such as α–hemolysin, which induce Ca^{2+} oscillations in host cells, thus ensuring bacterial virulence and facilitating bacterial adaptation to the host environment [13,38,39].

Consistent with these findings, our results showed increased Ca^{2+} levels in HaCaT cells ($[Ca^{2+}]_{in}$) cultured with *S. aureus*. Interestingly, cells infected with *S. aureus* for 3 h responded to bacterial invasion with a higher rise of cytosolic calcium than those infected for 6 h (Figure 3A). The long-term exposure to *S. aureus* could account for this dissimilarity. To establish bacterial infection, *S. aureus* must colonize the host cells and replicate [36]. Nevertheless, 6 h post-infection, in vitro bacterial replication could cease, and the stationary growth phase could be reached, thus attenuating bacterial virulence and calcium increase.

Intracellular calcium elevation ($[Ca^{2+}]_{in}$) has also been reported to exert antimicrobial activity. In particular, Ca^{2+} ions have been demonstrated to kill stationary-phase *S. aureus* cells [40]. $[Ca^{2+}]_{in}$ in cells cultured with *S. aureus* for 6 h and treated with HA (10 μM) was increased when compared with both control and *S. aureus* cultured cells (Figure 3A). Such a result supports what is reported above and suggests that HA may mediate antimicrobial effects by targeting bacterial pathogens (at a high concentration; see Figure 1) and/or mammalian host cells, influencing the host immune responses [34].

Cells infected with *S. aureus* for a shorter time (3 h) and then treated with HA also showed an increased $[Ca^{2+}]_{in}$ (Figure 3A), likely due to the ability of HA to regulate the host's innate immune response [41]. However, calcium accumulation was lower than in cells infected for 6 h (Figure 3A).

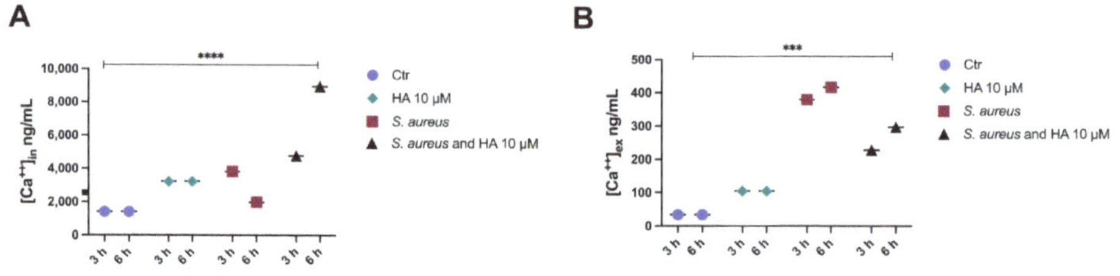

Figure 3. HA affects *S. aureus*-induced Ca^{2+} mobilization. HaCaT cells were infected with *S. aureus* or treated with HA 10 μM (after 90 min of bacterial exposure; *S. aureus* and HA), and cytosolic (**A**) as well as extracellular Ca^{2+} (**B**) were determined by Atomic Adsorption Spectroscopy after 3 or 6 h. Results are represented as means ± SD of three independent experiments, each performed in triplicate. Statistical significance was determined by one-way ANOVA followed by Bonferroni correction test (***, $p < 0.001$; ****, $p < 0.0001$). Statistical analysis was performed by comparing the above-reported experimental conditions (see legend) for each time of treatment.

Bacterial infections also impact the extracellular calcium concentration ($[Ca^{2+}]_{ex}$) [42] Furthermore, intracellular calcium accumulation often results in the extracellular calcium increase via transmembrane calcium fluxes. Nevertheless, extracellular calcium elevation may compromise the surrounding cell functions, triggering an exacerbated immune response through the NLRP3 inflammasome activation [42]. Intriguingly, HA was found to mitigate $[Ca^{2+}]_{ex}$ following *S. aureus* infection, compared with untreated cells (Figure 3B).

Taken together, these results indicate the valuable ability of HA to control *S. aureus* infections, by exerting a microbicidal action and/or supporting the host immune function against the pathogen, as well as to prevent a harmful inflammatory response.

In an attempt to investigate whether HA could hamper the host cell calcium oscillations, the culture medium of HaCaT cells was enriched with $CaCl_2$ and the extracellular Ca^{2+} levels were measured following HA treatment, using a colorimetric method. Compared with control cells, calcium levels were increased in the culture medium of cells supplied with $CaCl_2$ and, as expected, decreased in both supernatant and cytosol of cells treated with HA (Figure 4), indicating the capacity of HA to remove calcium ions—likely due to its chelating properties—and control cell calcium fluxes.

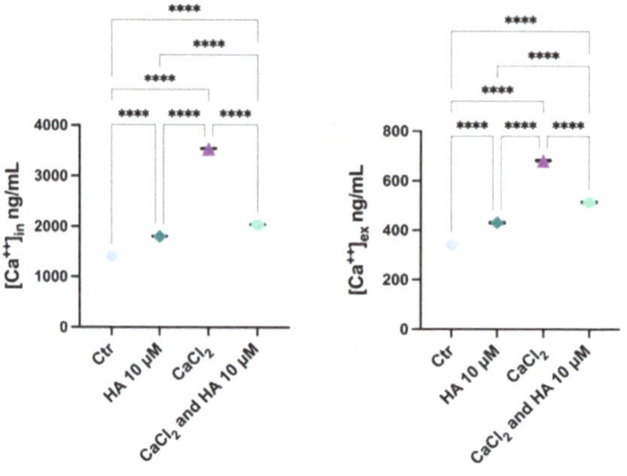

Figure 4. HA reduces $CaCl_2$-induced Ca^{2+} oscillation. HaCaT cells were cultured with $CaCl_2$ 1.8 mM or treated with HA 10 μM following 60 min of $CaCl_2$ exposure. (**A**) Cytosolic Ca^{2+} and (**B**) extracellular Ca^{2+} levels were determined by colorimetric assay. Results are represented as means ± SD of three independent experiments, each performed in triplicate. Statistical significance was determined by one-way ANOVA followed by Bonferroni correction test (****, $p < 0.0001$).

Therefore, the results revealed that HA may interfere with Ca(II) mobilization, not only in response to bacterial infections.

2.4. Coordination Properties of Harzianic Acid toward Ca^{2+}

Harzianic acid has been widely recognized as an efficient ligand of a variety of metal cations [30,31,43,44]. Since harzianic acid is a diprotic acid, the symbol H_2L is used in this section to indicate the fully protonated species, while HL^- and L^{2-} indicate deprotonated species whose dissociation constants were previously determined at 25 °C in 0.1 M $NaClO_4/(CH_3OH + H_2O$ 50/50 *w*/*w*) mixed solvent, the same solvent employed in this study [30].

Complex formation equilibria between harzianic acid toward the dipositive cation Ca^{2+} were studied using mass spectrometric, potentiometric, spectrophotometric, and nuclear magnetic resonance (NMR) techniques. A high-resolution mass spectrum (HRMS) of a solution consisting of $CaCl_2$ and HA was acquired (Section 4.11). The most abundant ions in the collected HRMS are reported in Table 1. Peaks corresponding to adducts of harzianic acid with hydrogen, sodium, and potassium were detected. Moreover, peaks related to ions containing both Ca^{2+} cation and harzianic acid in a 1:2 and 1:3 metal-to-ligand ratio were observed.

Table 1. Most abundant ions in high-resolution spectrum (HRMS) acquired by HPLC-ESI-HRMS on solutions of harzianic acid and Ca^{2+}.

Ion	Experimental Mass of Main Isotopic Peak (Da)	Formula	Exact Mass (Da)
	Harzianic acid + $CaCl_2$		
$[H_2L + H]^+$	366.1929	$C_{19}H_{28}NO_6$	366.1917
$[H_2L + Na]^+$	388.1750	$C_{19}H_{27}NO_6Na$	388.1736
$[H_2L + K]^+$	404.1404	$C_{19}H_{27}NO_6K$	404.1475
$[2H_2L - H + Ca]^+$	769.3243	$C_{38}H_{53}N_2O_{12}Ca$	769.3224
$[3H_2L - H + Ca]^+$	1134.5079	$C_{57}H_{80}N_3O_{18}Ca$	1134.5063

The chelating properties of HA towards the dipositive cation Ca^{2+} were also studied by collecting potentiometric and spectrophotometric data. In particular, the interaction between harzianic acid and calcium cations was monitored by acquiring UV–Vis spectra in a wide wavelength range (200–500 nm) at 25 °C of solutions of accurately known analytical concentrations of the metal cation (C_{Ca}, M) and of the ligand (C_{H_2L} M) in a 0.1 M $NaClO_4/(CH_3OH + H_2O$ 50/50 *w*/*w*) mixed solvent. The free proton concentration, $[H^+]$, was measured with a pH indicator glass electrode that was properly calibrated as is described in Materials and Methods, Section 4.12. By recording UV–Vis spectra as a function of pH at two molar metal/ligand ratios (Figure 5), it is evident that the spectral variations depend on the pH rather than on the molar metal/ligand ratio.

In order to evaluate the stoichiometry and formation constants between calcium metal ion and harzianic acid, the spectrophotometric data in Figure 5 were processed numerically by a Hyperquad program and the results are summarized in Table 2 [45].

Table 2. Summary of Ca^{2+}/harzianic acid (H_2L) formation constants. σ indicates the estimated standard deviation.

Equilibria	log (Formation Constant) ± 3σ
$Ca^{2+} + L^{2-} = CaL$	6.3 ± 0.1
$Ca^{2+} + 2L^{2-} = CaL_2^{2-}$	10.2 ± 0.1

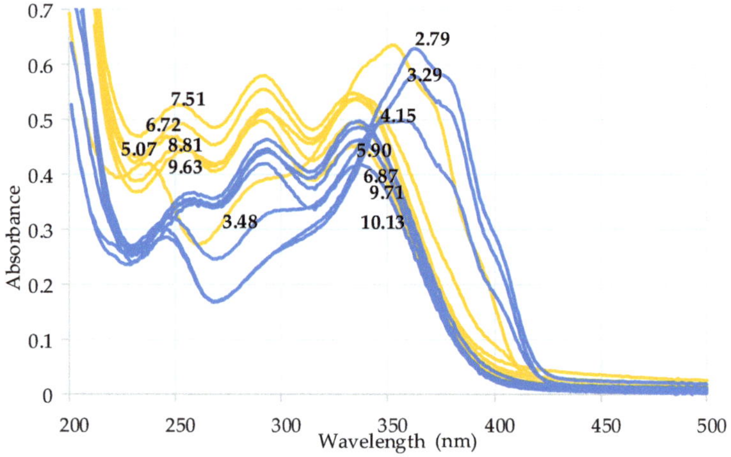

Figure 5. Raw UV–Vis spectra of solutions of Ca^{2+} and harzianic acid of accurately known analytical composition and pH in a 0.1 M $NaClO_4/(CH_3OH + H_2O$ 50/50 $w/w)$ mixed solvent. Absorption spectra define two groups differentiated by color; orange-colored spectra have been acquired on solutions with a concentration of the ligand nearly twice that of the calcium dipositive cation; blue-colored spectra have been acquired on solutions with concentration of ligand nearly twice that of the metal cation. Numerical labels on curves indicate the corresponding pH.

From the data in Table 2, distribution diagrams can be drawn (Figure 6A,B) showing the fraction of the total calcium concentration present in the form of each species (free Ca^{2+} or complexed $CaL/CaL_2{}^{2-}$) as a function of pH. Either in solutions containing equal concentrations of the cation and of the ligand (i.e., $C_{H_2L}/C_{Ca} = 1$, Figure 6A) or in solutions in which the ligand concentration is twice the concentration of the cation (i.e., $C_{H_2L}/C_{Ca} = 2$, Figure 6B), it can be seen that, at low pH, the prevailing species in the solution is the free Ca^{2+} due to the protonation of the bonding sites of harzianic acid [40]. At higher pH values, the mono complex CaL rises to about 90% when the $C_{H_2L}/C_{Ca} = 1$, as in Figure 6A. Moreover, the bis complex $CaL_2{}^{2-}$ is present in negligible concentration (about 5%).

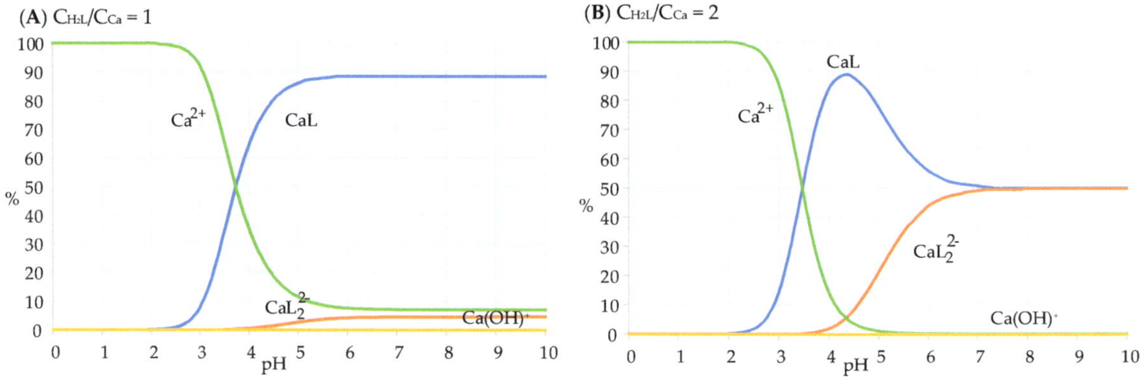

Figure 6. Distribution diagrams for Ca^{2+}–harzianic acid systems in the 0.1 M $NaClO_4/(CH_3OH + H_2O$ 50/50 $w/w)$ mixed solvent: (**A**) equal total concentrations (2.5×10^{-4} M) of harzianic acid and metal cations; (**B**) harzianic acid total concentration (5×10^{-4} M) twice the total concentration of metal cations.

In solutions in which the ligand concentration is twice the concentration of the cation (i.e., $C_{H_2L}/C_{Ca} = 2$, Figure 6B), the mono complex CaL is the prevailing species at pH $\approx$ 4, while at the highest pH investigated (pH > 7), the bis complex and mono complex species are equally present in solution.

NMR analysis of Ca^{2+}–HA solutions confirmed the chelating ability of the fungal metabolite. In fact, the comparison of the proton spectra of harzianic acid and the solution of Ca^{2+} and harzianic acids recorded in CD_3OD showed some significant shifts for the protons of the octadienoyl chain. In particular, the proton H–2, overlapped with H–3, resonated as a multiplet at δ 7.48–7.34, showing an upfield shift of Δδ 0.29. Moreover, protons H–3, H–4, and H–5 showed a downfield shift of Δδ 0.13, 0.07, and 0.27, respectively. The H–5′ proton of the pyrrolidine–2,4–dione ring resonated as a multiplet at δ 3.64–3.59, showing a downfield shift of Δδ 0.22. These data agree with those previously reported (Figure 7) [30,31].

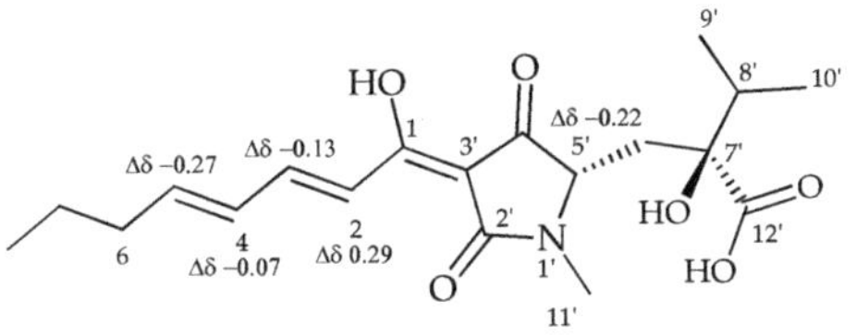

Figure 7. Main variations in chemical shifts observed by comparison of the ^{1}H NMR of harzianic acid and Ca^{2+}-harzianic acid complex recorded in CD_3OD at 400 MHz.

3. Conclusions

In this investigation, the effects of the fungal metabolite harzianic acid were evaluated against *S. aureus*, a causative agent of severe infections, especially in hospitalized patients. Harzianic acid activity was tested towards human keratinocytes infected with *S. aureus*. The results provide evidence about the capability of HA in controlling *S. aureus*, reducing the pathogen growth rate, and modulating the eukaryotic cell Ca^{2+} mobilization. Furthermore, the capability of HA to complex calcium divalent cations was investigated using mass spectrometric, potentiometric, spectrophotometric, and NMR techniques. The results demonstrate the ability of this natural compound to form stable neutral or negatively charged complexes in a calcium/harzianic acid ratio 1:1 or 1:2. The abundance of the species is dependent on the pH of the solution.

In conclusion, HA may modulate the host Ca^{2+} signaling pathway, thus showing beneficial effects, which could have implications in different diseases. However, further studies are needed to investigate the mechanisms underpinning the ability of HA to modulate the host immune response against *S. aureus* via Ca^{2+} mobilization interference. Moreover, the comprehensive understanding of HA characteristics as a chelator of multiple metal ions could provide new insight into the therapeutical role of HA in *S. aureus* infections, highlighting its clinical (beneficial and adverse) effects.

4. Materials and Methods

4.1. Harzianic Acid Production

Harzianic acid was obtained from *T. harzianum* M10 grown in liquid medium (PDB, HiMedia, Mumbai, India) for 21 days and purified following a previously described protocol with some modifications [25]. Briefly, culture filtrate was exhaustively extracted with ethyl acetate (EtOAc, Carlo Erba, Cornaredo, Milan, Italy), and the dry residue was resuspended in dichloromethane (DCM, Carlo Erba) and extracted with a 2M solution of sodium hydroxide (NaOH, Carlo Erba). The aqueous phase was acidified at pH = 2 with hydrochloric acid (HCl, Carlo Erba), and harzianic acid was obtained after vacuum filtration and precipitate wash with EtOAc. Harzianic acid identification was achieved by NMR and LC-MS analyses [30,31].

4.2. Cell Culture Conditions

Immortalized human keratinocytes (HaCaT cell line) were obtained from the Cell Lines Service (CLS, catalog number 300493). HaCaT cells were grown in Dulbecco's Modification of Eagle's Medium, high glucose (DMEM), supplemented with 10% fetal bovine serum (FBS), 1% penicillin/streptomycin, and 1% L–glutamine (all from Microtech, Naples, Italy) in a humidified atmosphere at 37 °C and 5% CO_2.

4.3. Staphylococcus aureus Growth Conditions

Starting from a frozen stock (−80 °C), *S. aureus* (ATCC 25923) was grown on Luria–Bertani (LB, Scharlab S.L., Barcelona, Spain) agar at 37 °C for 24 h. The next day, an isolated colony was transferred from the agar plate to the tube containing liquid LB medium. The tube was gently shaken to suspend bacterial cells and then incubated at 37 °C overnight on a shaker at 180 rpm.

4.4. Antibacterial Activity

Antimicrobial activity of HA against *S. aureus* was tested using the broth microdilution method [46]. HA was resuspended in LB medium containing 10% dimethyl sulfoxide (DMSO) and then diluted to obtain final concentrations used for the assay. In detail, four two-fold serially diluted concentrations of HA (1000 μM, 500 μM, 250 μM, 50 μM, and 5 μM) and three intermediate concentrations (100 μM, 10 μM, and 1 μM) were prepared in 15 mL sterile test tubes, using *S. aureus* growth medium (LB medium) as solvent. A final volume of 1 mL of each dilution (two times more concentrated than the above reported concentrations) was prepared using growth medium (LB) as diluent. Subsequently, the bacterial inoculum was prepared. In detail, the overnight culture was sub-cultured in fresh LB broth in order to reach the final concentration of 5×10^5 CFU mL^{-1}. An amount of 1 mL of the adjusted microbial suspension was added to each tube containing 1 mL of the sample and mixed. Finally, tubes were incubated at 37 °C on a shaker at 180 rpm for 16–18 h. The optical density at 600 nm (OD_{600}) was measured using a spectrophotometer (Smartspec Plus, Bio-Rad, Hercules, CA, USA). Bacterial culture grown in LB medium containing 10% DMSO and in the absence of HA was used as control, while LB medium containing 10% DMSO was used as blank.

4.5. Cell Viability Assay

Colorimetric MTT assay was performed to examine the cytotoxic effect of HA on HaCaT cells [47]. Cells were seeded in a 96-well plate at a density of 2×10^5 per well and incubated overnight at 37 °C and 5% CO_2. HA was resuspended in a mixture of cell culture medium (DMEM) and 10% DMSO, generating the stock solution. The stock solution was successively diluted, using cell culture medium, in order to prepare HA solutions at various concentrations used in the test (0.7–500 μM). The next day, culture medium was replaced with fresh medium containing different concentrations of HA (0.7–500 μM) and cells were further incubated for 24 h. After the incubation time, the medium containing the treatment under investigation was removed by aspiration, cells were washed with PBS, and fresh culture medium diluted with 3–(4, 5–dimethylthiazolyl–2)–2, 5–diphenyltetrazolium bromide solution (MTT; 1:10) was added to each well. Cells were further incubated for 3 h at 37 °C and 5% CO_2. The formed crystals were dissolved using DMSO and quantified using the Model 680 microplate reader (Bio-rad, Hercules, CA, USA) at 570 nm. The percentage of cell viability was calculated according to the following formula: $(ABS_{sample} - ABS_{blank})/(ABS_{control} - ABS_{blank}) \times 100$, where blank represents cells incubated with 10% DMSO in culture medium and control represents untreated cells. CC_{50} was calculated by GraphPad Prism software (version 9.1.1) using nonlinear regression analysis.

4.6. Infection by Staphylococcus aureus of Eukaryotic Cells

Infection of cells was performed following Stelzner et al. (2020) protocol with some modifications [36]. The day before the infection, 0.25×10^6 cells were seeded in a 24-well plate and incubated overnight at 37 °C and 5% CO_2. The next day an OD_{600} = 0.4 cell suspension was incubated at 37 °C for 1 h on a shaker at 180 rpm. When the exponential growth phase was reached, bacteria were centrifugated twice, at 6000× *g* for 10 min, and washed with Phosphate Buffer Solution (PBS; Microtech, Naples, Italy). Bacterial cells were then resuspended in DMEM with or without 10 µM HA and used to infect HaCaT cells (Multiplicity of Infection; MOI = 50). After 1 h of infection, extracellular bacteria were removed by lysostaphin treatment (20 µg mL^{-1} per well for 30 min). Finally, culture medium was removed, and cells were washed in PBS and restored with fresh medium containing 10 µM HA. After an additional 2 or 5 h of incubation, both culture medium and cells were collected and stored at –80 °C until calcium measurement.

4.7. Extracellular Ca^{2+} Supplementation

HaCaT cells were supplied with exogenous Ca^{2+}, to better investigate the role of HA in controlling calcium oscillations. Cells were seeded in a 24-well plate at a density of 0.25×10^6 per well and incubated at 37 °C and 5% CO_2 overnight. After cell attachment, the culture medium was renewed with a fresh one containing 1.8 mM $CaCl_2$ [36], with or without 10 µM HA, and incubated for 1 h. After the incubation time, cells were treated with 10 µM HA and further incubated. At 2 h after treatment, both culture medium and cells were collected and stored at –80 °C until calcium measurement.

4.8. Ca^{2+} Measurement by Atomic Adsorption Spectroscopy

Intracellular and extracellular calcium content was determined by Atomic Adsorption Spectroscopy, as reported by Fiorito et al. in 2021 [48]. For the analysis, an AA–6300 spectrophotometer (Shimadzu, Columbia, MD, USA) equipped with an ASC–6100 autosampler (Shimadzu, Columbia, MD, USA) and a GFA–EX7i graphite furnace atomizer (Shimadzu, Columbia, MD, USA) was used. Prior the analysis, a fine mist dispersion of cell culture medium or cell pellets was prepared, using a microwave digestion apparatus (MW–AD, Ethos EZ microwave digester, Mileston, Shelton, CT, USA). Samples were transferred into TFM®PTFE vessels, and 6 mL of ultra-pure concentrated HNO_3 (14.33 mol L^{-1}) and 1 mL of 30% H_2O_2 were added. The heating program for digestion was 160 °C for 5 min using 80% of microwave power, 190 °C for 10 min using 90% of microwave power, 50 °C for 11 min. Final solutions were diluted up to 25 mL with water and mineralized at 550 °C for 4 h. The analyte was detected according to the following working conditions: wavelength, 248.3 nm; slit width, 0.5 nm; lamp current, 5 mA; gas, Argon.

4.9. Ca^{2+} Measurement by Colorimetric Method

The concentration of free calcium ions was determined in order to assess whether HA can chelate cell Ca^{2+}, by colorimetric assay, using a calcium assay kit (Abcam, Cambridge, UK, #ab102505). Following Ca^{2+} supplementation and HA treatment (as reported above, Section 4.7), calcium concentration in both cells and cell medium was measured according to the manufacturer's instructions. Briefly, after sample preparation, the reaction mixture was added and incubated at room temperature for 5–10 min protected from light. The optical density was measured at 575 nm using a microplate reader (Model 680, Bio-rad, Hercules, CA, USA).

4.10. Reagents and Their Analysis

Stock solutions of calcium perchlorate for spectrophotometric and NMR measurements were prepared by dissolving its high-purity calcium carbonate anhydrous in concentrated perchloric acid (Merck, Darmstadt, Germany). The solution obtained was brought to a boil to remove the carbon dioxide produced, and then it was cooled. The exact concentration of metal solution was determined as described by Kolthoff et al. 1978 [49].

NMR spectra were recorded at 400 MHz in CD_3OD on a Bruker spectrometer (Ascend™400) (Bremen, Germany). The solvent was used as internal standard.

UV–Vis spectra were recorded by Cary model 5000 Spectrophotometer by Varian C. (Palo Alto, CA, USA), from 200 to 600 nm (optical path 0.2 cm) at 25.0 °C and under a constant flow of nitrogen.

4.11. HPLC-ESI-Q-TOF Analysis

HPLC-ESI-Q-TOF analysis was carried out on a quadrupole time-of-flight (Q–TOF) mass spectrometer (Agilent Technologies, Santa Clara, CA, USA), equipped with a Dual electrospray ionization source (Agilent Technologies) and coupled to a 1260 Infinity Series high-performance liquid chromatograph (Agilent Technologies). A solution consisting of $CaCl_2$ (2 mM, aqueous solution) and harzianic acid (1 mg mL^{-1}, methanolic solution) in a 1:1 (*v*/*v*) ratio was directly infused into the LC system. Elution, spectral, and all instrumental parameters were set following the method described by De Tommaso et al. [30]. Acquisition was achieved using Agilent MassHunter Data Acquisition Software, rev. B.05.01 (Agilent Technologies).

4.12. Preparation of Test Solutions for UV–Vis Spectrophotometric Measurements

The UV–Vis measurements of solutions of calcium cations and harzianic acid required the acquisition of spectra of solutions of accurately known pH (= $-\log[H^+]$); analytical compositions of metal ion C_{Ca} M, HA C_{H_2L} M, C_H M (analytical concentration of $HClO_4$); and C_{OH} M (analytical concentration of NaOH) in the 0.1 M $NaClO_4$/(CH_3OH + H_2O 50/50 *w*/*w*) mixed solvent. In particular, the spectra were collected to have the same ligand-to-metal ratio (i.e., C_{H_2L}/C_{Ca}= *constant*). The free hydrogen ionic concentration was measured with a potentiometric apparatus constituted by a multi-neck titration vessel equipped with a Metrohm AG (Herisau, Switzerland) 60102–100 pH sensitive glass electrode (GE) and an $Ag/AgCl_{(s)}$/0.1 M NaCl/(0.1 M $NaClO_4$/(CH_3OH + H_2O 50/50 *w*/*w*) double-junction reference electrode (RE).

The experiment started by introducing a fixed volume, V_H mL, of the $HClO_4$ stock solution in the titration vessel, which was kept in an air thermostat at 25 °C ± 0.1 °C. This realized a potentiometric cell, GE/Solution/RE, whose potential, E_G Volt, under the present conditions can be expressed by the following relation (1):

$$E_G(\text{Volt}) = E_G^0(\text{Volt}) + Slope \cdot \log[H^+] \tag{1}$$

The calibration constants, E_G^0, and *Slope* in Equation (1) were evaluated by preparing a solution in the potentiometric vessel, which was alkalimetrically titrated by stepwise addition of accurately measured volumes of the C_{OH}^0 M stock solution of NaOH. The alkalimetric titration ended when the same total volume, V_{OH}, of NaOH solution was added and the solution in the potentiometric vessel attained a fixed volume equal to $(V_H + V_{OH})$ mL. After this titration, accurately measured volumes of the C_{Ca}^0 M solution of Ca^{2+} and of the $C_{H_2L}^0$ M solution of harzianic acid were added to the $(V_H + V_{OH})$ mL of solution in the titration vessel. The added volumes of harzianic acid and metal solutions determined the ligand-to-metal ratio in the resulting solution. Hence, the solution was brought to its final pH by adding a measured volume of the C_{OH}^0 M solution of NaOH. The volume of the added NaOH solution determined the values of C_{Ca}, C_{H_2L}, and pH in the final solution, which was used for UV–Vis analyses; it did not change the ligand-to-metal ratio.

Subsequently, sufficient time was allowed for chemical equilibrium to be established and for the glass electrode potential, E_G, to achieve a constant value, which persisted for at least 15 min within ± 0.1 mV. Thus, the free proton concentration of the solution in the titration vessel was readily calculated from Equation (2) and the measured E_G, as follows:

$$E_G = E_G^0 + Slope \cdot \log[H^+] \rightarrow \text{pH} = -\log[H^+] = \frac{E_G^0 - E_G}{Slope} \tag{2}$$

Finally, appropriate volumes of solution were withdrawn from the titration vessel and submitted UV–Vis spectrophotometer at 25.0 °C.

In this way, using fixed volumes of the C^0_{Ca} M stock solution of Ca^{2+} and the $C^0_{H_2L}$ M stock solution of HA for each group of UV–Vis measurements, the ratio C_{H_2L}/C_{Ca} was kept the same in each group.

Spectrophotometric data were processed numerically by the Hyperquad program [45] to evaluate the stoichiometry and formation constants between the calcium metal ion and HA. The program for equilibrium data interpretation fits the experimental data by systematically modifying the equilibrium constants of an assumed set of species to minimize the sum of squared weighted residuals (U). In Equation (3), A_{iK} represents the absorbance measured at the k–*th* wavelength for the i–*th* solution, $(A_{iK})_c$ is the absorbance calculated for a fixed set of equilibrium constants, and the wk values are the weights assigned to each measurement. In the present work, we have assumed wk = 1.

$$U = \sum_i \sum_k (A_{ik} - A^c_{ik})^2 \quad (3)$$

4.13. Statistical Analysis

Statistical analysis was performed using GraphPad Prism Software version 9.1.1 (San Diego, CA, USA). Multiple comparisons were carried out using one-way or two-way ANOVA, followed by Bonferroni correction test. One-way ANOVA was used to compare two or more experimental conditions, while two-way ANOVA was used to compare two or more experimental conditions and two variables (factors). Data are represented as means ± SD resulting from three biological replicates and are considered statistically significant when p value is < 0.05.

Author Contributions: Conceptualization, F.V., R.C. and A.A.; methodology, M.M.S., A.S. and P.C.; software, G.D.T. and M.I.; validation, M.M.S., G.D.T. and A.A.; investigation, A.S., P.C. and G.C.T.; data curation, M.M.S. and P.C.; writing—original draft preparation, A.S. and P.C.; writing—review and editing, A.S., M.M.S. and P.C.; supervision, F.V., R.C. and A.A. All authors have read and agreed to the published version of the manuscript.

Funding: This study was carried out within the Agritech National Research Center and was funded by Bio Inspired Plant Protection project, PRIN 2020 2020T58TA3—CUP: B63C22000580001 and the European Union Next–Generation EU (PIANO NAZIONALE DI RIPRESA E RESILIENZA (PNRR)—MISSIONE 4 COMPONENTE 2, INVESTIMENTO 1.4—D.D. 1032 17/06/2022, CN00000022). This manuscript reflects only the authors' views and opinions neither the European Union nor the European Commission can be considered responsible for them.

Institutional Review Board Statement: Not applicable.

Informed Consent Statement: Not applicable.

Data Availability Statement: The data that support the findings of this study are available from the corresponding author upon reasonable request.

Conflicts of Interest: The authors declare no conflict of interest.

Sample Availability: Samples of harzianic acid are available from the authors.

References

1. Berridge, M.J.; Lipp, P.; Bootman, M.D. The versatility and universality of calcium signaling. *Nat. Rev. Mol. Cell* **2000**, *1*, 11–21. [CrossRef]
2. Edel, K.H.; Kudla, J. Increasing complexity and versatility: How the calcium signaling toolkit was shaped during plant land colonization. *Cell Calcium* **2015**, *57*, 231–246. [CrossRef]
3. Permyakov, E.A.; Kretsinger, R.H. Cell signaling, beyond cytosolic calcium in eukaryotes. *J. Inorg. Biochem.* **2009**, *103*, 77–86. [CrossRef]
4. Clapham, D.E. Calcium signaling. *Cell* **1995**, *80*, 259–268. [CrossRef]
5. Bose, J.; Pottosin, I.I.; Shabala, S.S.; Palmgren, M.G.; Shabala, S. Calcium efflux systems in stress signaling and adaptation in plants. *Front. Plant Sci.* **2011**, *2*, 85. [CrossRef]
6. Weiss, N.; Koschak, A. (Eds.) *Pathologies of Calcium Channels*; Springer: Berlin, Germany, 2014.
7. Tran Van Nhieu, G.; Dupont, G.; Combettes, L. Ca^{2+} signals triggered by bacterial pathogens and microdomains. *Biochim. Biophys. Acta Mol. Cell Res.* **2018**, *1865 Pt B*, 1838–1845. [CrossRef]

8. David, M.Z.; Daum, R.S. Treatment of *Staphylococcus aureus* Infections. In *Staphylococcus aureus. Current Topics in Microbiology and Immunology*; Bagnoli, F., Rappuoli, R., Grandi, G., Eds.; Springer: Berlin, Germany, 2017; Volume 409, pp. 325–383. [CrossRef]
9. Tong, S.Y.; Davis, J.S.; Eichenberger, E.; Holland, T.L.; Fowler, V.G., Jr. *Staphylococcus aureus* infections: Epidemiology, pathophysiology, clinical manifestations, and management. *Clin. Microbiol. Rev.* **2015**, *28*, 603–661. [CrossRef]
10. Olaniyi, R.; Pozzi, C.; Grimaldi, L.; Bagnoli, F. Staphylococcus aureus-Associated Skin and Soft Tissue Infections: Anatomical Localization, Epidemiology, Therapy and Potential Prophylaxis. In *Staphylococcus aureus. Current Topics in Microbiology and Immunology*; Bagnoli, F., Rappuoli, R., Grandi, G., Eds.; Springer: Berlin, Germany, 2016; Volume 409, pp. 199–227. [CrossRef]
11. Peraro, M.; van der Goot, F. Pore-forming toxins: Ancient, but never really out of fashion. *Nat. Rev. Microbiol.* **2016**, *14*, 77–92. [CrossRef]
12. Marchi, S.; Morroni, G.; Pinton, P.; Galluzzi, L. Control of host mitochondria by bacterial pathogens. *Trends Microbiol.* **2022**, *30*, 452–465. [CrossRef]
13. Eichstaedt, S.; Gäbler, K.; Below, S.; Müller, C.; Kohler, C.; Engelmann, S.; Hildebrandt, P.; Völker, U.; Hecker, M.; Hildebrandt, J.P. Effects of *Staphylococcus aureus*-hemolysin A on calcium signaling in immortalized human airway epithelial cells. *Cell Calcium* **2009**, *45*, 165–176. [CrossRef]
14. Singh, R.; Kumar, M.; Mittal, A.; Mehta, P.K. Microbial metabolites in nutrition, healthcare and agriculture. *3 Biotech* **2017**, *7*, 15. [CrossRef]
15. Ramírez-Rendon, D.; Passari, A.K.; Ruiz-Villafán, B.; Rodríguez-Sanoja, R.; Sánchez, S.; Demain, A.L. Impact of novel microbial secondary metabolites on the pharma industry. *Appl. Microbiol. Biotechnol.* **2022**, *106*, 1855–1878. [CrossRef]
16. Atanasov, A.G.; Zotchev, S.B.; Dirsch, V.M.; International Natural Product Sciences Taskforce; Supuran, C.T. Natural products in drug discovery: Advances and opportunities. *Nat. Rev. Drug Discov.* **2021**, *20*, 200–216. [CrossRef]
17. Lucke, M.; Correa, M.G.; Levy, A. The Role of Secretion Systems, Effectors, and Secondary Metabolites of Beneficial Rhizobacteria in Interactions with Plants and Microbes. *Front. Plant Sci.* **2020**, *11*, 589416. [CrossRef]
18. Sinno, M.; Ranesi, M.; Di Lelio, I.; Iacomino, G.; Becchimanzi, A.; Barra, E.; Molisso, D.; Pennacchio, F.; Digilio, M.C.; Vitale, S.; et al. Selection of Endophytic *Beauveria bassiana* as a Dual Biocontrol Agent of Tomato Pathogens and Pests. *Pathogens* **2021**, *10*, 1242. [CrossRef]
19. Harman, G.E.; Howell, C.R.; Viterbo, A.; Chet, I.; Lorito, M. *Trichoderma* species—Opportunistic, avirulent plant symbionts. *Nat. Rev. Microbiol.* **2004**, *2*, 43–56. [CrossRef]
20. Vinale, F.; Sivasithamparam, K.; Ghisalberti, E.L.; Marra, R.; Woo, S.L.; Lorito, M. Trichoderma–plant–pathogen interactions. *Soil Biol. Biochem.* **2008**, *40*, 1–10. [CrossRef]
21. Keswani, C.; Mishra, S.; Sarma, B.K.; Singh, S.P.; Singh, H.B. Unraveling the efficient applications of secondary metabolites of various *Trichoderma* spp. *Appl. Microbiol. Biotechnol.* **2014**, *98*, 533–544. [CrossRef]
22. Vinale, F.; Sivasithamparam, K. Beneficial effects of *Trichoderma* secondary metabolites on crops. *Phytother. Res.* **2020**, *34*, 2835–2842. [CrossRef]
23. Ramírez-Valdespino, C.A.; Casas-Flores, S.; Olmedo-Monfil, V. *Trichoderma* as a Model to Study Effector-Like Molecules. *Front. Microbiol.* **2019**, *10*, 1030. [CrossRef]
24. Vinale, F.; Nigro, M.; Sivasithamparam, K.; Flematti, G.; Ghisalberti, E.L.; Ruocco, M.; Varlese, R.; Marra, R.; Lanzuise, S.; Eid, A.; et al. Harzianic acid: A novel siderophore from *Trichoderma harzianum*. *FEMS Microbiol. Lett.* **2013**, *347*, 123–129. [CrossRef] [PubMed]
25. Vinale, F.; Flematti, G.; Sivasithamparam, K.; Lorito, M.; Marra, R.; Skelton, B.W.; Ghisalberti, E.L. Harzianic acid, an antifungal and plant growth promoting metabolite from *Trichoderma harzianum*. *J. Nat. Prod.* **2009**, *72*, 2032–2035. [CrossRef] [PubMed]
26. Dini, I.; Pascale, M.; Staropoli, A.; Marra, R.; Vinale, F. Effect of Selected *Trichoderma* Strains and Metabolites on Olive Drupes. *Appl. Sci.* **2021**, *11*, 8710. [CrossRef]
27. Manganiello, G.; Sacco, A.; Ercolano, M.R.; Vinale, F.; Lanzuise, S.; Pascale, A.; Napolitano, M.; Lombardi, N.; Lorito, M.; Woo, S.L. Modulation of tomato response to *Rhizoctonia solani* by *Trichoderma harzianum* and its secondary metabolite harzianic acid. *Front. Microbiol.* **2018**, *9*, 1966. [CrossRef]
28. Dini, I.; Graziani, G.; Fedele, F.L.; Sicari, A.; Vinale, F.; Castaldo, L.; Ritieni, A. Effects of *Trichoderma* Biostimulation on the Phenolic Profile of Extra-Virgin Olive Oil and Olive Oil By-Products. *Antioxidants* **2020**, *9*, 284. [CrossRef]
29. De Filippis, A.; Nocera, F.P.; Tafuri, S.; Ciani, F.; Staropoli, A.; Comite, E.; Bottiglieri, A.; Gioia, L.; Lorito, M.; Woo, S.L.; et al. Antimicrobial activity of harzianic acid against *Staphylococcus pseudintermedius*. *Nat. Prod. Res.* **2021**, *35*, 5440–5445. [CrossRef]
30. De Tommaso, G.; Salvatore, M.M.; Nicoletti, R.; DellaGreca, M.; Vinale, F.; Bottiglieri, A.; Staropoli, A.; Salvatore, F.; Lorito, M.; Iuliano, M.; et al. Bivalent Metal-Chelating Properties of Harzianic Acid Produced by *Trichoderma pleuroticola* Associated to the Gastropod *Melarhaphe neritoides*. *Molecules* **2020**, *25*, 2147. [CrossRef]
31. De Tommaso, G.; Salvatore, M.M.; Nicoletti, R.; DellaGreca, M.; Vinale, F.; Staropoli, A.; Salvatore, F.; Lorito, M.; Iuliano, M.; Andolfi, A. Coordination Properties of the Fungal Metabolite Harzianic Acid Toward Toxic Heavy Metals. *Toxics* **2021**, *9*, 19. [CrossRef]
32. Ouyang, X.; Hoeksma, J.; Beenker, W.A.G.; van der Beek, S.; den Hertog, J. *Harzianic Acid Has Multi-Target Antimicrobial Activity against Gram-Positive Bacteria*; Institute Biology Leiden, Leiden University: Leiden, The Netherlands, 2021; *to be submitted*.
33. Yendapally, R.; Hurdle, J.G.; Carson, E.I.; Lee, R.B.; Lee, R.E. N-substituted 3-acetyltetramic acid derivatives as antibacterial agents. *J. Med. Chem.* **2008**, *51*, 1487–1491. [CrossRef]

34. King, M.M.; Kayastha, B.B.; Franklin, M.J.; Patrauchan, M.A. Calcium Regulation of Bacterial Virulence. In *Calcium Signaling. Advances in Experimental Medicine and Biology*; Islam, M., Ed.; Springer: Cham, Switzerland, 2020; Volume 1131, pp. 827–855. [CrossRef]
35. McCaig, L.F.; McDonald, L.C.; Mandal, S.; Jernigan, D.B. *Staphylococcus aureus*-associated skin and soft tissue infections in ambulatory care. *Emerg. Infect. Dis.* **2006**, *12*, 1715–1723. [CrossRef]
36. Stelzner, K.; Winkler, A.C.; Liang, C.; Boyny, A.; Ade, C.P.; Dandekar, T.; Fraunholz, M.J.; Rudel, T. Intracellular *Staphylococcus aureus* perturbs the host cell Ca^{2+} homeostasis to promote cell death. *mBio* **2020**, *11*, e02250-20. [CrossRef] [PubMed]
37. Cheung, G.Y.C.; Bae, J.S.; Otto, M. Pathogenicity and virulence of *Staphylococcus aureus*. *Virulence* **2021**, *12*, 547–569. [CrossRef] [PubMed]
38. Menestrina, G.; Dalla Serra, M.; Comai, M.; Coraiola, M.; Viero, G.; Werner, S.; Colin, D.A.; Monteil, H.; Prévost, G. Ion channels and bacterial infection: The case of beta-barrel pore-forming protein toxins of *Staphylococcus aureus*. *FEBS Lett.* **2003**, *552*, 54–60. [CrossRef] [PubMed]
39. Tengholm, A.; Hellman, B.; Gylfe, E. Mobilization of Ca^{2+} stores in individual pancreatic β-cells permeabilized or not with digitonin or α-toxin. *Cell Calcium* **2000**, *27*, 43–51. [CrossRef] [PubMed]
40. Xie, Y.; Yang, L. Calcium and magnesium ions are membrane-active against stationary-phase *Staphylococcus aureus* with high specificity. *Sci. Rep.* **2016**, *6*, 20628. [CrossRef]
41. Büchau, A.S.; Gallo, R.L. Innate immunity and antimicrobial defense systems in psoriasis. *Clin. Dermatol.* **2007**, *25*, 616–624. [CrossRef]
42. Rossol, M.; Pierer, M.; Raulien, N.; Quandt, D.; Meusch, U.; Rothe, K.; Schubert, K.; Schöneberg, T.; Schaefer, M.; Krügel, U.; et al. Extracellular Ca^{2+} is a danger signal activating the NLRP3 inflammasome through G protein-coupled calcium sensing receptors. *Nat. Commun.* **2012**, *3*, 1329. [CrossRef]
43. De Tommaso, G.; Salvatore, M.M.; Siciliano, A.; Staropoli, A.; Vinale, F.; Nicoletti, R.; DellaGreca, M.; Guida, M.; Salvatore, F.; Iuliano, M.; et al. Interaction of the Fungal Metabolite Harzianic Acid with Rare-Earth Cations (La^{3+}, Nd^{3+}, Sm^{3+}, Gd^{3+}). *Molecules* **2022**, *27*, 1959. [CrossRef]
44. Salvatore, M.M.; Siciliano, A.; Staropoli, A.; Vinale, F.; Nicoletti, R.; DellaGreca, M.; Guida, M.; Salvatore, F.; Iuliano, M.; Andolfi, A.; et al. Interaction of the Fungal Metabolite Harzianic Acid with Rare-Earth Cations (Pr^{3+}, Eu^{3+}, Ho^{3+}, Tm^{3+}). *Molecules* **2022**, *27*, 6468. [CrossRef]
45. Gans, P.; Sabatini, A.; Vacca, A. Investigation of equilibria in solution. Determination of equilibrium constants with the HYPERQUAD suite of programs. *Talanta* **1996**, *43*, 1739–1753. [CrossRef]
46. Balouiri, M.; Sadiki, M.; Ibnsouda, S.K. Methods for in vitro evaluating antimicrobial activity: A review. *J. Pharm. Anal.* **2016**, *6*, 71–79. [CrossRef] [PubMed]
47. Cuomo, P.; Medaglia, C.; Allocca, I.; Montone, A.M.I.; Guerra, F.; Cabaro, S.; Mollo, E.; Eletto, D.; Papaianni, M.; Capparelli, R. Caulerpin Mitigates *Helicobacter pylori*-Induced Inflammation via Formyl Peptide Receptors. *Int. J. Mol. Sci.* **2021**, *22*, 13154. [CrossRef] [PubMed]
48. Fiorito, F.; Irace, C.; Nocera, F.P.; Piccolo, M.; Ferraro, M.G.; Ciampaglia, R.; Tenore, G.C.; Santamaria, R.; De Martino, L. MG-132 interferes with iron cellular homeostasis and alters virulence of bovine herpesvirus 1. *Res. Vet. Sci.* **2021**, *137*, 1–8. [CrossRef] [PubMed]
49. Kolthoff, I.M.; Elving, P.J.; Meehan, E.J. *Treatise on Analytical Chemistry*; Wiley: Hoboken, NJ, USA, 1978; ISBN 978-0-471-80647-9.

toxins

Article

Biological Activity of Naphthoquinones Derivatives in the Search of Anticancer Lead Compounds

Alexandra G. Durán [1], Nuria Chinchilla [1], Ana M. Simonet [1], M. Teresa Gutiérrez [2], Jorge Bolívar [2], Manuel M. Valdivia [2], José M. G. Molinillo [1] and Francisco A. Macías [1,*]

[1] Allelopathy Group, Department of Organic Chemistry, Institute of Biomolecules (INBIO), Campus de Excelencia Internacional (ceiA3), School of Science, University of Cadiz, 11510 Puerto Real, Cádiz, Spain; alexandra.garcia@uca.es (A.G.D.); nuria.chinchilla@uca.es (N.C.); ana.simonet@uca.es (A.M.S.); chema.gonzalez@uca.es (J.M.G.M.)

[2] Department of Biomedicine, Biotechnology and Public Health-Biochemistry and Molecular Biology, Institute of Biomolecules (INBIO), University of Cádiz, República Saharaui 7, 11510 Puerto Real, Cádiz, Spain; mariateresa.gutierrez@gm.uca.es (M.T.G.); jorge.bolivar@uca.es (J.B.); manuel.valdivia@uca.es (M.M.V.)

* Correspondence: famacias@uca.es

Abstract: Naphthoquinones are a valuable source of secondary metabolites that are well known for their dye properties since ancient times. A wide range of biological activities have been described highlighting their cytotoxic activity, gaining the attention of researchers in recent years. In addition, it is also worth mentioning that many anticancer drugs possess a naphthoquinone backbone in their structure. Considering this background, the work described herein reports the evaluation of the cytotoxicity of different acyl and alkyl derivatives from juglone and lawsone that showed the best activity results from a etiolated wheat coleoptile bioassay. This bioassay is rapid, highly sensitive to a wide spectrum of activities, and is a powerful tool for detecting biologically active natural products. A preliminary cell viability bioassay was performed on cervix carcinoma (HeLa) cells for 24 h. The most promising compounds were further tested for apoptosis on different tumoral (IGROV-1 and SK-MEL-28) and non-tumoral (HEK-293) cell lines by flow cytometry. Results reveal that derivatives from lawsone (particularly derivative **4**) were more cytotoxic on tumoral than in non-tumoral cells, showing similar results to those obtained with of etoposide, which is used as a positive control for apoptotic cell death. These findings encourage further studies on the development of new anticancer drugs for more directed therapies and reduced side effects with naphthoquinone skeleton.

Keywords: naphthoquinones; cytotoxic activity; juglone; lawsone; flow cytometry

Key Contribution: Derivative 4 showed high selectivity on ovarian carcinoma cells with a 46.7% of viable cells in comparison with melanoma cells, where it did not show significant activity (74.5% of viable cells). Moreover, its cytotoxicity on non-tumoral cells was similar to the positive control (63.6% and 66.9% of viable cells, respectively).

Citation: Durán, A.G.; Chinchilla, N.; Simonet, A.M.; Gutiérrez, M.T.; Bolívar, J.; Valdivia, M.M.; Molinillo, J.M.G.; Macías, F.A. Biological Activity of Naphthoquinones Derivatives in the Search of Anticancer Lead Compounds. *Toxins* **2023**, *15*, 348. https://doi.org/10.3390/toxins15050348

Received: 27 April 2023
Revised: 15 May 2023
Accepted: 18 May 2023
Published: 20 May 2023

1. Introduction

Cancer represents an important cause of morbidity and mortality worldwide, where 19.3 million new cases and 10 million cancer deaths were estimated in 2020. Additionally, a 47% increase in new cancer cases is expected in 2040 [1,2]. In Spain, this disease constitutes the second leading cause of death (25.2%) after those caused by diseases of the circulatory system (26.4%) in 2021 [3]. Nowadays, there is still a continuous effort in the search for more selective approaches and with reduced side effects to fight this illness.

Naphthoquinones have been known since ancient times due to their dye properties and their use in traditional medicine as wound-healing agents. Interest in these compounds has increased recently, owing to their broad range of biological activities, particularly their cytotoxic effects [4–7]. This cytotoxicity has been mainly ascribed to the ability of naphthoquinones to generate reactive oxygen species (ROS) as well as the electrophilicity of the quinone moiety to react with different biological targets through 1,4-Michael addition by the nucleophilic thiol species, proteins, DNA and RNA [8–10]. Other mechanisms of action have also been described, including the regulation of the tumor suppressor factor p53, inhibition of topoisomerase II, induction of apoptosis via ERS (endoplasmic reticulum stress) or Aurora-kinase inhibitors [11–13].

These natural products are widespread in nature and are characterized by possessing two carbonyl groups at positions 1,4 on the naphthalene ring, and more rarely at positions 1,2. Despite being isomers, these two different arrangements show different pharmacological actions due to their different physicochemical properties [14].

Nowadays, many drugs based on natural products that contain a 1,4-naphthoquinone backbone in their chemical structure are used as anticancer agents, such as doxorubicin, daunorubicin, mitoxantrone and aclacinomycin A (Figure 1) [14–16]. In the search for new effective and selective chemotherapy approaches, naphthoquinones could play a crucial role.

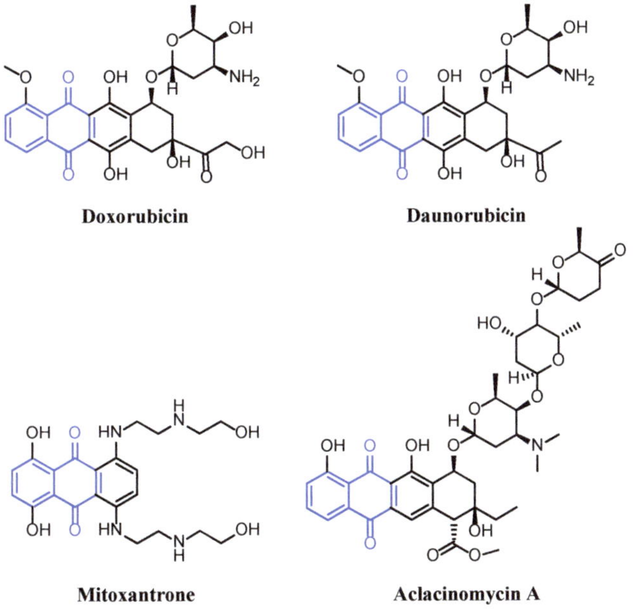

Figure 1. Examples of anticancer drugs that contain a 1,4-naphthoquinone skeleton in their structure.

In previous studies, a quantitative structure–activity relationship (QSAR) study was performed with two biologically active naphthoquinones, juglone (5-hydroxy-1, 4-naphthoquinone (**1**)) and lawsone (2-hydroxy-1,4-naphthoquinone (**2**)). A correlation between the transport phenomena and the bioactivity of compounds was assessed to determine the optimal transport conditions [17]. These structures allow for easy chemical modifications that make themself suitable scaffolds for the study of their physicochemical properties in the search for more active compounds. A total of 44 synthesized *O*-acyl and *O*-alkyl derivatives were evaluated in a general activity bioassay named wheat coleoptile bioassay. This is an easy and rapid test (24 h) that is highly sensitive to a wide range of biological activities [18]. Different behaviors could be observed for each family of compounds, which are the modifications introduced at position 5 of the naphthoquinone backbone being more active.

The work described here concerns the evaluation of the cytotoxicity of the most active naphthoquinones derivatives from the previous wheat coleoptile bioassay study [17]. A preliminary cell viability bioassay was performed on cervix carcinoma (HeLa) cells for

24 h. The most promising compounds were further tested on different tumoral (ovarian carcinoma (IGROV-1) and human melanoma (SK-MEL-28)) and non-tumoral (human embryonic kidney 293 (HEK-293)) cell lines by flow cytometry.

2. Results and Discussion

Ten naphthoquinones (**3–12**) selected from the wheat coleoptile bioassay (Figure 2) were evaluated in a first screening of cytotoxicity on HeLa cells at 100 μM for 24 h using the Trypan blue dye exclusion method. An untreated control (cells treated with 0.1% DMSO) and a positive control (cells treated with etoposide at 100 μM) were also included and evaluated for 24 h.

This is a simple, rapid, economic, and widely used method to assess cell viability after treatment with desired compounds [19]. Cells with damaged membranes are stained, while live cells with intact cell membranes are excluded and do not take up dye; however, this technique has two issues, and the results should be interpreted with caution. One of these concerns is that viability is being determined indirectly from cell membrane integrity, thus cell membrane integrity may be abnormal, yet the cell may be able to repair itself and become fully viable, but it would be determined as nonviable. On the other hand, dye uptake is assessed subjectively; small amounts of dye uptake indicative of cell injury may go unnoticed [20]. On the other hand, this method cannot explain the cause of cell death. Therefore, after completion of this first screening, the most active compounds were further evaluated by flow cytometry to detect apoptosis.

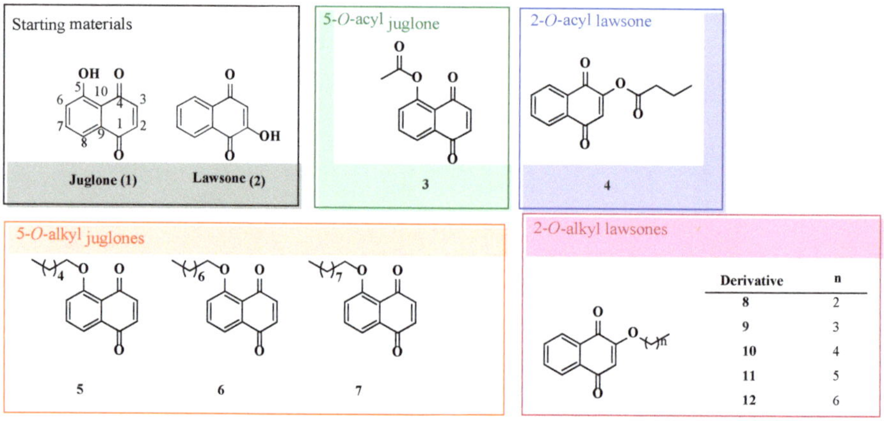

Figure 2. Naphthoquinones selected from the previous wheat coleoptile bioassay to perform the cytotoxicity study.

2.1. *First Screening of Cytotoxicity on HeLa Cells by Trypan Blue Dye Exclusion Method*

An *in vitro* cytotoxicity study on HeLa cells was used as a preliminary bioassay for screening of natural products with potential anticancer activity. Results of the ten naphthoquinones selected from the wheat coleoptile bioassay were assayed on HeLa cells for 24 h. are illustrated in Figure 3. These lead naphthoquinones are 5-acetoxy-1,4-naphthoquinone (**3**), 2-butanoyloxy-1,4-naphthoquinone (**4**), 5-*O*-alkyl juglones (chains of six, eight and nine carbon atoms, respectively) (**5–7**), and 2-*O*-alkyl lawsones (from three to seven carbon atoms) (**8–12**) (Figure 2). All the derivatives tested were more active than the corresponding starting materials, and most of them showed better growth inhibition than the positive control (etoposide), except for compounds **8**, **9** and **12**. It is also worth noting that an improvement of the activity could be observed for 2-*O*-alkyl lawsones with increase of side chain reaching the optimal value for derivative **10** (with 5 carbon atoms) and a loss of the activity with an increment in chain length. Taking into account each target backbone, the greatest activity values were noted for derivatives **3**, **4**, **6** and **10** with cell viability values lower than 30%.

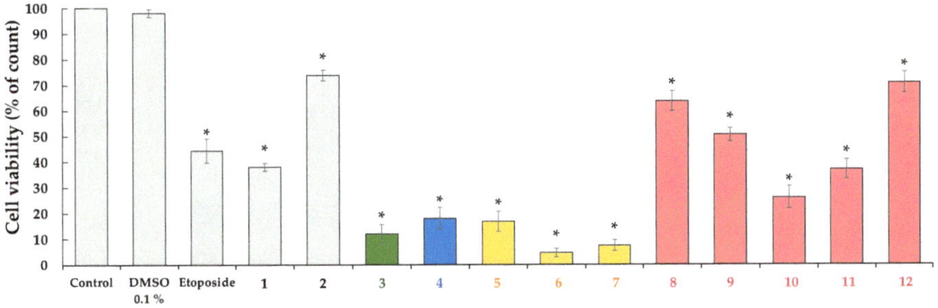

Figure 3. Cell viability by dye exclusion against cervical carcinoma cells (HeLa). Starting materials (**1** and **2**), products (**3–12**) classified by skeleton using different colors, and positive control (etoposide) were evaluated at 100 μM for 24 h. Experiments were performed in triplicate, and data are expressed as mean ± SD, $n = 3$, * $p < 0.05$ vs. untreated cells (DMSO 0.1%).

2.2. Flow Cytometry Analysis of Cell Apoptosis on Ovarian Carcinoma (IGROV-1) Cells

Cancer is considered one of the main causes of morbidity and mortality in millions of people worldwide. Ovarian cancer is the seventh most common malignant tumor worldwide and the eighth cause of mortality in women [21]. Usually, most women are diagnosed with advanced stage cancer with a poor prognosis (with a 5-year survival rate of only 17% for a patient at an advanced stage), which is partly driven by delay in diagnosis and unequal access to quality care. Globally, around 428,000 new ovarian cancer cases and 307,000 deaths are predicted to occur in 2040 [22,23].

To date, one of the main drugs used in chemotherapy against this pathology is cisplatin. However, cisplatin resistance constitutes one of the main problems in antitumor therapy [24]. Despite the great therapeutic advances made in this area, there is not yet effective treatment that provides acceptable success rates and reduce the adverse effects. Therefore, there is still a pressing need to develop less harmful and cost-effective therapeutic alternatives; the discovery of novel anticancer drugs based in natural products is a key research field that has attracted a great interest in recent years.

Apoptosis, or programmed cell death, is characterized by numerous morphological and biochemical changes to the cellular architecture. It is well known that inappropriate apoptosis is implicated in many diseases, including neurodegenerative, ischemic, autoimmune disorders, and several forms of cancer [25]. One of the earlier events of apoptosis includes the translocation of membrane phosphatidylserine (PS) from the inner side of the plasma membrane to the surface, leading to the loss of plasma membrane asymmetry. On the other hand, PS translocation also precedes the loss of membrane integrity in later stages of cell death resulting from either apoptotic or necrotic processes (Figure 4a). Annexin V (a Ca^{2+}-dependent phospholipid-binding protein) possesses high affinity for this phospholipid. Therefore, fluorochrome-labelled Annexin V can be used by flow cytometry in the detection of exposed phosphatidylserine at the outer leaflet of the plasma membrane, which is an indicator ofthe apoptotic death. Moreover, a vital dye, such as propidium iodide (PI), is typically used in conjunction with Annexin V for identification of early and late apoptotic cells. Viable cells with intact membranes exclude PI, whereas cell membranes or damaged cells are permeable to PI [26,27].

Therefore, a flow cytometric assay of Annexin V/PI was conducted to quantify the apoptotic profile in quinone-treated IGROV-1 cells. Naphthoquinones **3**, **4**, **6** and **10**, and etoposide (positive control) were tested at 100 μM for 24 h. Untreated cells (negative control) were also included in the experiment. These results are shown in dot plots, where the LL quadrant represents viable cells (both Annexin V and PI negative), the LR quadrant represents unviable cells (PI positive and Annexin V negative), the UL quadrant represents cells in early apoptosis/cell apoptosis (Annexin V positive and PI negative) and UR quadrant represents cells that are in late apoptosis or necrosis (both Annexin V and PI positive) (Figure 4b).

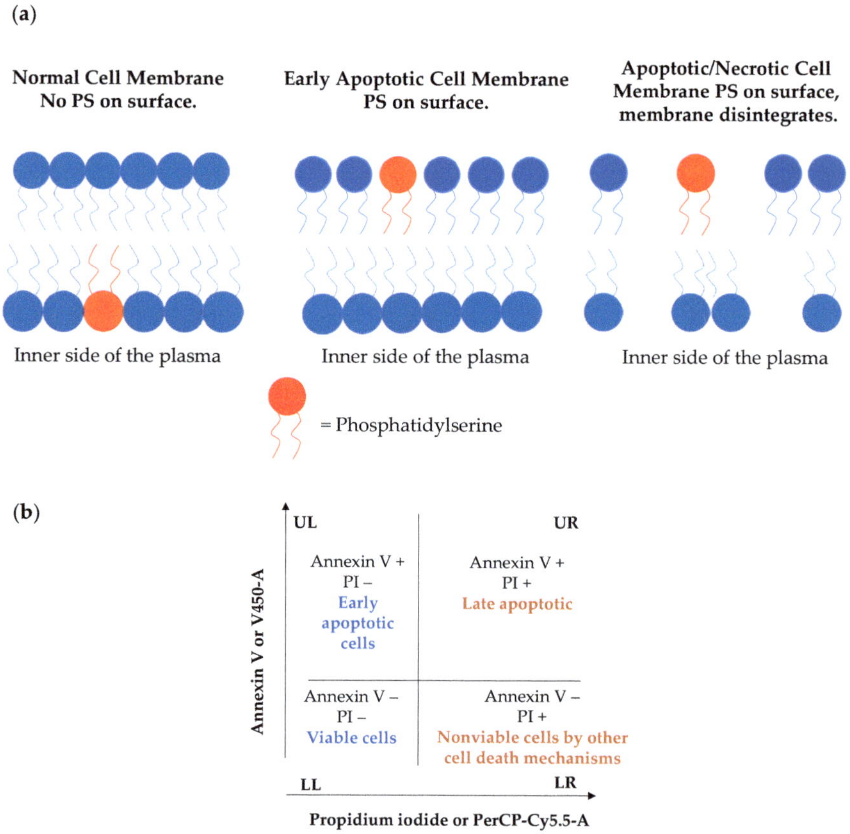

Figure 4. (**a**) Phosphatidylserine translocation and loss of membrane integrity in later stages of cell death; (**b**) plot illustrating flow cytometry analysis with AnnexinV-450 labelling apoptotic cells and 7-AAD (7-amino-actinomycin D) for cell death. Live cells are indicated in blue and death cells in orange.

In the negative control (untreated cells), most of the cells were viable (99.0%) and showed to be non-apoptotic. In contrast, significant differences could be observed after the treatment of the naphthoquinones (Figure 5). A remarkable increase in apoptotic cell number (UL + UR quadrants) was observed compared to the untreated cells. It is worth highlighting that derivatives **4**, **6**, and **10** produced a significant increase in early and late apoptotic cells (52–81%) while the population of nonviable cells by other death mechanisms scarcely increased (0.4–2.5%). Moreover, derivative **3** caused an increase in apoptotic or dead cells from untreated to treated cells (0.1% to 66.4%, respectively), together with a lesser increase in the early apoptotic cell populations (2.4%) with only 16.8% of viable cells.

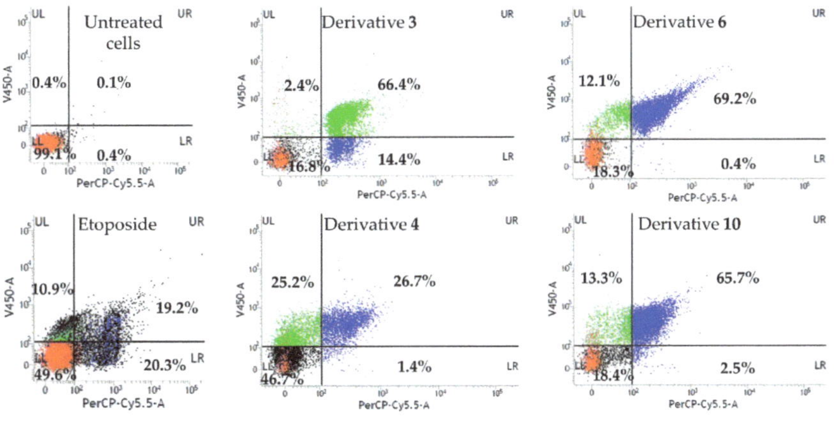

Figure 5. Flow cytometry results for the derivatives **3**, **4**, **6** and **10** on IGROV-1 cells at 100 µM for 24 h. Etoposide was used as positive control.

In view of the results outlined above, derivative **3** was selected to perform a time course study over various concentrations in IGROV-1 cell line by cell viability assay to find the optimal conditions for its evaluation by flow cytometry in order to know if the early apoptotic cell population would increase. A concentration range from 3.125 to 50 µM and a time range of 3–48 h were evaluated. Results indicated that compound **3** inhibited the IGROV-1 cell growth after 24 h of incubation in a dose-dependent manner (Figure 6).

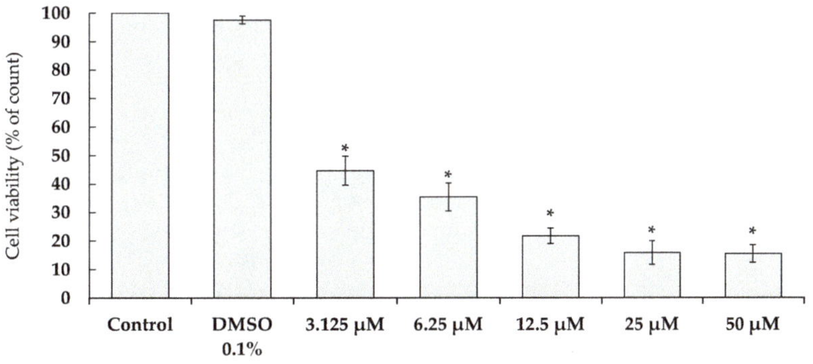

Figure 6. Cell viability by dye exclusion against ovarian carcinoma cells (IGROV-1) of compound **3** from 3.125 to 50 µM for 24 h. Etoposide and untreated cells (0.1% DMSO) were used as a positive and negative control, respectively. Experiments were performed in triplicate, and data are expressed as mean ± SD, $n = 3$, * $p < 0.05$ vs. untreated cells (DMSO 0.1%).

Two concentrations were selected from the study over time (3.125 and 6.25 µM), which showed values of 55.3 and 64.7% of growth inhibition, respectively, in ovarian carcinoma cells for 24 h. Results obtained with these concentrations in a time range of 3–48 h are illustrated in Figures S1 and S2. A 46.4% growth inhibition was reached at 3.125 µM for 24 h, therefore these conditions were considered optimal for their study by flow cytometry due to the less pronounced decrease in cell viability over time. Flow cytometry analysis under these optimal conditions for derivative **3** is shown in Figure 7. In this case, the number of viable cells increased to 54.8% in comparison to the previous experiment with a 16.8% of viable cells at 100 µM. Therefore, the drastic conditions and high cell death decreased. Moreover, a 5.2% of early apoptotic cells, 21% of apoptotic cells and 19% of nonviable cells were observed. Although an increase in the number of viable cells under these conditions (3.125 μM and 24 h) had been achieved, the number of early apoptotic cells was similar to that of 100 μM and 24 h (5.2% and 2.4%, respectively), and even the number of nonviable cells by other cell death mechanisms was higher in this last case with the optimal conditions (19.0%).

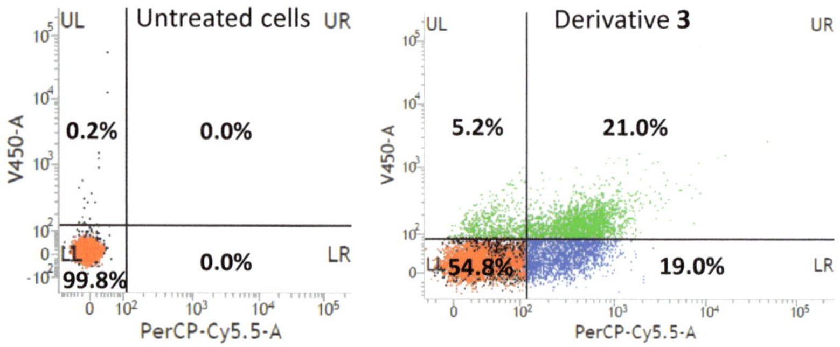

Figure 7. Flow cytometry results for the derivative **3** on IGROV-1 cells at 3.125 μM for 24 h. Apoptosis was quantitatively assessed after cells were stained with Annexin V-450 and 7-AAD.

Nevertheless, taking into account the results obtained for the other three naphthoquinone derivatives (**4**, **6**, and **10**), it is worth mentioning that the number of nonviable cells by other cell mechanisms different to apoptosis is very small (0.4–2.5%), and the number of early and late apoptotic cells was increased (52–81%), making apoptosis the primary cell death mechanism. These findings propose these structures as candidates to find more oriented therapies. To gain further insight into the apoptosis cell death, these naphthoquinones were further evaluated on human melanoma cells (SK-MEL-28) and non-tumoral human embryonic kidney 293 (HEK-293) cells.

2.3. Flow Cytometry Analysis of Cell Apoptosis on Human Melanoma (SK-MEL-28) and Non-Tumoral Human Embryonic Kidney 293 (HEK-293) Cells

Derivatives with the most promising results (2-butanoyloxy-1,4-naphthoquinone (**4**); 5-octoxy-1,4-naphthoquinone (**6**); and 2-pentoxy-1,4-naphthoquinone (**10**)) that trigger cell death by apoptotic processes were evaluated on a different tumoral (human melanoma) and non-tumoral (human embryonic kidney 293) cells (Figures 8 and 9).

The overall prevalence and incidence of both non-melanoma (basal cell and squamous cell carcinomas) and melanoma skin cancers have increased over the past decades. It is estimated that between 2 and 3 million non-melanoma skin cancers and 132,000 melanoma skin cancers occur globally each year. Surgical excision of these malignancies remains the traditional mainstay of treatment as well as topical treatments with semisolid formulations (with 5-fluorouracil, diclofenac, and imiquimod) and photodynamic therapy, among others. Despite the remarkable progress in cancer treatment over the last decades, the survival rate of many patients remains slow. Additionally, owing to the difficulties in clinical trials, there is no FDA (Food and Drug Administration) registered topical treatments of skin cancer so far [28–31].

The human embryonic kidney 293 (HEK 293) cell line was developed in 1977 from the sheared Adenovirus 5 (Ad5) DNA transformation of the human embryonic kidney cell [32]. HEK-293 cells are relatively easy to transfect and widely used to study a large variety of biological processes [33]. These cells are considered one among the widely used standards for non-tumoral human cells [34]. For these reasons, the HEK-293 cell line was chosen to gain better insights into the selectivity of the lead compound against tumoral and non-tumoral cells [35].

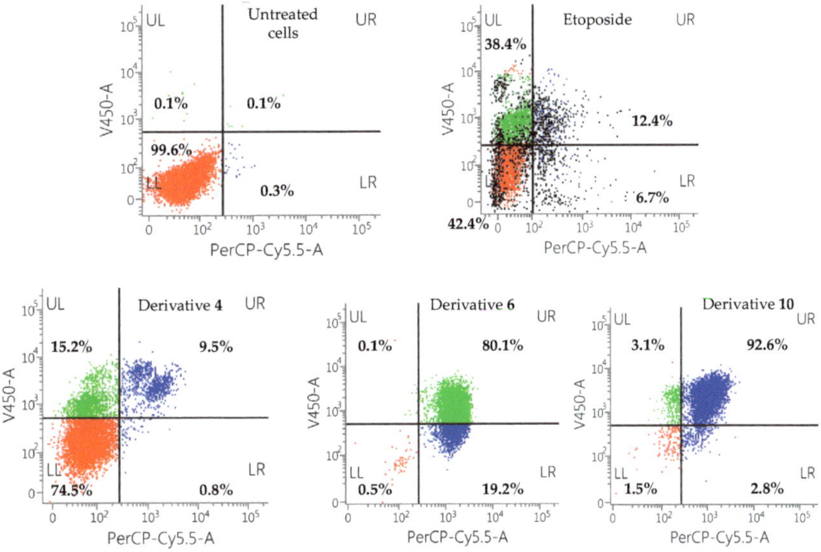

Figure 8. Flow cytometry results for the derivatives **4**, **6**, and **10** on SK-MEL-28 cells at 100 µM for 24 h. Etoposide was used as positive control.

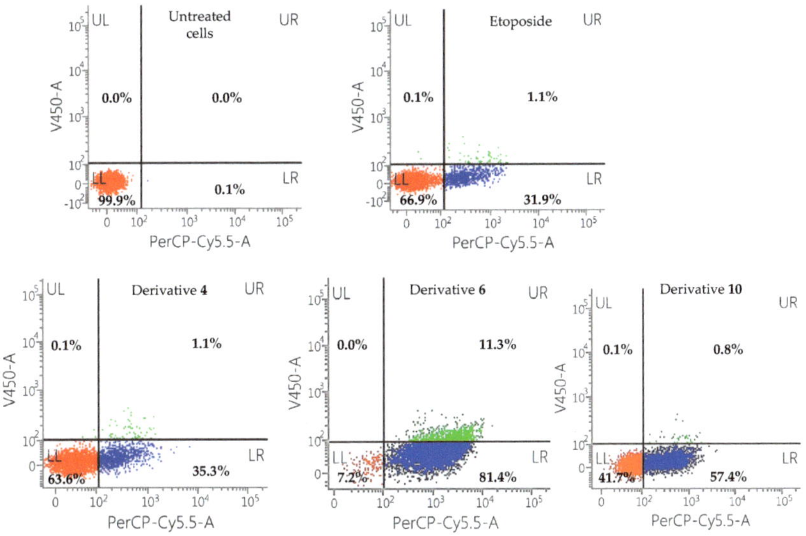

Figure 9. Flow cytometry results for the derivatives **4**, **6**, and **10** on HEK-293 cells at 100 µM for 24 h. Etoposide was used as positive control.

In view of the results obtained, it can be drawn that the most cytotoxic naphthoquinone derivative in all the cell lines tested is the derivative 5-*O*-acyl juglone (**6**), with a percentage of viable cells of 18.3%, 0.5%, and 7.2% on IGROV-1, SK-MEL-28, and HEK-293 cells, respectively. On the other hand, naphthoquinones modified at position 2 of the naphthoquinone backbone (2-*O*-acyl lawsone (**4**) and 2-*O*-alkyl lawsone (**10**), showed certain selectivity among the different cell lines assayed.

2-butanoyloxy-1,4-naphthoquinone (**4**) showed significant cytotoxic activity on ovarian carcinoma cells, with 51.9% of apoptotic cells (UL + UR quadrants) and 46.7% of viable cells, showing better results than the positive control etoposide (30.1% of apoptotic cells and 49.6% of viable cells). Nevertheless, it did not show a significant cytotoxic activity on melanoma cells, with 74.5% of viable cells and 24.7% of apoptotic cells. It is worth highlighting that 63.6% of viable cells were observed on non-tumoral HEK-293 cells, with similar cytotoxic values showed by the positive control (66.9% of viable cells). These results highlight the higher toxicity on IGROV-1 than in SK-MEL-28 tumoral cells and in non-tumoral human embryonic kidney cells (HEK-293) at 100 μM for 24 h.

On the other hand, derivative **10** (2-pentoxy-1,4-naphthoquinone) showed high cytotoxicity in the two tumoral cell lines tested, reaching activity values better than etoposide (18.4% of viable cells and 79% of apoptotic cells on IGROV-1 and 1.5% of viable cells and 95.2% of apoptotic cells on SK-MEL-28 cells). Regarding the cytotoxicity on non-tumoral cells, it showed 41.7% of viable cells.

It has been demonstrated that different substitution patterns on the naphthoquinone moiety, as well as the position of the hydroxyl groups, may play a crucial role in the activity observed, since it affects the redox potentials and pro-oxidant activities [36]. Thus, there are several studies that describe this fact. Ali and co-workers evaluated the effect of antileishmanial activity of a series of naphthoquinones, including simple, oxygenated in the aromatic or quinonoid ring, dimeric and furanonaphthoquinones. Leishmanicidal activity was strongly dependent on the nature and position of these substituents. The most active compounds were those with hydroxylation at C-5 and dihydroxy substitution at C-5 and C-8 on the napththoquinone ring. In contrast, 2-hydroxynaphthoquinones were less active [36]. Another study performed by Wang and co-workers, describes the preparation of a series of 2-position and 3-position lipophilic-substituted lawsone and juglone derivatives to evaluate their anticancer activity in vitro. Most of the more active compounds with better activity values were those with 2-*O*-alkyl-, or 3-*C*-alkyl- derivatives synthesized from lawsone, which are 2-hydroxy-3-farnesyl-1,4-naphthoquinone, the most cytotoxic compound against the cell lines tested [4]. Likewise, a SAR study of the cytotoxicity of a series of 1,4-naphthoquinones was performed by Shen and co-workers, where the high cytotoxicity was observed for juglone derivatives [37].

Moreover, one of the main disadvantages described for this kind of compounds is its high cytotoxicity and its low therapeutic selectivity. Nevertheless, these results reveal certain selectivity, especially for derivative **4** with strong cytotoxicity on ovarian carcinoma cells and non-significant toxicity on non-tumoral HEK-293 cells, with values similar to the positive control etoposide. Furthermore, it was noted that modifications performed at position 2 of the naphthoquinone backbone were more cytotoxic on tumoral cells than in non-tumoral (2-*O*-acyl and 2-*O*-alkyl derivatives) in comparison to 5-*O*-acyl and 5-*O*-alkyl derivatives.

The starting materials, juglone (found in leaves, roots, husks, and barks of several species of walnut trees) and lawsone (isolated from the leaves and shoots of henna, *Lawsonia inermis* L.) have shown cytotoxicity against a wide range of human cancer cell lines [38–41]. Regarding the analogues investigated, cytotoxic properties for derivatives **4**, **6** and **10**, are described for the first time. In contrast, the cytotoxic properties of derivative **3** (5-acetoxy-1,4-naphthoquinone) have been previously reported in the literature. It has shown strong cytotoxicity on human oral epidermoid carcinoma (KB) cell line with an IC_{50} value of 1.39 μM [37], and it has also shown cytotoxicity against L-60 (leukemia), MDA-MB-435 (melanoma), SF-295 (brain) and HCT-8 (colon), human cancer cell lines [41]. In our experiments, an IC_{50} value of 7.54 μM for derivative **3** was obtained for ovarian carcinoma (IGROV-1) cells.

3. Conclusions

Naphthoquinones have been known for a long time to show cytotoxic properties [4]. These effects are mainly ascribed to the ability of these scaffolds to generate ROS and also to react with different biological targets, such as DNA topoisomerase [42]. However, they have been considered as PAINS (pan-assay interference compounds) in high-throughput screenings and are therefore considered as notorious troublemakers by the scientific community [14]. Nevertheless, these kind of compounds have been used for many medicinal traditional uses since ancient times and a great number of approved drugs or that are in preclinical trials even possess a naphthoquinone skeleton. Moreover, these compounds possess multitarget activity, which can be employed as synergic polypharmacology in chemotherapies treatments and also to fight resistant tumoral cells. It has been previously reported that a large number of naphthoquinones have shown high efficacy in tumoral cell lines resistant to drugs or chemotherapeutic agents [14,43,44].

A series of 1,4-naphthoquinone derivatives have been evaluated on different tumoral (HeLa, IGROV-1, and SK-MEL-28) and non-tumoral (HEK-293) cell lines. Results denoted that derivatives from lawsone showed more selectivity against tumoral cells, while their cytotoxicity on non-tumoral cells were similar to the positive control etoposide. On the other hand, those derivatives from juglone result to be more cytotoxic against all the cell lines tested. Therefore, the number of apoptotic cells was quantified and assayed by flow cytometry. Derivatives **4** (2-butanoyloxy-1,4-naphthoquinone) and **10** (2-pentoxy-1,4-naphthoquinone) cause apoptosis to be the primarily cell death mechanism. These findings encourage further studies on the development of new anticancer drugs with a naphthoquinone backbone, with improved selectivity, avoiding the induction of drug resistance and reduce toxicity. Cytotoxicity of derivatives **4**, **6**, and **10** is described for the first time.

4. Materials and Methods

4.1. Chemicals and General Experimental Procedures

5-Hydroxy-1,4-naphthoquinone (juglone, technical grade, 97%) and 2-hydroxy-1,4-naphthoquinone (lawsone, 98%) were supplied by Alfa Aesar (Heysham, UK) and Acros Organics (Morris Plains, NJ, USA), respectively.

Dimethyl sulfoxide was supplied by Panreac Quimica SAU (Castellar del Vallés, Barcelona, Spain). Dulbecco's Modified Eagle's Medium (DMEM) was supplied by Lonza (Verviers, Belgium), premixed phosphate-buffered saline solution (PBS, 10×) was supplied by Roche (Steinheim, Germany), fetal bovine serum, penicillin/streptomycin, L-glutamine, sodium pyruvate, trypsin, and minimum essential medium non-essential amino acids (MEM NEAA), were purchased from Gibco (Paisley, UK). BD Annexin V: FITC Apoptosis Detection Kit I was supplied by BD Biosciences (Madrid, Spain).

4.2. Cell lines and Cell Cultures

HeLa (human cervix carcinoma), IGROV-1 (human ovarian carcinoma), SK-MEL-28 (human melanoma), and HEK-293 (human embryonic kidney 293) cells were cultured as monolayers in DMEM (GIBCO) supplemented with 10% fetal bovine serum, 5% glutamine, 5% non-essential amino acids, 5% penicillin–streptomycin, and 5% sodium pyruvate. Cells were maintained in a Hera Cell 150i (Thermo Scientific, Waltham, MA, USA) incubator at 37 °C, 5% CO_2 and 95% humidity. For all assays, cells were allowed to attach until 70% confluence was reached prior to treatment.

4.3. Cell Viability Assays

The different cell lines were sterile cultured in 6-well plates (VWR, Darmstadt, Germany) each to 70% confluence during at least 48 h. Cell lines were treated for 24 h with the corresponding naphthoquinone derivative in DMSO (0.1% *v/v*) at a concentration of 100 μM. In addition, concentration ranges from 3.125 μM to 50 μM and treatments ranging from 3 h to 48 h of product **3** were also evaluated. Control cultures, including cells treated with 0.1% DMSO and positive control of cells treated with etoposide at 100 μM, were also included in each experiment.

Trypan blue solution (0.4% Sigma Aldrich, Steinheim, Germany) was mixed 1:1 with a sample of control or treated cells. After incubation for 2 min, a fraction of blue-stained cells was assessed using an Automated Cell Counter T20 (Bio-Rad, Hercules, CA, USA).

Experiments were performed in triplicate; data are expressed as the mean of triplicate measurements (mean ± SD).

$$\% \text{ viability} = (\text{Total number of viable cells}/\text{Total number of viable and non-viable cells}) \times 100$$

4.4. Flow Cytometry and Data Analysis

Detection of apoptosis was performed using the kit Annexin V FITC assay, which contains Annexin V-FITC, propidium iodide staining solution, and Annexin V binding buffer.

The fluorescence of single cells was measured by a FACSVerse™ bench top flow cytometer equipped with blue (488 nm), red (640 nm) and violet (405 nm) lasers. Amplification of signals were carried out at logarithmic scale and measurements of events were plotted on forward light scatter (FSC), side light scatter (SSC), violet fluorescence to detect Annexin-V 450 and red fluorescence for 7-AAD. A gating strategy was used to distinguish the fluorescently labelled cell population from unstained populations. A total of 10,000 events as defined by gates were counted and cell counts were expressed as percentage. The data were analyzed using BD Assurity Linc™ Software v 1.0.

After treatment with the products, cell culture medium was collected into 15 mL tubes, and each well was cleaned with PBS (1 mL). Accutase was added to each well, enough to cover the surface (300 µL) and incubated for 1–2 min at room temperature. Then, 2 mL of PBS was added to each well, and the contents transferred to the 15 mL tubes. They were centrifuged, and the supernatant was discarded. Cells were transferred to an eppendorf and washed with cold PBS in triplicate. They were resuspended in 1×X Binding buffer (100 µL), and then Annexin V-450 (5 µL) and 7-AAD (7-amino-actinomycin D, 2.9 µL) were added. They were diluted again with 400 µL of 1× binding buffer, and the cells were mixed and incubated for 15 min at room temperature in the dark prior to analysis. Measurements were done within 1 h.

4.5. Statistical Analysis

The results are presented as the mean ± standard deviation (SD) of at least three independent experiments. Data were evaluated with GraphPad Prism® Version 5.00 software (San Diego, CA, USA) and analyzed using one-way ANOVA. Values were considered to be statistically significant when $p < 0.05$. Additionally, an IC_{50} value for derivative **3** was determined using the same software.

Supplementary Materials: The following supporting information can be downloaded at: https://www.mdpi.com/article/10.3390/toxins15050348/s1, Figure S1: Cell viability by dye exclusion of derivative **3** on ovarian carcinoma cells (IGROV-1) at 3.125 µM; Figure S2: Cell viability by dye exclusion of derivative **3** on ovarian carcinoma cells (IGROV-1) at 6.25 µM.

Author Contributions: Conceptualization, A.G.D., J.M.G.M. and J.B.; methodology, A.G.D., M.T.G. and J.B.; validation, A.G.D. and M.T.G.; formal analysis, A.G.D., N.C. and A.M.S.; investigation, A.G.D., M.T.G., J.B. and M.M.V.; resources, M.M.V. and F.A.M.; data curation, A.G.D.; writing—original draft preparation, A.G.D.; writing—review and editing, A.G.D., N.C., A.M.S., M.T.G., J.B., M.M.V., J.M.G.M. and F.A.M.; visualization, A.G.D.; supervision, J.B., M.M.V., J.M.G.M. and F.A.M.; project administration, A.G.D.; funding acquisition, F.A.M. and J.M.G.M. All authors have read and agreed to the published version of the manuscript.

Funding: This work was financially supported by the Ministerio de Economía y Competitividad (Project PID2020-115747RB-I00), Spain.

Institutional Review Board Statement: Not applicable.

Informed Consent Statement: Not applicable.

Data Availability Statement: Not applicable.

Acknowledgments: The authors would like to thank to Servicios Centrales de Investigación Científica y Tecnológica (University of Cádiz) and the Centro Nacional de Investigaciones Oncológicas' (CNIO, Madrid) for supplying the cell lines.

Conflicts of Interest: The authors declare no conflict of interest.

References

1. Sung, H.; Ferlay, J.; Siegel, R.L.; Laversanne, M.; Soerjomataram, I.; Jemal, A.; Bray, F. Global Cancer Statistics 2020: GLOBOCAN Estimates of Incidence and Mortality Worldwide for 36 Cancers in 185 Countries. *CA Cancer J. Clin.* **2021**, *71*, 209–249. [CrossRef] [PubMed]
2. Yadav, P.; Yadav, R.; Jain, S.; Vaidya, A. Caspase-3: A Primary Target for Natural and Synthetic Compounds for Cancer Therapy. *Chem. Biol. Drug Des.* **2021**, *98*, 144–165. [CrossRef] [PubMed]
3. Deaths According to Cause of Death. Available online: https://www.ine.es/en/prensa/edcm_2021_en.pdf (accessed on 27 April 2023).
4. Wang, S.-H.; Lo, C.-Y.; Gwo, Z.-H.; Lin, H.-J.; Chen, L.-G.; Kuo, C.-D.; Wu, J.-Y. Synthesis and Biological Evaluation of Lipophilic 1,4-Naphthoquinone Derivatives against Human Cancer Cell Lines. *Molecules* **2015**, *20*, 11994–12015. [CrossRef]
5. Wellington, K.W. Understanding Cancer and the Anticancer Activities of Naphthoquinones—A Review. *RSC Adv.* **2015**, *5*, 20309–20338. [CrossRef]
6. Ravichandiran, P.; Athinarayanan, J.; Premnath, D.; Periasamy, V.S.; Alshatwi, A.A.; Vasanthkumar, S. Synthesis, Molecular Docking and Biological Evaluation of Novel 6-(4-(4-Aminophenylsulfonyl)Phenylamino)-5H-Benzo[a]Phenothiazin-5-One Derivatives. *Spectrochim. Acta A Mol. Biomol. Spectrosc.* **2015**, *139*, 477–487. [CrossRef] [PubMed]
7. Ravichandiran, P.; Premnath, D.; Vasanthkumar, S. Synthesis, Molecular Docking and Antibacterial Evaluation of 2-(4-(4-Aminophenylsulfonyl)Phenylamino)-3-(Thiophen-2-Ylthio)Naphthalene-1,4-Dione Derivatives. *Front. Chem. Sci. Eng.* **2015**, *9*, 46–56. [CrossRef]
8. Bhasin, D.; Chettiar, S.N.; Etter, J.P.; Mok, M.; Li, P.-K. Anticancer Activity and SAR Studies of Substituted 1,4-Naphthoquinones. *Bioorganic Med. Chem.* **2013**, *21*, 4662–4669. [CrossRef]
9. Ravichandiran, P.; Subramaniyan, S.A.; Kim, S.-Y.; Kim, J.-S.; Park, B.-H.; Shim, K.S.; Yoo, D.J. Synthesis and Anticancer Evaluation of 1,4-Naphthoquinone Derivatives Containing a Phenylaminosulfanyl Moiety. *ChemMedChem* **2019**, *14*, 532–544. [CrossRef]
10. Ravichandiran, P.; Jegan, A.; Premnath, D.; Periasamy, V.S.; Vasanthkumar, S. Design, Synthesis, Molecular Docking as Histone Deacetylase (HDAC8) Inhibitors, Cytotoxicity and Antibacterial Evaluation of Novel 6-(4-(4-Aminophenylsulfonyl)Phenylamino)-5H-Benzo[a]Phenoxazin-5-One Derivatives. *Med. Chem. Res.* **2015**, *24*, 197–208. [CrossRef]
11. Pereyra, C.E.; Dantas, R.F.; Ferreira, S.B.; Gomes, L.P.; Silva-Jr, F.P. The Diverse Mechanisms and Anticancer Potential of Naphthoquinones. *Cancer Cell Int.* **2019**, *19*, 207. [CrossRef]
12. Furqan, M.; Fayyaz, A.; Firdous, F.; Raza, H.; Bilal, A.; Saleem, R.S.Z.; Shahzad-ul-Hussan, S.; Wang, D.; Youssef, F.S.; al Musayeib, N.M.; et al. Identification and Characterization of Natural and Semisynthetic Quinones as Aurora Kinase Inhibitors. *J. Nat. Prod.* **2022**, *85*, 1503–1513. [CrossRef] [PubMed]
13. Kavaliauskas, P.; Opazo, F.S.; Acevedo, W.; Petraitiene, R.; Grybaitė, B.; Anusevičius, K.; Mickevičius, V.; Belyakov, S.; Petraitis, V. Synthesis, Biological Activity, and Molecular Modelling Studies of Naphthoquinone Derivatives as Promising Anticancer Candidates Targeting COX-2. *Pharmaceuticals* **2022**, *15*, 541. [CrossRef] [PubMed]
14. Qiu, H.-Y.; Wang, P.-F.; Lin, H.-Y.; Tang, C.-Y.; Zhu, H.-L.; Yang, Y.-H. Naphthoquinones: A Continuing Source for Discovery of Therapeutic Antineoplastic Agents. *Chem. Biol. Drug Des.* **2018**, *91*, 681–690. [CrossRef]
15. Aminin, D.; Polonik, S. 1,4-Naphthoquinones: Some Biological Properties and Application. *Chem. Pharm. Bull. (Tokyo)* **2020**, *68*, 46–57. [CrossRef] [PubMed]
16. Verma, R.P. Anti-Cancer Activities of 1,4-Naphthoquinones: A QSAR Study. *Anticancer Agents Med. Chem.* **2006**, *6*, 489–499. [CrossRef] [PubMed]
17. Durán, A.G.; Chinchilla, N.; Molinillo, J.M.G.; Macías, F.A. Influence of Lipophilicity in O -acyl and O -alkyl Derivatives of Juglone and Lawsone: A Structure–Activity Relationship Study in the Search for Natural Herbicide Models. *Pest Manag. Sci.* **2018**, *74*, 682–694. [CrossRef]
18. García, B.; Torres, A.; Macías, F. Synergy and Other Interactions between Polymethoxyflavones from Citrus Byproducts. *Molecules* **2015**, *20*, 20079–20106. [CrossRef]
19. Diana, E.J.; Mathew, T.V. Synthesis and Characterization of Surface-Modified Ultrafine Titanium Dioxide Nanoparticles with an Antioxidant Functionalized Biopolymer as a Therapeutic Agent: Anticancer and Antimicrobial Evaluation. *Colloids Surf. B Biointerfaces* **2022**, *220*, 112949. [CrossRef]
20. Strober, W. Trypan Blue Exclusion Test of Cell Viability. *Curr. Protoc. Immunol.* **2015**, *111*, A3.B.1–A3.B.3. [CrossRef]
21. Gaona-Luviano, P.; Medina-Gaona, L.A.; Magaña-Pérez, K. Epidemiology of Ovarian Cancer. *Chin. Clin. Oncol.* **2020**, *9*, 47. [CrossRef]
22. Cabasag, C.J.; Fagan, P.J.; Ferlay, J.; Vignat, J.; Laversanne, M.; Liu, L.; van der Aa, M.A.; Bray, F.; Soerjomataram, I. Ovarian Cancer Today and Tomorrow: A Global Assessment by World Region and Human Development Index Using GLOBOCAN 2020. *Int. J. Cancer* **2022**, *151*, 1535–1541. [CrossRef]
23. Huang, J.; Chan, W.C.; Ngai, C.H.; Lok, V.; Zhang, L.; Lucero-Prisno, D.E.; Xu, W.; Zheng, Z.-J.; Elcarte, E.; Withers, M.; et al. Worldwide Burden, Risk Factors, and Temporal Trends of Ovarian Cancer: A Global Study. *Cancers* **2022**, *14*, 2230. [CrossRef] [PubMed]

24. Tossetta, G.; Fantone, S.; Montanari, E.; Marzioni, D.; Goteri, G. Role of NRF2 in Ovarian Cancer. *Antioxidants* **2022**, *11*, 663. [CrossRef] [PubMed]
25. Cohen, G.M. Caspases: The Executioners of Apoptosis. *Biochem. J.* **1997**, *326*, 1–16. [CrossRef]
26. Vermes, I.; Haanen, C.; Steffens-Nakken, H.; Reutelingsperger, C. A Novel Assay for Apoptosis Flow Cytometric Detection of Phosphatidylserine Early Apoptotic Cells Using Fluorescein Labelled Expression on Annexin V. *J. Immunol. Methods* **1995**, *184*, 39–51. [CrossRef] [PubMed]
27. Kupcho, K.; Shultz, J.; Hurst, R.; Hartnett, J.; Zhou, W.; Machleidt, T.; Grailer, J.; Worzella, T.; Riss, T.; Lazar, D.; et al. A Real-Time, Bioluminescent Annexin V Assay for the Assessment of Apoptosis. *Apoptosis* **2019**, *24*, 184–197. [CrossRef]
28. Urban, K.; Mehrmal, S.; Uppal, P.; Giesey, R.L.; Delost, G.R. The Global Burden of Skin Cancer: A Longitudinal Analysis from the Global Burden of Disease Study, 1990–2017. *JAAD Int.* **2021**, *2*, 98–108. [CrossRef]
29. Khan, N.H.; Mir, M.; Qian, L.; Baloch, M.; Ali Khan, M.F.; Rehman, A.-; Ngowi, E.E.; Wu, D.-D.; Ji, X.-Y. Skin Cancer Biology and Barriers to Treatment: Recent Applications of Polymeric Micro/Nanostructures. *J. Adv. Res.* **2022**, *36*, 223–247. [CrossRef]
30. Cullen, J.K.; Simmons, J.L.; Parsons, P.G.; Boyle, G.M. Topical Treatments for Skin Cancer. *Adv. Drug Deliv. Rev.* **2020**, *153*, 54–64. [CrossRef]
31. Simões, M.C.F.; Sousa, J.J.S.; Pais, A.A.C.C. Skin Cancer and New Treatment Perspectives: A Review. *Cancer Lett.* **2015**, *357*, 8–42. [CrossRef]
32. Shen, C.; Gu, M.; Song, C.; Miao, L.; Hu, L.; Liang, D.; Zheng, C. The Tumorigenicity Diversification in Human Embryonic Kidney 293 Cell Line Cultured in Vitro. *Biologicals* **2008**, *36*, 263–268. [CrossRef] [PubMed]
33. Cusick, J.K.; Mustian, A.; Goldberg, K.; Reyland, M.E. RELT Induces Cellular Death in HEK 293 Epithelial Cells. *Cell. Immunol.* **2010**, *261*, 1–8. [CrossRef]
34. Liu, X.; Shan, K.; Shao, X.; Shi, X.; He, Y.; Liu, Z.; Jacob, J.A.; Deng, L. Nanotoxic Effects of Silver Nanoparticles on Normal HEK-293 Cells in Comparison to Cancerous HeLa Cell Line. *Int. J. Nanomed.* **2021**, *16*, 753–761. [CrossRef]
35. Gutiérrez, M.T.; Durán, A.G.; Mejías, F.J.R.; Molinillo, J.M.G.; Megias, D.; Valdivia, M.M.; Macías, F.A. Bio-Guided Isolation of Acetogenins from *Annona Cherimola* Deciduous Leaves: Production of Nanocarriers to Boost the Bioavailability Properties. *Molecules* **2020**, *25*, 4861. [CrossRef]
36. Ali, A.; Assimopoulou, A.; Papageorgiou, V.; Kolodziej, H. Structure/Antileishmanial Activity Relationship Study of Naphthoquinones and Dependency of the Mode of Action on the Substitution Patterns. *Planta Med.* **2011**, *77*, 2003–2012. [CrossRef] [PubMed]
37. Shen, C.-C.; Afraj, S.N.; Hung, C.-C.; Barve, B.D.; Kuo, L.-M.Y.; Lin, Z.-H.; Ho, H.-O.; Kuo, Y.-H. Synthesis, Biological Evaluation, and Correlation of Cytotoxicity versus Redox Potential of 1,4-Naphthoquinone Derivatives. *Bioorg. Med. Chem. Lett.* **2021**, *41*, 127976. [CrossRef] [PubMed]
38. Karki, N.; Aggarwal, S.; Laine, R.A.; Greenway, F.; Losso, J.N. Cytotoxicity of Juglone and Thymoquinone against Pancreatic Cancer Cells. *Chem. Biol. Interact.* **2020**, *327*, 109142. [CrossRef]
39. Pradhan, R.; Dandawate, P.; Vyas, A.; Padhye, S.; Biersack, B.; Schobert, R.; Ahmad, A.; Sarkar, F.H. From Body Art to Anticancer Activities: Perspectives on Medicinal Properties of Henna. *Curr. Drug Targets* **2012**, *13*, 1777–1798. [CrossRef]
40. López López, L.I.; Nery Flores, S.D.; Silva Belmares, S.Y.; Sáenz Galindo, A. Naphthoquinones: Biological Properties and Synthesis of Lawsone and Derivates—A Structured Review. *Vitae* **2014**, *21*, 248–258. [CrossRef]
41. Montenegro, R.C.; Araújo, A.J.; Molina, M.T.; Filho, J.D.B.M.; Rocha, D.D.; Lopéz-Montero, E.; Goulart, M.O.F.; Bento, E.S.; Alves, A.P.N.N.; Pessoa, C.; et al. Cytotoxic Activity of Naphthoquinones with Special Emphasis on Juglone and Its 5-O-Methyl Derivative. *Chem. Biol. Interact.* **2010**, *184*, 439–448. [CrossRef]
42. Rahman, M.M.; Islam, M.R.; Akash, S.; Shohag, S.; Ahmed, L.; Supti, F.A.; Rauf, A.; Aljohani, A.S.M.; Al Abdulmonem, W.; Khalil, A.A.; et al. Naphthoquinones and Derivatives as Potential Anticancer Agents: An Updated Review. *Chem. Biol. Interact.* **2022**, *368*, 110198. [CrossRef] [PubMed]
43. Feldmann, C.; Miljković, F.; Yonchev, D.; Bajorath, J. Identifying Promiscuous Compounds with Activity against Different Target Classes. *Molecules* **2019**, *24*, 4185. [CrossRef] [PubMed]
44. Tandon, V.K.; Kumar, S. Recent Development on Naphthoquinone Derivatives and Their Therapeutic Applications as Anticancer Agents. *Expert Opin. Ther. Pat.* **2013**, *23*, 1087–1108. [CrossRef] [PubMed]

toxins

MDPI

Article

Effects of Sesquiterpene Lactones on Primary Cilia Formation (Ciliogenesis)

Marina Murillo-Pineda [1], Juan M. Coto-Cid [2,3], María Romero [1], Jesús G. Zorrilla [2,4], Nuria Chinchilla [2], Zahara Medina-Calzada [1], Rosa M. Varela [2], Álvaro Juárez-Soto [1], Francisco A. Macías [2,*] and Elena Reales [1,2,*]

[1] Research Unit, Biomedical Research and Innovation Institute of Cádiz (INiBICA), Department of Urology, University Hospital of Jerez de la Frontera, 11407 Jerez, Spain; marina.murillo@inibica.es (M.M.-P.); maria.romero@inibica.es (M.R.); zahara.medina@inibica.es (Z.M.-C.); alvaro.juarez.sspa@juntadeandalucia.es (Á.J.-S.)

[2] Allelopathy Group, Department of Organic Chemistry, Institute of Biomolecules (INBIO), School of Science, University of Cadiz, Campus de Excelencia Internacional (ceiA3), 11510 Puerto Real, Spain; jcoto@us.es (J.M.C.-C.); jesus.zorrilla@uca.es (J.G.Z.); nuria.chinchilla@uca.es (N.C.); rosa.varela@uca.es (R.M.V.)

[3] Department of Organic Chemistry, University of Seville, 41012 Seville, Spain

[4] Department of Chemical Sciences, University of Naples Federico II, Complesso Universitario Monte S. Angelo, Via Cinthia 4, 80126 Naples, Italy

* Correspondence: famacias@uca.es (F.A.M.); elena.reales@uca.es (E.R.)

Abstract: Sesquiterpene lactones (SLs), plant-derived metabolites with broad spectra of biological effects, including anti-tumor and anti-inflammatory, hold promise for drug development. Primary cilia, organelles extending from cell surfaces, are crucial for sensing and transducing extracellular signals essential for cell differentiation and proliferation. Their life cycle is linked to the cell cycle, as cilia assemble in non-dividing cells of G_0/G_1 phases and disassemble before entering mitosis. Abnormalities in both primary cilia (non-motile cilia) and motile cilia structure or function are associated with developmental disorders (ciliopathies), heart disease, and cancer. However, the impact of SLs on primary cilia remains unknown. This study evaluated the effects of selected SLs (grosheimin, costunolide, and three cyclocostunolides) on primary cilia biogenesis and stability in human retinal pigment epithelial (RPE) cells. Confocal fluorescence microscopy was employed to analyze the effects on primary cilia formation (ciliogenesis), primary cilia length, and stability. The effects on cell proliferation were evaluated by flow cytometry. All SLs disrupted primary cilia formation in the early stages of ciliogenesis, irrespective of starvation conditions or cytochalasin-D treatment, with no effect on cilia length or cell cycle progression. Interestingly, grosheimin stabilized and promoted primary cilia formation under cilia homeostasis and elongation treatment conditions. Thus, SLs have potential as novel drugs for ciliopathies and tumor treatment.

Keywords: sesquiterpene lactones; grosheimin; costunolide; primary cilia; ciliogenesis

Key Contribution: Natural compounds grosheimin; costunolide and α-, β- and γ-cyclocostunolides can modify primary cilia formation and represent an interesting possibility as drugs for the treatment of ciliopathies and/or tumors.

Citation: Murillo-Pineda, M.; Coto-Cid, J.M.; Romero, M.; Zorrilla, J.G.; Chinchilla, N.; Medina-Calzada, Z.; Varela, R.M.; Juárez-Soto, Á.; Macías, F.A.; Reales, E. Effects of Sesquiterpene Lactones on Primary Cilia Formation (Ciliogenesis). *Toxins* **2023**, *15*, 632. https://doi.org/10.3390/toxins15110632

Received: 6 September 2023
Revised: 22 October 2023
Accepted: 25 October 2023
Published: 27 October 2023

1. Introduction

The primary cilium (PC) is a single nonmotile organelle that projects from the cell surface in nearly all cell types [1,2]. It is made up of the ciliary membrane that surrounds a microtubule-based structure, the axoneme, which is nucleated from the basal body [3]. Analogous to an antenna, the cilium transduces chemical and mechanical external signals through membrane receptors localized in the ciliary membrane. Signaling pathways dependent on primary cilia include Sonic Hedgehog (Shh), Wingless/Int (WNT), and

Transforming Growth Factor-β (TGF-β), which are essential for proper tissue development and cell homeostasis [4]. The presence of cilium is regulated by the cell cycle, as PC emerges on G_0 (quiescent) or the early G_1 phase, and it is maintained until cells enter mitosis, being resorbed during G_2/M transition [5]. The formation of primary cilia (ciliogenesis) in non-polarized cells is a process highly regulated. Briefly, it starts with the attachment of the distal end of the mother centriole to a ciliary vesicle, which is mediated by the centriolar distal appendages. After docking, the ciliary vesicle grows with the axoneme and gives rise to the ciliary sheath, whose fusion with the plasma membrane results in the emergence of the cilium in the extracellular environment [6,7]. Once primary cilium is a mature surface-exposed cilium, the activation of cellular pathways that regulate the ciliary length and cilia assembly and disassembly are activated [5,8]. Thus, the PC is a result of coordinated trafficking, docking, and fusion of vesicle events that will define the unique composition of the ciliary membrane and the membrane domain at the base of the cilia. Many molecular details of these pathways remain unresolved.

Defects in PC and motile cilia function or formation are associated with a growing list of human developmental and degenerative disorders, collectively referred to as ciliopathies, that include Nephronophthisis (NPHP), Retinitis Pigmentosa (RP), Lebel Congenital Amaurosis (LCA), Bardet-Biedl Syndrome (BBS), Joubert Syndrome (JBTS), Primary Ciliary Dyskinesia (PCD), and Polycystic Kidney Disease (PKD) [9,10]. These ciliopathies present with diverse etiologies that include kidney disease, lung disorders, and loss of vision. Additionally, ciliary dysfunction is also associated with several types of cancer. It has been shown that in breast, prostate, and other cancer types, cilia loss is required for tumor progression; instead, in medulloblastoma and basal cell carcinoma, cilia retention or active ciliation is required [11,12]. Highly metastatic astroglioma cells have internal cilium precursors that fail to protrude, which may allow cancer cells to evade regulatory checkpoints [13]. Thus, there is a growing need to find new active compounds able to modify PC function to provide novel strategies for their treatment.

Natural products are important leads in drug discovery. Sesquiterpene lactones (SLs) constitute a large and diverse group of biologically active secondary metabolite plant chemicals [14,15]. They are terpenoids with a basic structure of 15 carbons, and their usual feature is a γ-lactonic ring that can also contain α-methylene groups, hydroxyls, esterified hydroxyls, or epoxides rings [16]. SLs and their derivatives show a promising role in drug development as they have promising anticancer and anti-inflammatory effects, antifungal, analgesic, antimalarial, and antimicrobial activities, among others, or they can be used in combination therapy as sensitizing agents to enhance the action of drugs in clinical use [15,17]. There are several structure–activity relationship analyses showing that several SLs react with thiols via rapid Michael-type addition. These reactions are mediated by the α- and β-unsaturated carbonyl systems and depend on the geometry of the molecule, although additionally, other factors such as lipophilicity and chemical environment may also influence the activity [18]. Although it has been described that SLs possess a broad spectrum of biological activities, the effect on PC formation or function has not been studied yet. Here, we report the capacity of the SLs grosheimin, costunolide, and α-, β-, and γ-cyclocostunolide to perturb primary cilium biogenesis in human retinal pigment epithelial (RPE) cells, a model of non-polarized retinal cells. Ciliogenesis can be induced by cell starvation during 24 h or accelerated by actin destabilization via cytochalasin D treatment. We observed a reduction in cilia percentage in RPE cells after treatment with all products tested under both cilia induction conditions without affecting cell cycle progression or cilia length. Interestingly, grosheimin showed an increase in cilia formation at the late stages of ciliogenesis, where cell pathways for cilia stabilization are activated. Altogether, we propose the potential of SLs to be investigated as drugs for the treatment of ciliopathies and/or tumors.

2. Results and Discussion

From a small library of plant allelochemicals synthesized previously in our lab and based on previous biological studies in human cells [19], two sesquiterpene lactones were selected to elucidate their function in cilia formation: grosheimin [20] isolated from a leaf extract from *Cynara scolymus*, and costunolide [21] isolated from a root extract from *Saussurea lappa*. From the former, three eudesmanolide-type sesquiterpene lactones were also obtained by cyclization reaction using *p*-TsOH (para-toluenesulfonic acid), generating three cyclocostunolides with a characteristic double bound located in different positions (α,β,γ) [22] (Figure 1), which are likewise natural products isolated from plants [23,24].

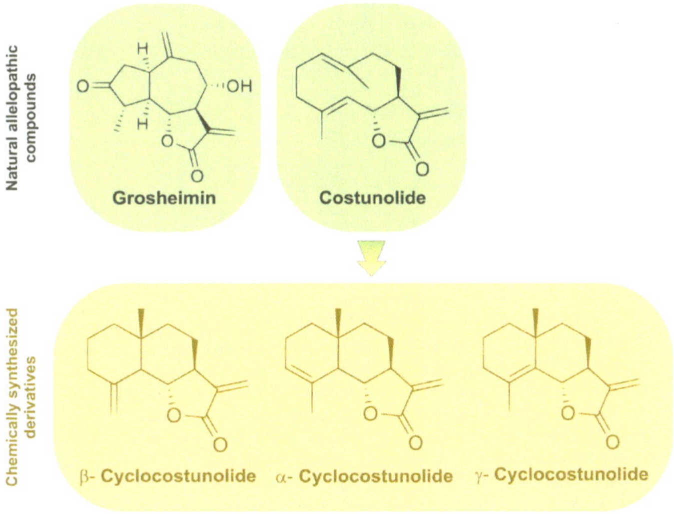

Figure 1. Test compounds used in this study. Natural sesquiterpene lactones isolated from plants are indicated at the top. From costunolide, the three plant-derived eudesmanolides shown at the bottom were synthetized.

2.1. *Effect of Sesquiterpene Lactones on Cell Viability and Cell Cycle Progression*

First, we evaluated the cytotoxicity of the products in telomerase-immortalized retinal pigment epithelial (RPE-1) cells, a well-known human cell line used to study primary cilia formation in non-polarized cells [25,26]. For determining the cell viability after treatment with the compounds, we used the crystal violet assay [27], a simple and widely used method to assess the impact of molecules on cell survival and growth inhibition. As crystal violet dye binds to proteins and DNA, it stains only living cells that are attached in the culture, and we can obtain the % of surviving cells under diverse stimulated conditions. RPE cells at high confluency (90–100%) were treated with SLs ranging from 1 to 25 μM final concentration for 24 h in a serum-free media, and cell viability was scored using the crystal violet assay. Treatment with solvent 0.1% DMSO was used as a control. All compounds tested showed no effect on cell viability at 10 μM concentration or below. Grosheimin (G), costunolide (C), and β-cyclocostunolide (β-C) were also innocuous at 25 μM, while α- and γ-cyclocostunolides (α-C; γ-C) showed around 60% viability decrease (Figure 2A). Most products displayed toxicity in RPE cells at concentrations exceeding 50 μM. For the rest of the experiments, 10 μM final concentration was selected to address effects on cell cycle and primary cilia formation, in order to maintain the highest cell viability in our ciliogenesis assays.

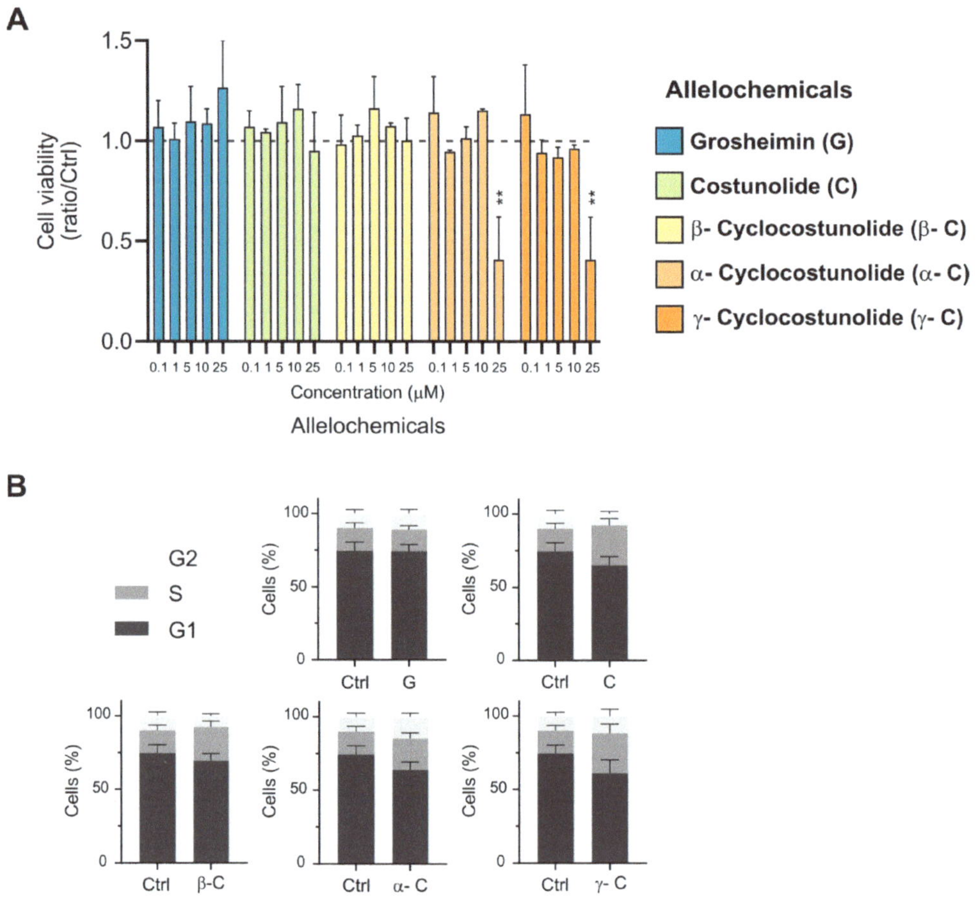

Figure 2. Effect of sesquiterpene lactones on cell viability and cell cycle progression in RPE cell line. (**A**) Effect of increasing concentration of the SLs on viability measured by crystal violet assay. On the right, color code and abbreviation panel indicating selected allelochemicals. Graph shows mean and SEM of 3 independent experiments of the viability ratio compared to control (DMSO-solvent 0.1%). Two-way ANOVA was performed, and significant differences are indicated when $p < 0.01$ (**). (**B**) SLs' effect on cell cycle progression in cells treated with products at 10 μM final concentration for 24 h in medium containing 0.5% serum. Propidium iodide-stained cells were analyzed by flow cytometry. Graph shows mean and SEM of 3 independent experiments. Multiple *t*-test analysis was performed, and no significant differences were detected.

The primary cilia life cycle is tightly coupled with the cell cycle. Cilia assemble in non-dividing quiescent or post-mitotic differentiated cells ($G0_0/G_1$ phases) and disassemble before entering mitosis [28]. Although the connection between the cell cycle and primary cilia is still under exploration, there appears to be a bidirectional crosstalk between cilium formation and cell division, as improper division can result in abnormal cilia formation and failure to form a cilium can regulate the cell cycle. For example, over-proliferative cancer cell lines generally lack cilia, and cells that cannot properly form a cilium undergo inappropriate cell division [29]. In addition, several studies have documented changes in cell cycle progression in the context of cancer cells under the effect of some SLs in the search for therapeutic anti-tumoral treatments. Such is the documented case for alantolactone or eremanthin, compounds that affect cell cycle progression, arresting cancer cells at the G_2 phase [30,31].

To test if the selected SLs have an effect on cell cycle progression in non-tumoral cells, we analyzed the cell cycle status of RPE cells treated with the test compounds for 24 h by flow cytometry analysis (Figure 2B). Cells were stained with the intercalating DNA dye propidium iodide, which allows the detection of cellular DNA content. Via flow cytometry, the DNA staining generates a histogram of fluorescence intensity that represents the distribution of cells in the different phases of the cell cycle (G_0/G_1, S, and G_2/M). Cell cycle analysis showed that the treatment with all the compounds tested in RPE cells during 24 h does not affect cell cycle progression. As compounds were added in a starvation medium which inhibits cell proliferation, cells were mostly arrested in the G_1 phase. These data indicate that incubation with the SLs grosheimin (G), costunolide (C), and α-, β-, and γ-cyclocostunolide at 10 μM does not perturb the cell cycle progression at tested conditions. The fact that the SLs under study in this work do not affect cell cycle progression suggests that any perturbation over ciliogenesis detected would be independent from the cell cycle.

2.2. *Effect of Sesquiterpene Lactones on Early Steps of Primary Cilia Formation*

PC formation in RPE cells can be induced by the absence of serum in the cell culture for at least 24–48 h [32]. Via live cell imaging, it has been described that newly forming and elongating internal cilia happen around the first 2–4 h after inducing cilia formation by starvation [25]. Once internal cilia are formed, it will fuse with the plasma membrane. Mature external primary cilia elongation and composition are maintained via different membrane trafficking pathways in the cell until it is disassembled to start a new cell cycle [33]. To determine the effect of the selected SLs on the early steps of ciliogenesis, RPE cells were serum starved by incubation for 24 h with a medium containing 0.5% serum to induce cilia formation, and tested compounds were added at the same time at 10 μM final concentration. PC (percentage and length) was analyzed using confocal immunofluorescence microscopy. Acetylated α-tubulin and γ-tubulin were used as a ciliary marker and centrosome marker, respectively. DAPI (4′,6-diamidino-2-phenylindole) fluorescent stain, which binds to DNA, was used for nucleus labeling. The addition of all SLs further affected early cilia formation in RPE cells. Grosheimin was the one with a percentage of primary cilia closer to control levels, and costunolide, β-cyclocostunolide and α-cyclocostunolide were the most dramatic ones showing less than 5% ciliated cells (Figure 3A,B). γ-cyclocostunolide showed a bimodal response as sometimes cells were similar to control levels (0.1% DMSO), and sometimes cells were not ciliated at all and even showed some DAPI phenotype indicative of cell damage (Figure 3A,B). We also measured the length of primary cilia, and there were no significant differences compared to the control condition for all tested compounds (Figure 3B), indicating that although cells treated with SLs can ciliate less in serum starvation conditions, the cells that manage to ciliate produce a normal-length cilium. No differences were observed for the centrosome labeling, except for cells treated with γ-cyclocostunolide, in which the centrosome has dispersed labeling, probably associated with cell damage or cytoskeleton damage. Further studies need to be conducted to know the reason for this phenotype.

Together, these findings described that the natural compounds grosheimin (G), costunolide (C), and α-, β-, and γ-cyclocostunolide are able to interrupt cilia formation in non-polarized and non-tumoral cells, without affecting the cell cycle progression (as shown in Figure 2B). Further work will be important to investigate the molecular target of the tested SLs and/or signaling pathways affected.

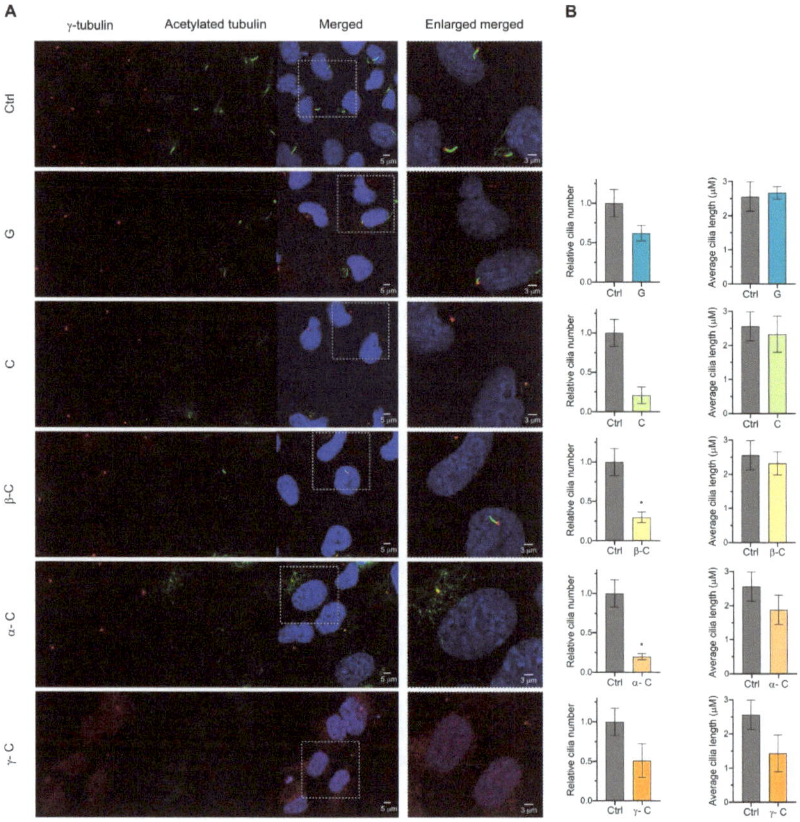

Figure 3. Effect of sesquiterpene lactones on primary cilia formation on RPE cell line. (**A**,**B**) RPE cells were incubated for 24 h with a medium containing 0.5% serum to induce cilia formation, and compounds at 10 μM final concentration were added at the same time. Ctrl: 0.1% DMSO. Immunofluorescence was performed using acetylated α-tubulin to label primary cilia and γ-tubulin to visualize the centrosome. Representative images for each condition are shown (**A**). Graph shows mean and SEM of 4 independent experiments of the ratio of ciliated cells and the average cilia length (**B**). Mann–Whitney test analysis was performed, and significant differences are indicated when $p < 0.05$ (*).

2.3. *Effect of Sesquiterpene Lactones on Primary Cilia Formation Induced by Cytochalasin D*

PC can also be induced by the actin polymerization inhibitor cytochalasin D (CytD), which facilitates ciliogenesis and promotes cilium elongation independently of serum starvation [32,34]. Cytochalasin D induces ciliogenesis at doses that do not affect stress fiber formation, excluding the possibility of global actin cytoskeleton rearrangement in ciliogenesis control. To examine the effect of the selected SLs on ciliogenesis induced by CytD and on actin dynamics, we treated RPE cells with CytD for 18 h together with the SLs grosheimin, costunolide, or α-, β-, and γ-cyclocostunolide. As expected, the addition of CytD and DMSO at the same time increased ciliated cells compared to DMSO-only treated cells (Figure 4A,B). The addition of all the SLs further affected cilia formation in a similar way as cilia-induced starvation conditions (Figure 3). Grosheimin showed less effect, while all the other compounds showed a decrease in the ratio to 0.4–0.5 (Figure 4B). The variability associated with γ-cyclocostunolide was not detected in this treatment, pointing to a cellular defect due to the addition of the compound under starvation conditions. We further measured the length of primary cilia, and we observed that there were no significant differences compared to the control condition (CytD and DMSO) for all tested compounds (Figure 4B). We also analyzed the cell cycle progression in CytD treatment conditions in RPE cells. It has been reported that CytD treatment inhibits the cell cycle progression from G_0 to S phase and also mitosis during cytokinesis [35,36]. Therefore, treatment of RPE cells with CytD for 18 h (control) showed an increase in the population with DNA content = 2, as cytokinesis blockage leads to the accumulation of tetraploid cells that in G_1 will have the same amount of DNA as diploid G_2 cells. Nevertheless, incubations with the allelochemicals plus CytD resulted in no effect on the profile compared to the control condition (Figure 4C).

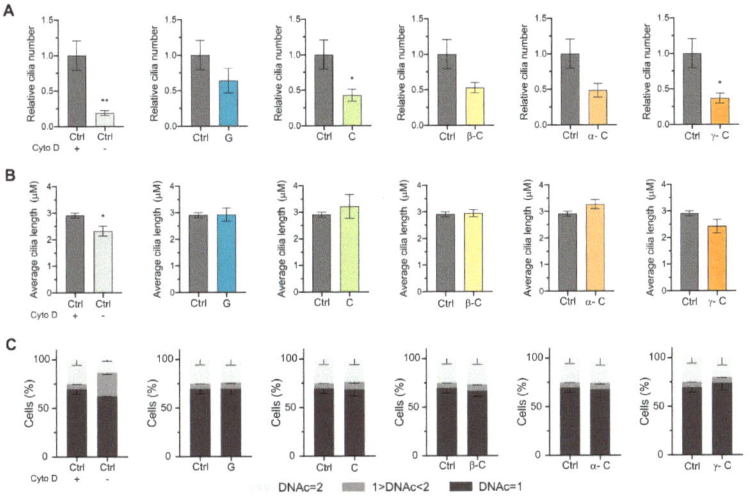

Figure 4. Effect of sesquiterpene lactones on primary cilia induced by cytochalasin D. (**A–C**) RPE cells were incubated for 18 h with cytochalasin D at 200 nM final concentration to induce primary cilia formation. Compounds at 10 µM final concentration were added at the same time. (**A**,**B**) Immunofluorescence was performed as in Figure 2. Graph shows mean and SEM of 6 independent experiments of the ratio of ciliated cells (**A**) or the average cilia length (**B**). Mann–Whitney test analysis was performed, and significant differences are indicated when $p < 0.05$ (*) or 0.01 (**). (**C**) Sesquiterpene lactones' effect on cell cycle under cytochalasin D treatment. Propidium iodide-stained cells were analyzed by flow cytometry. Graph shows mean and SEM of 3 independent experiments. Cytochalasin D blocks cytokinesis after chromosome divergence in anaphase of mitosis; therefore, cell cycle stage and DNAc are not unequivocally linked (ex. DNAc = 2 will contain G_2 and mitotic cells but also tetraploid cells that will be entering G_1).

Blocking actin assembly facilitates ciliogenesis by stabilizing a pericentrosomal preciliary compartment (PPC), a transient tubular and vesicular compartment in charge of sorting transmembrane proteins destined for cilia during the early ciliogenesis. It is observed after initiation of ciliogenesis (4 h after starvation) and disappears after 24 h serum starvation from the ciliary base. Previous studies have shown that CytD-treated cells promote PPC formation (in 2 h), facilitating both axoneme assembly and ciliary membrane biogenesis [32]. Because SLs block ciliogenesis induced by CytD and starvation, it is therefore tempting to speculate that the allelochemicals tested in this study may interfere in the formation and stabilization of the preciliary compartment, a process that involves fusion of transport of vesicles at the base of the cilia, via the recruitment of lipid and membrane proteins that enables the biogenesis of ciliary membrane and axoneme assembly.

2.4. Effect of Sesquiterpene Lactones on Late Steps of Ciliogenesis

Ciliogenesis requires enormous coordination of cell cycle regulatory signaling and the recruitment of ciliary proteins with proper stoichiometry. The final step of ciliogenesis is the extension of the ciliary axoneme and ciliary membrane. Its regulation is orchestrated by intracellular trafficking, intraflagellar transport (IFT), and autophagy, among others [37,38]. Because primary cilia are formed in quiescent cells and resorbed during the G_2/M transition, the coordination of these two processes must be highly robust. It has been shown that ciliary resorption is related to stress responses [39], cell cycle progression, and cell differentiation [28]. To see if SLs have an effect in maintaining the equilibrium between cilia assembly and disassembly and cilia extension, we also analyzed the effect of the compounds on the late phases of ciliogenesis, where primary cilia are already facing the extracellular media, axoneme is assembled, and ciliary membrane formed. Cells were serum-starved for 24 h to induce primary cilia formation, and compounds were added for an additional 24 h in the serum-starved medium. In these conditions, the grosheimin compound showed an increase in the ratio of total ciliated cells and α-cyclocostunolide and γ-cyclocostunolide a decrease (Figure 5A,B). For the latter products, α-cyclocostunolide and γ-cyclocostunolide, the reduction in cilia percentage was more than half compared to control. Cilia length was also evaluated (Figure 5B), and α-cyclocostunolide showed a reduction in the cilia length, while grosheimin, costunolide, and β-cyclocostunolide showed an increase, and γ-cyclocostunolide showed any difference. For γ-cyclocostunolide, we again detected significant differences among replicates ranging from no difference in cilia percentage to almost a 35% decrease (Figure 5B), indicating variability when cells are under the action of this product. The reason for this variability needs to be further studied.

The increase in the ciliated cells ratio and ciliary length found in cells treated with grosheimin at late stages of ciliogenesis, together with the decrease in percentage detected at early steps, suggests that grosheimin has a positive effect on the assembly and/or length of the primary cilia, promoting a higher rate of elongation and ciliary-assembly pathways than ciliary-disassembly ones. Given that grosheimin incubation does not affect cell viability or cell cycle progression, this could be a promising compound to specifically promote ciliogenesis. It could be studied in ciliopathies that result from abnormally short cilia or impaired ciliogenesis, such as Bardet-Biedl syndrome (BBS), Nephronophthisis (NPHP), Meckel syndrome (MKS), Joubert syndrome (JBTS), short-rib polydactyly syndrome, and cranioectodermal dysplasia syndrome [9]. Although investigations in primary cilia and disease have been conducted mainly in ciliopathies, some documented changes in ciliation have also been shown in cancer initiation and progression. Differences in ciliation between cancer cells and cells from the tumor microenvironment contribute to the growth of the tumor. In some cancer types, a loss of ciliation promotes oncogenesis and cancer-related signaling [40,41]. Cilia loss occurs during the early stages of breast, prostate, pancreatic, and other cancer types [29]. Knockdown of the gene encoding tubulin monoglycylase (TTLL3), which reduces the number of primary cilia and increases the proliferation of colon epithelial cells, strongly promotes the development of colorectal carcinomas in a mouse model [42]. In these types of tumors, grosheimin could be considered being studied as a new drug for treating tumors, increasing ciliogenesis, and reducing cell proliferation.

α-cyclocostunolide showed a reduction in both the ciliated cell ratio and cilia length compared to the control condition. This indicates a strong effect on the cilia elongation process and makes this compound an interesting tool to test in ciliopathy models such as asphyxiating thoracic dystrophy, where increased ciliogenesis is observed, as well as ciliopathies characterized by excessively long cilia such as juvenile cystic kidney disease [43] and tuberous sclerosis [44]. Following the same idea, treatment with α-cyclocostunolide that shows opposite effects might be interesting in conditions where cilia reduction is needed. For example, Sonic Hedgehog (SHH) signaling at primary cilia drives the proliferation and progression of a subset of medulloblastomas [45].

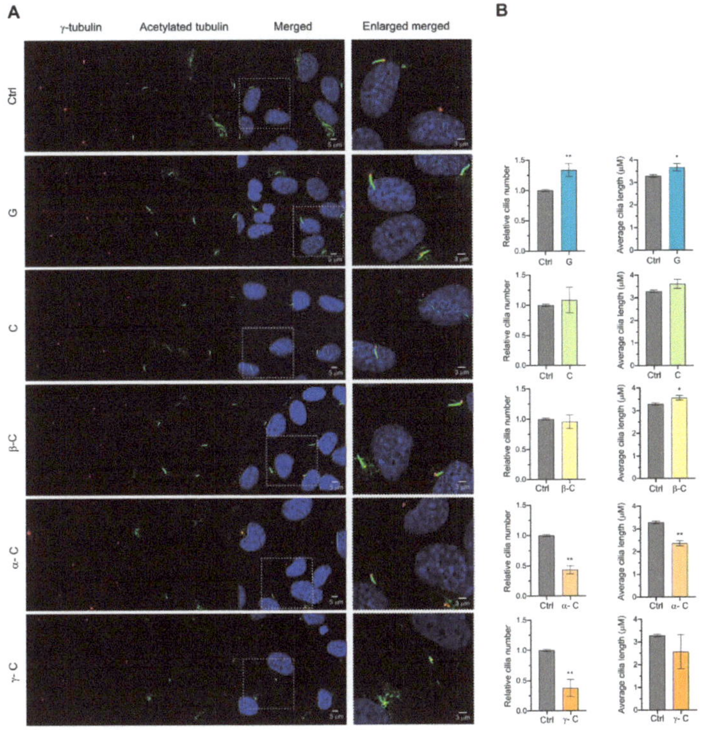

Figure 5. Effect of sesquiterpene lactones on assembled primary cilia. (**A**,**B**) RPE cells were incubated for 24 h in a medium containing 0.5% serum to induce primary cilia formation; then, compounds at 10 μM final concentration were added for an additional 24 h in a medium still containing 0.5% serum. Immunofluorescence was performed as in Figure 3. Representative images for each condition are shown (**A**). Graph shows mean and SEM of 5 independent experiments of the ratio of ciliated cells and the average cilia length (**B**). Mann–Whitney test analysis was performed, and significant differences are indicated when $p < 0.05$ (*), 0.01 (**).

3. Conclusions

The major function of primary cilia is to sense a variety of external stimuli, including flow, ligands, and light, to regulate cell homeostasis, proliferation, and differentiation. Ciliation varies during organismal development, and cells oscillate between ciliated and non-ciliated stages in cycling cells, where the presence of cilia antagonizes cell cycle progression [37]. Abnormalities in ciliogenesis result in cancer, pleiotropic disorders, and denominated ciliopathies, and no treatment options are currently available for the latter. In this study, we demonstrate for the first time that the sesquiterpene lactones grosheimin, costunolide, and α-, β-, and γ-cyclocostunolide can modify primary cilium formation in a cellular model of human normal non-polarized cells, RPE. The activity exhibited by SLs serves as a promising and expanding strategy for the treatment of diseases related to primary cilium dysfunction.

We propose that grosheimin, costunolide, and α-, β-, and γ-cyclocostunolide are able to block ciliogenesis via targeting proteins that are implicated in the early stages of ciliogenesis, where trafficking and docking of ciliary membranes to the mother centriole happens (Figure 6). Growing evidence indicates that some oncogenic signaling pathways induce ciliation while others repress it. Finding new chemicals capable of blocking cilia formation would be useful in tumors where tumor cell growth is dependent on ciliary signaling. The new function of SLs on cilia formation, shown in this work, encourages further studies on the development of new anticancer drugs with a γ-lactone ring that had primary cilia as a target. Further work is needed to identify the SL targets and effects on tumor cells.

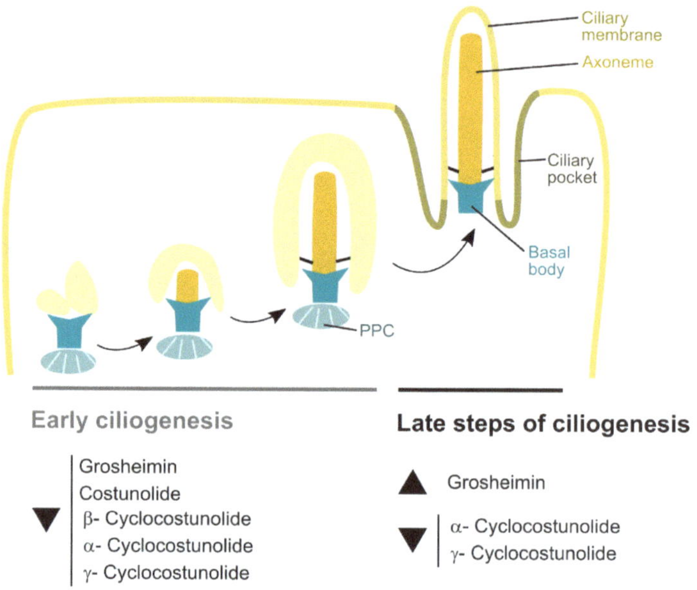

Figure 6. Model of action of SLs on ciliogenesis. The image depicts the SLs that decrease or increase the process of ciliogenesis in RPE cells after 24 h treatment. In early ciliogenesis, products are added at the same time as primary cilia induction by serum starvation or CytD treatment. In the late steps of ciliogenesis, products are added to the cell culture after 24 h of cilia induction by serum starvation.

Interestingly, at the late steps of ciliogenesis, where axoneme and ciliary membrane stabilization and elongation happens, the effect of grosheimin is the opposite, promoting ciliogenesis and elongation of primary cilium in normal cells (Figure 6). This suggests a specific effect of grosheimin in promoting cilia assembly against disassembly, pointing out a cellular function specific to the molecule, perhaps related to the -thiols group on its structure. Primary cilium dysfunction diseases exhibit little genotype–phenotype relationship. Mutations in a single gene can be implicated in multiple distinct ciliopathies affecting multiple organs with variable manifestations. Compounds that target disease-associated symptoms or cilia biogenesis are developed as an alternative therapeutic approach. This preliminary result showing that grosheimin promotes cilia assembly encourages further studies with this compound to be tested in cellular models of disease and to be studied as a therapy to treat ciliopathies and tumor growth.

Ciliopathies and diseases exhibiting affected ciliary function are increasing, and identifying modulators of ciliogenesis to connect ciliogenesis with other basic cellular processes assumes increasing importance. Much more work is required to address SL molecular targets and solubility in order to increase our knowledge of primary cilium function and structure and create new therapies for ciliary dysfunction diseases, an emerging field of study.

4. Materials and Methods

4.1. Plant Material and Extraction and Isolation of Test Compounds

Reactions were quality assessed via analytical thin layer chromatography on precoated silica gel 60 F254 glass plates (Merck, Rahway, NJ, USA) in the normal phase and

60 RP-18 F254S (Merck) in the reverse phase. Compound detection was carried out via exposition to UV (λ = 254 nm) using oil (CH_3COOH: H_2O: H_2SO_4 4:20:1) and thermic treatment (250 °C).

Product purification was conducted via (i) column chromatography with silica gel Merck 60 (pore size 0.063–0.0200 mm, 0.040–0.063 mm) using gravity elution with the indicated compounds; (ii) semi-preparative HPLC using LiChrospher (Torrance, CA, USA) 100 RP-18 (10 μm) in reverse phase in Merck-Hitachi with refraction index detector equipment; and (iii) solid phase extraction (SPE) using StraraTM-X (Não-Me-Toque, Brazil) (33 μm Polimeric Reverse Phase, 200 mg/3 mL). Organic solvents and reagents were obtained from Fisher Chemical® (Waltham, MA, USA), VWR, Panreac® (Castellar del Vallès, Spain), and Sigma-Aldrich® (St. Louis, MO, USA). Synthesized compounds were identified using NMR spectra in chloroform-d using AGILENT®-500 MHz equipment (Santa Clara, CA, USA). Spectra obtained were one-dimensional ^{1}H-RMN and ^{13}C-RMN and two-dimensional ^{1}H-COSY (^{1}H-^{1}H correlation) and HSQC (^{1}H-^{13}C correlation).

Costunolide ((3a*S*,6*E*,10*E*,11a*R*)-6,10-dimethyl-3-methylene-3a,4,5,8,9,11a-hexahydro cyclodeca[*b*]furan-2(3*H*)-one) was isolated from a root extract from *Saussurea lappa* purchased from Pierre Chauvet S.A. (Seillans, France). A total of 50 g of *S. lappa* root extract was dissolved in CH_2Cl_2 and fractioned by column chromatography using *n*-hexane (0.6 mL) as first eluent, and then a mixture of *n*-hexane/AcOEt 95:5 (6 L) [46]. Those fractions containing costunolide, according to thin-layer chromatography analysis, were further purified by column chromatography using *n*-hexane/AcOEt 95:5 to obtain costunolide in a total amount of 2.3 g (4.6%). Spectroscopy data were in agreement with those already reported for costunolide [47].

Grosheimin ((3a*S*,6a*R*,9*S*,9a*R*,9b*R*)-9-methyl-3,6-dimethyleneoctahydroazuleno[4,5-*b*]furan-2,8(3*H*,4*H*)-dione) was isolated from a leaf extract from Cynara scolymus. An amount of 12.5 g of C. scolymus leaf extract was dissolved in EtOAc. Colum chromatography separation with hexane/acetone 70:30 to 20:80 was performed and the eluted fraction containing the lactones was separated again using n-hexane/acetone 60:40. The fraction were monitored with analytical thin layer chromatography using H_2O:acetone 60:40 and the fraction with less polar products was extracted by SPE using H_2O:acetone 35% obtaining grosheimin (9.2 mg and 0.07%). Spectroscopy data were in agreement with those already reported for grosheimin [48].

4.2. Semi-Synthesis

Isolated costunolide (120 mg, 0.517 mmol) was stirred in CH_2Cl_2 (5 mL), and p-TsOH (para-toluenesulfonic acid; 24.3 mg, 0.141 mmol) was added for cyclization reaction at room temperature for 4 h [49]. The crude mixture was diluted with CH_2Cl_2 (20 mL) and treated with $NaHCO_3$-saturated aqueous solution (25 mL). The organic phase was separated, and the aqueous phase was washed with CH_2Cl_2 (3 × 25 mL). The organic phases were pulled together for neutralization with the NaCl aqueous solution (100 mL). The organic phase was separated again, and aqueous residues were removed with Na_2SO_4 addition. The solution was gravity-filtered and concentrated under reduced pressure before purification by column chromatography. The eluant used was n-hexane/AcOEt 95:5. Products by elution order are as follows: γ-cyclocostunolide (8.2 mg, 7% yield: (3a*S*,5a*R*,9b*S*)-5a,9-dimethyl-3-methylene-3a,4,5,5a,6,7,8,9b-octahydronaphtho[1,2-*b*]furan-2(3*H*)-one)), α-cyclocostunolide (42.0 mg, 35% yield: (3a*S*,5a*R*,9b*S*)-5a,9-dimethyl-3-methylene-3a,4,5,5a,6,7,9a,9b-octahydronaph tho[1,2-*b*]furan-2(3*H*)-one)), and β-cyclocostunolide (65.9 mg, 55% yield: (3a*S*,5a*R*,9b*S*)-5a-methyl-3,9-dimethylenedecahydronaphtho[1,2-*b*]furan-2(3*H*)-one)). Spectroscopy data were in agreement with those already reported for α-, β-, and γ-cyclocostunolide [49].

4.3. Cell Culture Conditions and Biological Assays

The human cell line used was hTERT-immortalized retinal pigment epithelial cells (hTERT RPE-1) provided by Dr. Fernando Balestra at Cabimer, Seville, Spain. Cells were grown at 37 °C, 5% CO_2 in DMEM/F-12 containing L-glutamine and 15 mM HEPES cell culture media. Media was supplemented with 10% FBS, 100 U/mL penicillin, 100 μg/mL streptomycin, and 3 μg/mL ciprofloxacin (NORMON laboratories).

For cilia experiments, cells were seeded at a density of 70,000 cells/well in 12-well plates, and the following day, cilia were induced by incubating cells for 24 h with media supplemented only with 0.5% FBS. In experiments aimed to see the effect of test compounds in cilia formation, test compounds were added at the same time as the 0.5% FBS media at a final concentration of 10 μM. In experiments aimed to see the effect of test compounds in established cilia, after incubating cells for 24 h in 0.5% FBS media, test compounds were added for an additional 24 h in 0.5% FBS media at a final concentration of 10 μM. For all experiments, DMSO was added as the control condition (as test compounds are diluted in DMSO stock solution). For cytochalasin D treatment, cells were seeded as above, and the following day, cilia were induced by incubating cells for 18 h with 200 nM cytochalasin D. Test compounds were added at the same time at a final concentration of 10 μM. DMSO was added as the control condition. For cell viability, cells were seeded at a density of 15,000 cells/well in 96-well plates, and the following day, media was changed to media supplemented only with 0.5% FBS and test compounds at different final concentrations or DMSO as a control. After incubating for 24 h, cells were washed with 1X PBS and fixed with 1% glutaraldehyde (in 1X PBS) for 20–30 min. Then, after another 1X PBS wash, crystal violet 0.1% (in H_2O) solution was added for another 20–30 min. Finally, after one wash with H_2O, plates were left to dry. To quantify % of cell viability, stained fixed cells were resuspended with 10% acetic acid (CH_3COOH) solution, and absorbance was measured at 590 nm in a plate reader (sometimes samples were additionally diluted 1/10 in 10% acetic acid to obtain values within the range of the plate reader). Cell viability was calculated as a percentage of the viability of control cells treated with DMSO.

4.4. *Immunofluorescence (IF)*

Cells were seeded onto coverslips in 12-well plates, and cilia experiments were performed as indicated above. For IF, coverslips were fixed with −20 °C cold methanol for 10 min at −20 °C, washed with 1X PBS, and blocked for 1h at RT in IF blocking buffer (5% [*wt/vol*] BSA, 0.05% [*vol/vol*] Tween in 1X PBS). Cells were incubated with primary antibody diluted in IF blocking buffer overnight at 4 °C. Coverslips were washed three times for 5 min at room temperature in 1X PBS containing 0.05% (*vol/vol*) Tween and incubated with secondary fluorescent antibody diluted in blocking buffer for 1h at RT. Coverslips were washed three times again, incubated with DAPI (Sigma), washed with 1X PBS, and mounted in the glycerol-based 2.5% [*wt/vol*] PVA-DABCO mounting medium for imaging. Primary antibodies used for staining: γ-tubulin (at concentration 1:1000) from Sigma T3559 and acetylated-tubulin (1:2000) from Sigma T7451; Secondary antibodies: Alexa (San Fancisco, CA, USA) 488 conjugated anti-mouse A32723 from Invitrogen (Waltham, MA, USA) and Alexa 568 conjugated anti-rabbit A11011 from Invitrogen. Both were used at 1:500. DAPI was used as a final concentration of 5 μg/mL for 5 min.

4.5. *Microscopy*

Images were collected at room temperature on a Zeiss (Oberkochen, Germany) LSM 900 inverted confocal microscope using a 40X 1.3 NA oil-immersion objective controlled with Zeiss ZEN software 3.2. Images were collected as 0.5-μm z sections. Images presented in the figures are maximum intensity projections. Fluorophores imaged are those conjugated to secondary antibodies listed above. Images were z-stacked and changed to jpg format using Fiji software 1.53c [27] and subsequently analyzed for cilia proportion and cilia length both manually using Fiji software 1.53c and semi-automatized ACDC software_v0.93 [28] run in MATLAB R2016b (Windows OS). A >4 times magnification of the image is also included for better visualization of the cilia and/or centrosome.

4.6. Cell Cycle Analysis and Flow Cytometry

For cell cycle analysis, after the indicated treatments, cells were collected and fixed in cold 70% ethanol for at least 30 min at 4 °C. Then, cells were centrifuged, washed with 1X PBS, centrifuged, and treated with RNAse in 1X PBS at a final concentration of 100 µg/mL for at least 1 h at 37 °C. Finally, propidium iodide was added at a final concentration of 50 µg/mL and incubated, protected from light for at least 1 h before cytometry. Cells were analyzed in a BD FACS Celesta SORP (Franklin Lakes, NJ, USA) with Diva software 9.0. Forward scatter (FS) and side scatter (SS) were used to identify single cells, and PI was visualized using the yellow/green laser with excitation at 561 nm (PI maximum emission 605 nm). Cell cycle analysis was performed using the cell cycle tool of FlowJo software v10.8.1.

4.7. Statistical Analysis

All experiments were performed at least in triplicates (when $n > 3$, it is indicated in figure legend), and in each experiment for each condition, around 100 cells were analyzed. Data are expressed as a ratio between the mean values compared to the DMSO control and the standard deviation of the mean (SEM). Data statistics were analyzed in GraphPad Prism. We used Mann–Whitney test analysis to identify any difference between two means (test condition and control) that is greater than the expected standard error. For cell viability experiments, we performed a two-way ANOVA analysis, and for cell cycle experiments, a multiple *t*-test analysis comparing G_1-S-G_2 values for each test condition versus control. The p values are indicated within the figures.

Author Contributions: Conceptualization, E.R., M.M.-P. and F.A.M.; methodology, M.M.-P. and E.R.; validation, M.M.-P. and E.R.; formal analysis, M.M.-P., M.R. and E.R.; investigation, M.M.-P., J.M.C.-C., M.R. and J.G.Z.; resources, N.C., R.M.V. and Z.M.-C.; data curation, M.M.-P. and E.R.; writing—original draft preparation, M.M.-P. and E.R.; writing—review and editing, M.M.-P., E.R., J.M.C.-C., J.G.Z., N.C. and F.A.M.; visualization, M.M.-P. and E.R.; supervision, E.R. and F.A.M.; project administration, E.R., Á.J.-S. and F.A.M.; funding acquisition, E.R. and Á.J.-S. All authors have read and agreed to the published version of the manuscript.

Funding: This work has been co-financed by (1) the European Union under the 2014-2020 ERDF Operational Programme and by the Department of Economic Transformation, Industry, Knowledge and Universities of the Regional Government of Andalusia. Project reference: FEDER-UCA18-108266 and (2) by the Integrated Territorial Initiative 2014-2020 for the Province of Cádiz, ITI-FEDER Funds (ITI-0020-2019). M.R. was the recipient of a grant for young researchers within the Operational Programme for young employability POEJ 2014-2020 and the young employability initiative YEI (POEJ-TU 2021).

Institutional Review Board Statement: Not applicable.

Informed Consent Statement: Not applicable.

Data Availability Statement: Not applicable.

Acknowledgments: The authors would like to thank INiBICA and the members of the Allelopathy lab at the University of Cadiz for helping in the compound synthesis. We are very grateful to Balestra at CABIMER for providing us with the cell line RPE. J.G.Z. thanks to the University of Cadiz for the postdoctoral support with the Margarita Salas fellowship (2021-067/PN/MS-RECUAL/CD), funded by the NextGenerationEU programme of the European Union.

Conflicts of Interest: The authors declare no conflict of interest.

References

1. Sung, C.H.; Leroux, M.R. The roles of evolutionarily conserved functional modules in cilia-related trafficking. *Nat. Cell Biol.* **2013**, *15*, 1387–1397. [CrossRef] [PubMed]
2. Mill, P.; Christensen, S.T.; Pedersen, L.B. Primary cilia as dynamic and diverse signalling hubs in development and disease. *Nat. Rev. Genet.* **2023**, *24*, 421–441. [CrossRef] [PubMed]
3. Pedersen, L.B.; Schroder, J.M.; Satir, P.; Christensen, S.T. The ciliary cytoskeleton. *Compr. Physiol.* **2012**, *2*, 779–803. [CrossRef] [PubMed]

4. Kiseleva, A.A.; Korobeynikov, V.A.; Nikonova, A.S.; Zhang, P.; Makhov, P.; Deneka, A.Y.; Einarson, M.B.; Serebriiskii, I.G.; Liu, H.; Peterson, J.R.; et al. Unexpected Activities in Regulating Ciliation Contribute to off-target Effects of Targeted Drugs. *Clin. Cancer Res.* **2019**, *25*, 4179–4193. [CrossRef] [PubMed]
5. Goto, H.; Inaba, H.; Inagaki, M. Mechanisms of ciliogenesis suppression in dividing cells. *Cell. Mol. Life Sci.* **2017**, *74*, 881–890. [CrossRef] [PubMed]
6. Shakya, S.; Westlake, C.J. Recent advances in understanding assembly of the primary cilium membrane. *Fac. Rev.* **2021**, *10*, 16. [CrossRef] [PubMed]
7. Goetz, S.C.; Anderson, K.V. The primary cilium: A signalling centre during vertebrate development. *Nat. Rev. Genet.* **2010**, *11*, 331–344. [CrossRef] [PubMed]
8. Rivera-Molina, F.E.; Xi, Z.; Reales, E.; Wang, B.; Toomre, D. Exocyst complex mediates recycling of internal cilia. *Curr. Biol.* **2021**, *31*, 5580–5589.e5. [CrossRef]
9. Hildebrandt, F.; Benzing, T.; Katsanis, N. Ciliopathies. *N. Engl. J. Med.* **2011**, *364*, 1533–1543. [CrossRef]
10. Focsa, I.O.; Budisteanu, M.; Balgradean, M. Clinical and genetic heterogeneity of primary ciliopathies (Review). *Int. J. Mol. Med.* **2021**, *48*, 176. [CrossRef]
11. Liu, H.; Kiseleva, A.A.; Golemis, E.A. Ciliary signalling in cancer. *Nat. Rev. Cancer* **2018**, *18*, 511–524. [CrossRef]
12. Khan, N.A.; Garg, A.D.; Agostinis, P.; Swinnen, J.V. Drug-induced ciliogenesis in pancreatic cancer cells is facilitated by the secreted ATP-purinergic receptor signaling pathway. *Oncotarget* **2018**, *9*, 3507–3518. [CrossRef] [PubMed]
13. Moser, J.J.; Fritzler, M.J.; Rattner, J.B. Primary ciliogenesis defects are associated with human astrocytoma/glioblastoma cells. *BMC Cancer* **2009**, *9*, 448. [CrossRef] [PubMed]
14. Macias, F.A.; Fernandez, A.; Varela, R.M.; Molinillo, J.M.; Torres, A.; Alves, P.L. Sesquiterpene lactones as allelochemicals. *J. Nat. Prod.* **2006**, *69*, 795–800. [CrossRef] [PubMed]
15. Cheikh, I.A.; El-Baba, C.; Youssef, A.; Saliba, N.A.; Ghantous, A.; Darwiche, N. Lessons learned from the discovery and development of the sesquiterpene lactones in cancer therapy and prevention. *Expert Opin. Drug Discov.* **2022**, *17*, 1377–1405. [CrossRef] [PubMed]
16. Sut, S.; Maggi, F.; Nicoletti, M.; Baldan, V.; Dall Acqua, S. New Drugs from Old Natural Compounds: Scarcely Investigated Sesquiterpenes as New Possible Therapeutic Agents. *Curr. Med. Chem.* **2018**, *25*, 1241–1258. [CrossRef]
17. Coricello, A.; Adams, J.D.; Lien, E.J.; Nguyen, C.; Perri, F.; Williams, T.J.; Aiello, F. A Walk in Nature: Sesquiterpene Lactones as Multi-Target Agents Involved in Inflammatory Pathways. *Curr. Med. Chem.* **2020**, *27*, 1501–1514. [CrossRef] [PubMed]
18. Bosco, A.; Golsteyn, R.M. Emerging Anti-Mitotic Activities and Other Bioactivities of Sesquiterpene Compounds upon Human Cells. *Molecules* **2017**, *22*, 459. [CrossRef]
19. Mejias, F.J.R.; Duran, A.G.; Zorrilla, J.G.; Varela, R.M.; Molinillo, J.M.G.; Valdivia, M.M.; Macias, F.A. Acyl Derivatives of Eudesmanolides to Boost their Bioactivity: An Explanation of Behavior in the Cell Membrane Using a Molecular Dynamics Approach. *ChemMedChem* **2021**, *16*, 1297–1307. [CrossRef]
20. Mejias, F.J.R.; Fernandez, I.P.; Rial, C.; Varela, R.M.; Molinillo, J.M.G.; Calvino, J.J.; Trasobares, S.; Macias, F.A. Encapsulation of Cynara Cardunculus Guaiane-type Lactones in Fully Organic Nanotubes Enhances Their Phytotoxic Properties. *J. Agric. Food Chem.* **2022**, *70*, 3644–3653. [CrossRef]
21. Cardenas, D.M.; Mejias, F.J.R.; Molinillo, J.M.G.; Macias, F.A. Synthesis of Vlasouliolides: A Pathway toward Guaiane-Eudesmane C(17)/C(15) Dimers by Photochemical and Michael Additions. *J. Org. Chem.* **2020**, *85*, 7322–7332. [CrossRef] [PubMed]
22. Choodej, S.; Pudhom, K.; Mitsunaga, T. Inhibition of TNF-alpha-Induced Inflammation by Sesquiterpene Lactones from Saussurea lappa and Semi-Synthetic Analogues. *Planta Med.* **2018**, *84*, 329–335. [CrossRef] [PubMed]
23. Masoodi, R.H.a.M.H. Saussurea lappa: A Comprehensive Review on its Pharmacological Activity and Phytochemistry. *Curr. Tradit. Med.* **2020**, *6*, 13–23. [CrossRef]
24. Toyota, M.; Nagashima, F.; Asakawa, Y. Labdane type diterpenoids from the liverwort Frullania hamachiloba. *Phytochemistry* **1998**, *27*, 1789–1793. [CrossRef]
25. Lu, Q.; Insinna, C.; Ott, C.; Stauffer, J.; Pintado, P.A.; Rahajeng, J.; Baxa, U.; Walia, V.; Cuenca, A.; Hwang, Y.S.; et al. Early steps in primary cilium assembly require EHD1/EHD3-dependent ciliary vesicle formation. *Nat. Cell Biol.* **2015**, *17*, 228–240. [CrossRef] [PubMed]
26. Kukic, I.; Rivera-Molina, F.; Toomre, D. The IN/OUT assay: A new tool to study ciliogenesis. *Cilia* **2016**, *5*, 23. [CrossRef] [PubMed]
27. Feoktistova, M.; Geserick, P.; Leverkus, M. Crystal Violet Assay for Determining Viability of Cultured Cells. *Cold Spring Harb. Protoc.* **2016**, *2016*, 343–346. [CrossRef] [PubMed]
28. Plotnikova, O.V.; Golemis, E.A.; Pugacheva, E.N. Cell cycle-dependent ciliogenesis and cancer. *Cancer Res.* **2008**, *68*, 2058–2061. [CrossRef]
29. Kiseleva, A.A.; Nikonova, A.S.; Golemis, E.A. Patterns of Ciliation and Ciliary Signaling in Cancer. *Rev. Physiol. Biochem. Pharmacol.* **2023**, *185*, 87–105. [CrossRef]
30. Liu, T.; Zhao, X.; Song, D.; Liu, Y.; Kong, W. Anticancer activity of Eremanthin against the human cervical cancer cells is due to G2/M phase cell cycle arrest, ROS-mediated necrosis-like cell death and inhibition of PI3K/AKT signalling pathway. *J. BUON* **2020**, *25*, 1547–1553.

31. Zhang, Y.; Zhao, Y.; Ran, Y.; Guo, J.; Cui, H.; Liu, S. Alantolactone exhibits selective antitumor effects in HELA human cervical cancer cells by inhibiting cell migration and invasion, G2/M cell cycle arrest, mitochondrial mediated apoptosis and targeting Nf-kB signalling pathway. *J. BUON* **2019**, *24*, 2310–2315. [PubMed]
32. Kim, J.; Lee, J.E.; Heynen-Genel, S.; Suyama, E.; Ono, K.; Lee, K.; Ideker, T.; Aza-Blanc, P.; Gleeson, J.G. Functional genomic screen for modulators of ciliogenesis and cilium length. *Nature* **2010**, *464*, 1048–1051. [CrossRef] [PubMed]
33. Pugacheva, E.N.; Jablonski, S.A.; Hartman, T.R.; Henske, E.P.; Golemis, E.A. HEF1-dependent Aurora A activation induces disassembly of the primary cilium. *Cell* **2007**, *129*, 1351–1363. [CrossRef]
34. Smith, C.E.L.; Lake, A.V.R.; Johnson, C.A. Primary Cilia, Ciliogenesis and the Actin Cytoskeleton: A Little Less Resorption, a Little More Actin Please. *Front. Cell Dev. Biol.* **2020**, *8*, 622822. [CrossRef] [PubMed]
35. Ohta, T.; Takasuka, T.; Ishibashi, S.; Ide, T. Cytochalasin D inhibits the progression from the Go to S phase at the mid-prereplicative stage in GC-7 cells stimulated with serum. *Cell Struct. Funct.* **1985**, *10*, 37–46. [CrossRef]
36. Trendowski, M. Using cytochalasins to improve current chemotherapeutic approaches. *Anticancer Agents Med. Chem.* **2015**, *15*, 327–335. [CrossRef] [PubMed]
37. Avasthi, P.; Marshall, W.F. Stages of ciliogenesis and regulation of ciliary length. *Differentiation* **2012**, *83*, S30–S42. [CrossRef]
38. Pedersen, L.B.; Rosenbaum, J.L. Intraflagellar transport (IFT) role in ciliary assembly, resorption and signalling. *Curr. Top. Dev. Biol.* **2008**, *85*, 23–61. [CrossRef]
39. Luo, M.; Cao, M.; Kan, Y.; Li, G.; Snell, W.; Pan, J. The phosphorylation state of an aurora-like kinase marks the length of growing flagella in Chlamydomonas. *Curr. Biol.* **2011**, *21*, 586–591. [CrossRef]
40. Hassounah, N.B.; Nagle, R.; Saboda, K.; Roe, D.J.; Dalkin, B.L.; McDermott, K.M. Primary cilia are lost in preinvasive and invasive prostate cancer. *PLoS ONE* **2013**, *8*, e68521. [CrossRef]
41. Hassounah, N.B.; Nunez, M.; Fordyce, C.; Roe, D.; Nagle, R.; Bunch, T.; McDermott, K.M. Inhibition of Ciliogenesis Promotes Hedgehog Signaling, Tumorigenesis, and Metastasis in Breast Cancer. *Mol. Cancer Res.* **2017**, *15*, 1421–1430. [CrossRef] [PubMed]
42. Rocha, C.; Papon, L.; Cacheux, W.; Marques Sousa, P.; Lascano, V.; Tort, O.; Giordano, T.; Vacher, S.; Lemmers, B.; Mariani, P.; et al. Tubulin glycylases are required for primary cilia, control of cell proliferation and tumor development in colon. *EMBO J.* **2014**, *33*, 2247–2260. [CrossRef]
43. Sohara, E.; Luo, Y.; Zhang, J.; Manning, D.K.; Beier, D.R.; Zhou, J. Nek8 regulates the expression and localization of polycystin-1 and polycystin-2. *J. Am. Soc. Nephrol.* **2008**, *19*, 469–476. [CrossRef] [PubMed]
44. DiBella, L.M.; Park, A.; Sun, Z. Zebrafish Tsc1 reveals functional interactions between the cilium and the TOR pathway. *Hum. Mol. Genet.* **2009**, *18*, 595–606. [CrossRef] [PubMed]
45. Conduit, S.E.; Ramaswamy, V.; Remke, M.; Watkins, D.N.; Wainwright, B.J.; Taylor, M.D.; Mitchell, C.A.; Dyson, J.M. A compartmentalized phosphoinositide signaling axis at cilia is regulated by INPP5E to maintain cilia and promote Sonic Hedgehog medulloblastoma. *Oncogene* **2017**, *36*, 5969–5984. [CrossRef] [PubMed]
46. Zorrilla, J.G.; Rial, C.; Varela, R.M.; Molinillo, J.M.G.; Macías, F.A. Facile synthesis of anhydrojudaicin and 11,13-dehydroanhydrojudaicin, two eudesmanolide-skeleton lactones with potential allelopathic activity. *Phytochem. Lett.* **2019**, *31*, 229–236. [CrossRef]
47. Rao Vadaparthi, P.R.; Kumar, K.; Sarma, V.U.; Hussain, Q.A.; Babu, K.S. Estimation of Costunolide and Dehydrocostus Lactone in Saussurea lappa and its Polyherbal Formulations followed by their Stability Studies Using HPLC-DAD. *Pharmacogn. Mag.* **2015**, *11*, 180–190. [CrossRef]
48. Yayli, N.; Baltaci, C.; Gök, Y.; Aydin, E.; Üçüncü, O. Sesquiterpene lactones from Centaurea helenioides Boiss. *Turk. J. Chem.* **2006**, *30*, 229–233.
49. Cala, A.; Zorrilla, J.G.; Rial, C.; Molinillo, J.M.G.; Varela, R.M.; Macias, F.A. Easy Access to Alkoxy, Amino, Carbamoyl, Hydroxy, and Thiol Derivatives of Sesquiterpene Lactones and Evaluation of Their Bioactivity on Parasitic Weeds. *J. Agric. Food Chem.* **2019**, *67*, 10764–10773. [CrossRef]

toxins

MDPI

Review

Bioactive Metabolite Production in the Genus *Pyrenophora* (Pleosporaceae, Pleosporales)

Marco Masi [1,†], Jesús García Zorrilla [1,2,†] and Susan Meyer [3,*,†]

1 Department of Chemical Sciences, University of Naples "Federico II", Complesso Universitario Monte S. Angelo, Via Cintia 4, 80126 Napoli, Italy
2 Allelopathy Group, Department of Organic Chemistry, Facultad de Ciencias, Institute of Biomolecules (INBIO), University of Cadiz, C/Avenida República Saharaui, s/n, 11510 Puerto Real, Spain
3 Shrub Sciences Laboratory, U.S. Forest Service Rocky Mountain Research Station, 735 North 500 East, Provo, UT 84606, USA
* Correspondence: susan.meyer@usda.gov
† These authors equally contributed to this work.

Abstract: The genus *Pyrenophora* includes two important cereal crop foliar pathogens and a large number of less well-known species, many of which are also grass pathogens. Only a few of these have been examined in terms of secondary metabolite production, yet even these few species have yielded a remarkable array of bioactive metabolites that include compounds produced through each of the major biosynthetic pathways. There is little overlap among species in the compounds identified. *Pyrenophora tritici-repentis* produces protein toxin effectors that mediate host-specific responses as well as spirocyclic lactams and at least one anthraquinone. *Pyrenophora teres* produces marasmine amino acid and isoquinoline derivatives involved in pathogenesis on barley as well as nonenolides with antifungal activity, while *P. semeniperda* produces cytochalasans and sesquiterpenoids implicated in pathogenesis on seeds as well as spirocyclic lactams with phytotoxic and antibacterial activity. Less well-known species have produced some unusual macrocyclic compounds in addition to a diverse array of anthraquinones. For the three best-studied species, in silico genome mining has predicted the existence of biosynthetic pathways for a much larger array of potentially toxic secondary metabolites than has yet been produced in culture. Most compounds identified to date have potentially useful biological activity.

Keywords: *Pyrenophora*; toxins; biological activity; phytotoxicity; pathogenicity; biomolecules

Key Contribution: (1) Review of the biology, pathogenicity, and toxic metabolites produced by the most relevant *Pyrenophora* species; (2) classification of the toxic metabolites in a table according to their structures, with descriptions of the main agronomic and pharmacological activities reported for them.

Citation: Masi, M.; Zorrilla, J.G.; Meyer, S. Bioactive Metabolite Production in the Genus *Pyrenophora* (Pleosporaceae, Pleosporales). *Toxins* **2022**, *14*, 588. https://doi.org/10.3390/toxins14090588

Received: 22 July 2022
Accepted: 23 August 2022
Published: 27 August 2022

1. Introduction

Species of the fungal ascomycete genus *Pyrenophora* are known to produce a spectacular array of secondary metabolites, but, to date, there has been no published effort to integrate the large volume of information available on this topic. In this review of bioactive metabolites produced by members of the genus, the goal is to present this information in a format that will be useful for agronomists studying plant disease and researchers in chemical ecology, as well as natural products chemists and applied scientists seeking novel compounds for diverse uses.

Pyrenophora is a genus of approximately 190 currently recognized species in the Dothidiomycete family Pleosporaceae [1]. Both the family Pleosporaceae and the genus *Pyrenophora* are well supported as monophyletic groups based on molecular phylogenetic analysis, and the *Drechslera* anamorphs traditionally associated with *Pyrenophora* species are also supported as genetically similar to their teleomorphs and conspecific with them [2–4]. Most *Pyrenophora* species are foliar pathogens of grasses, but some are also known as endophytes, as foliar pathogens of dicots, and in at least one case, as a seed pathogen.

For many species, little information beyond a species description is available, but two economically important cereal crop foliar pathogens, *P. tritici-repentis* and *P. teres*, have been well-studied [5–7]. A third well-studied species is *P. semeniperda*, a seed pathogen under consideration as a possible biocontrol for weedy annual bromes [8,9]. This review covers the literature from 1934 through 2022. The toxic metabolites discovered in each of the three well-studied species are presented, along with a few reports from additional species, and their isolation, structure determination, and biological activities are discussed.

2. Biology, Pathogenicity, and Toxin Production of *Pyrenophora* spp.

2.1. *Pyrenophora teres*

2.1.1. Biology and Pathogenicity of *Pyrenophora teres*

Pyrenophora teres is the causal agent of net blotch on barley, which is an economically important foliar disease that can cause up to 40% yield reduction and also lowers grain quality [7]. It reproduces sexually on standing barley at the end of the growing season and overwinters on crop residues. There are multiple cycles of asexual reproduction via conidia during the growing season. This pathogen can also infect developing seeds and be moved as seed-borne inoculum. It has long been known that there are two forms that are morphologically identical but that cause quite different disease symptoms on barley leaves. The net form *P. teres* f. *teres* (Ptt) causes longitudinal dark brown necrotic lesions that can later become chlorotic, while the spot form *P. teres* f. *maculata* (Ptm) causes circular or elliptical spots that are dark brown and are associated with chlorosis on the surrounding leaf tissues. The two forms are genetically distinct and may represent different species [10]. They can be induced to hybridize under laboratory conditions, but hybrids under natural conditions are extremely rare. The two forms also differ in the growth rate, symptom development, and toxin production in culture.

P. teres can infect a wide range of cereal and native grass hosts, but rarely, if ever, causes significant disease on these hosts [11]. This makes wild grass species an unlikely source of inoculum. Disease levels on different barley cultivars appear to be mediated by gene-for-gene interactions, but toxins specifically produced by these virulence genes have not yet been identified [6,12]. Many of the toxins produced by this fungus in culture can induce some level of disease symptoms on barley leaves, but these effects are not strain- or host genotype-specific.

Genome mining has identified a large number of predicted biosynthetic gene clusters that could mediate the production of novel toxins in *P. teres* [13]. The total number is greater for Ptt (36 to 82 depending on strain) than for Ptm (45–47, two strains). The majority of these (15–53) are NRPS (non-ribosomal peptide synthase) loci, with 12–15 PKS (polyketide synthase) loci, 2–9 PKS-NRPS hybrid loci, and 4–6 terpene biosynthase loci. There is a high probability that further research can unravel the identity of toxic effectors and their specificity in the gene-for-gene interactions that have been documented genetically and phenotypically in this pathosystem, whether the effectors are secondary metabolites or proteins [6].

2.1.2. Phytotoxins Produced by *Pyrenophora teres*

Chemically diverse toxins have been isolated from cultures of *P. teres*. These compounds belong to different classes according to their structures, including amino acid derivatives of the marismine class, nonenolides, spirocyclic lactones, isoquinolines, and an anthraquinone (Figure 1). As reviewed in this section, many of them are phytotoxic, whereas other types of biological activities of agronomic or pharmacological interest have been described for some of them.

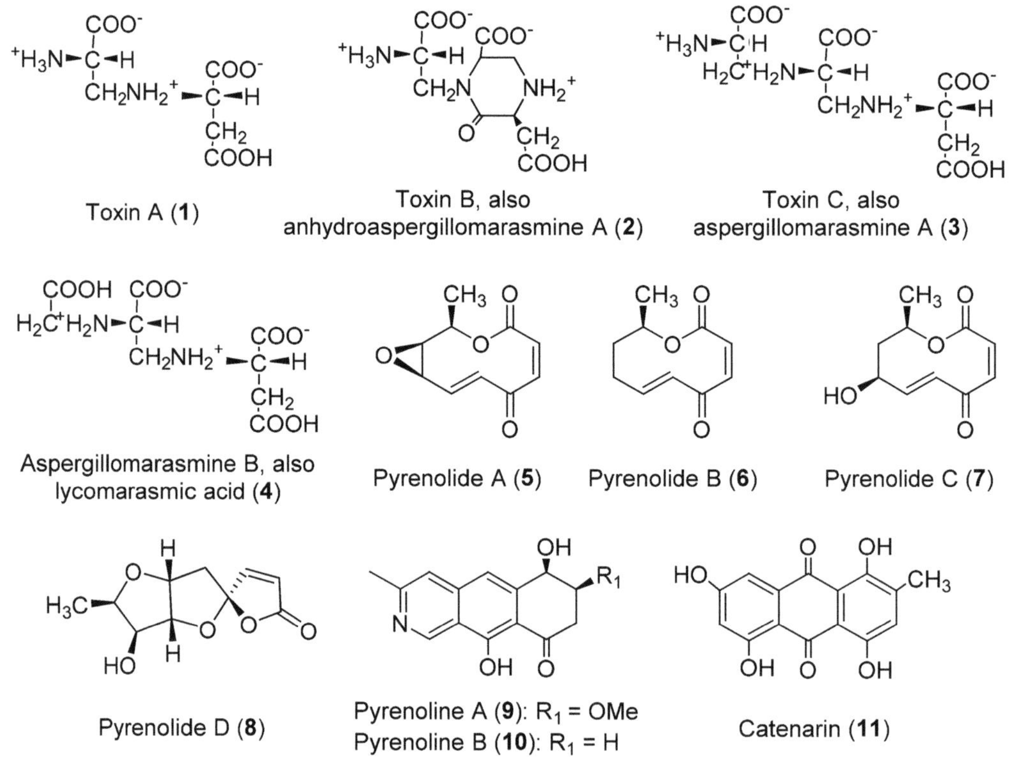

Figure 1. Structures of the toxins produced by *P. teres*.

Amino acid derivatives (**1–4**, Figure 1) in a family that belongs to the marasmine class are among the phytotoxins produced by *P. teres*. All of these were obtained from cultures grown in Fries' liquid medium. Toxins A and B (**1** and **2**), isolated for the first time from culture filtrates of *P. teres* collected from barley leaves, were the first to be discovered from this family [14]. Their structures were described in a later study, with toxin A (**1**) being characterized as *N*-(2-amino-2-carboxyethyl)aspartic acid, and toxin B (**2**) as 1-(2-amino-2-carboxyethyl)-6-carboxy-3-carboxymethyl-2-piperazinone [15]. Toxin B (**2**) is also known as anhydroaspergillomarasmine A [16]. Compounds **1** and **2** showed phytotoxic effects on barley, provoking chlorosis and collapse of tissues [14]. It was suggested that toxins A and B (**1** and **2**) play a key role in the disease syndrome of net-spot blotch of barley, also contributing to the virulence of individual isolates of *P. teres* [14]. The same study that provided the characterization of compounds **1** and **2** [15] also reported the first isolation of toxin C (**3**) from *P. teres*. The structure of this compound, also known as aspergillomarasmine A, corresponded with that of *N*-[2-(2-amino-2-carboxyethylamino)-2-carboxyethyl]aspartic acid, an already-known fungal compound previously described from *Fusarium oxysporum*, *Colletotrichum gloeosporioides*, *Aspergillus flavus-oryzae*, and *Paecilomyces* species [16–18]. Toxin A (**1**) was suggested as a precursor of toxin C (**3**) in cultures of *P. teres*, whereas toxin C (**3**) generates toxin B (**2**) by a non-enzymatic mechanism [16]. Different strategies for the synthesis of compound **3** are available in the literature [19–23]. As for toxins A and B (**1** and **2**), toxin C (**3**) has phytotoxic activity on barley, and it has been suggested that compound **3** plays a major role in the pathological changes associated with the barley net-spot blotch disease [16]. Compound **3** also possesses pharmacological interest due to its activity against some factors that generate resistance in Gram-negative pathogens. In fact, it is a potent inactivator of metallo-β-lactamases and has proven to reverse carbapenem resistance in vivo [24]. The inhibition of metallo-β-lactamases by compound **3** would occur via the selective sequestering of Zn^{2+} [25]. Of interest for the development of drugs, it could be worth highlighting that the structure of compound **3** proved to be tolerant of changes in the stereochemistry at positions 3, 6, and 9 regarding the activity against the metallo-β-lactamase NDM-1 [20].

It is interesting to note the study by Weiergang et al. (2002) [26] on the phytotoxicity of toxins A–C (**1**–**3**) on barley leaves, which showed the different activity profiles of these compounds. It was found that toxin A (**1**) generates chlorotic symptoms and little necrosis, whereas toxin C (**3**) provokes distinct necrotic symptoms and chlorosis, and toxin B (**2**) is weakly toxic. It was concluded that the interaction of barley with toxins A and C (**1** and **3**) is correlated with that observed with *P. teres* (both *f. teres* and *f. maculata*). This suggested that these toxins may be used to select resistant barley lines in the early stages of breeding programs [26].

Aspergillomarasmine B (**4**), also known as lycomarasmic acid, is a toxin identified as a product of *P. teres* in 2008 [27]. This compound, similar to the closely related compound **3**, had been previously found in the fungal species *A. flavus-oryzae*, *C. gloeosporioides*, and *Paecilomyces* [17,18,28]. Its isolation from *C. gloeosporioides*, the pathogen of olive crops (*Olea europaea* L.), represented its first report as a toxin produced by a plant pathogen [28]. Compound **4** showed remarkable phytotoxic activity, whose mechanism may be based on a chelation process that forms toxic iron chelates [27].

The family of pyrenolides (**5**–**8**, Figure 1) constitutes a group of bioactive toxins also produced by *P. teres* that are compounds with antifungal activity [29] isolated from cultures grown in malt-dextrose medium. Structurally, pyrenolides **5**–**7** are nonenolides formed by a 10-membered lactone ring with different substituents. Pyrenolide A (**5**) was first isolated from *P. teres* [30]. It was later found in *Ascochyta hyalospora* [31], and some hydroxylated derivatives were isolated from a marine-derived *Curvularia* species [32]. Pyrenolides B and C (**6** and **7**) were isolated in a later study [29]. The synthesis of pyrenolide B (**6**) was reported in different studies [33–35], though not as an enantiomerically pure product. It is worth highlighting that Suzuki et al. (1987) [34] proved that synthetic (±)-pyrenolide B shows significant antimicrobial activity (against *Aspergillus niger* and *Cochliobolus miyabeanus*) and phytotoxicity. The synthesis of (±)-pyrenolide C by Wasserman and Prowse (1992) [36] was the first reported for this compound, also allowing the establishment of its stereochemistry.

The structure of pyrenolide D (**8**) differs from those of the previously described pyrenolides A–C (**5**–**7**), showing a tricyclic spiro-γ-lactone scaffold of five-membered rings instead of the nonenolide scaffold. Pyrenolide D (**8**) was isolated for the first time from *P. teres* [37]. The same study reported that this compound possesses cytotoxic activity (against HL-60 cells), whereas antifungal activity was not found, unlike pyrenolides A–C. The synthesis of pyrenolide D (**8**) was the focus of later studies, as a result of which this toxin was obtained as an enantiomerically pure product [38–42].

Two isoquinolines, named pyrenolines A and B (**9** and **10**, Figure 1), were also reported as phytotoxins isolated from *P. teres* [43]. Both compounds showed phytotoxic activity on different plant species, including barley. Pyrenoline A (**9**) required lower concentrations to generate the phytotoxic effects evaluated. Pyrenoline A (**9**) did not show host specificity regarding monocot and dicot species. The kinetics of production of pyrenolines A and B (**9** and **10**) by *P. teres* were studied in later research. It was found that their concentration in the culture medium varies in time following a repetitive cycle of production and degradation, with pyrenoline B always being produced in higher quantities than pyrenoline A [44].

Catenarin (**11**) is a red anthraquinone pigment isolated from *Drechslera teres* [45] and other fungal species including *Helminthosporium gramineum*, *Pyrenophora tritici-repentis*, and *Conoideocrella krungchingensis* [46–48]. The culture medium employed for its isolation from *P. teres* is potato dextrose agar (PDA), unlike compounds **1**–**10**, for which a liquid medium (Fries, Malt-Dextrose or M1D) was used. Its synthesis was reported in the middle of the last century [48,49]. With regard to its biological activities, catenarin (**11**) induces necrosis on wheat in a non-specific manner [50] and inhibits, to some extent, the growth of the mycelium of *D. teres*, but not the germination of conidia [45]. Compound **11** also possesses a remarkable antibacterial profile. It significantly inhibits *B. subtilis* (at low concentrations of <0.1 μM) [45], as well as other Gram-positive bacteria and fungal species [46,50]. It is also cytotoxic against NCI-H187 cancer cells (IC_{50} = 8.21 μg/mL), and inactive against the non-cancerous line tested in the same assay [47]. Moreover, antidiabetic activity was described for catenarin (**11**), though few studies have been performed in this regard [51].

2.2. *Pyrenophora tritici-repentis*

2.2.1. Biology and Pathogenicity of *P. tritici-repentis*

Pyrenophora tritici-repentis is the causal agent of the foliar disease tan spot of wheat [5]. It also occurs on related cereal crops and some native grasses but is not known to cause serious disease on these hosts. It is a necrotrophic pathogen that can survive saprophytically and increase its inoculum through sexual reproduction on crop residues over winter. Recent research on this disease has focused on the role of host-specific toxins (HSTs) in the pathogenesis of different cultivars of wheat. HST genes interact with host sensitivity genes in a manner that is essentially the inverse of the interaction of avirulence genes in biotrophic fungi with host resistance genes. In biotrophs, the host resistance gene product can recognize the pathogen avirulence gene product and initiate defense measures, including programmed cell death, that prevent further tissue colonization by the pathogen. However, for necrotrophic pathogens, programmed cell death is the opening that enables successful infection; thus, recognition by the host actually increases pathogen virulence. There are currently three HSTs known to be produced by this pathogen on wheat, and the combination of these in any pathogen strain and their complementary sensitivity genes in the host determines which wheat cultivars are susceptible to a given strain.

Tan spot disease has long been endemic in wheat but was considered a minor pathogen until quite recently. It has emerged as an economically important disease of wheat worldwide only in the last 60–80 years [52]. The advent of no-till agriculture is one probable contributor to its recent ascendance as a major disease of wheat. However, the major factor, as discussed below, that has increased its virulence on wheat involved a recent horizontal gene transfer from a related wheat pathogen, *Stagonospora nodorum* [53]. Both organisms produce PtrToxA, a host-specific toxin (HST) that causes severe disease in wheat cultivars that possess the corresponding sensitivity gene *Tsn1*. PtrToxA-producing strains have now become the prevalent strains in wheat-producing regions across most of the world (e.g., [54]). Even more recently, there appears to have been a second horizontal gene transfer of the PtrToxA gene from *P. tritici-repentis* to *P. teres*, which has enabled this barley pathogen to effectively expand its host range to include wheat [55]. Horizontal gene transfer is difficult to demonstrate conclusively, but the evidence *for PtrToxA* horizontal gene transfer into *P. tritici-repentis* is quite strong.

P. tritici-repentis also produce toxins that are not host-specific, but there has been little research on the role of these toxins in disease development in wheat. A genome-mining exercise for this pathogen revealed the presence of >30 putative genes or gene clusters that are likely responsible for the biosynthesis of some of these other toxins [5]. These included both NRPS (non-ribosomal peptide synthase) and PKS (polyketide synthase) loci as well as two NRPS-PKS hybrid loci. More recently, a more comprehensive genome mining exercise identified a similar number of these biosynthesis gene clusters in *P. tritici-repentis*, as well as a number of terpene synthesis clusters [13]. The NRPS-PKS biosynthesis gene cluster responsible for triticone (spirostaphylotrichin) biosynthesis has been specifically identified [56].

2.2.2. Phytotoxins Produced by *Pyrenophora tritici-repentis*

For the species *P. tritici-repentis*, a collection of toxins, mostly with protein- and spirocyclic lactam-like structures (Figure 2), has been isolated and studied.

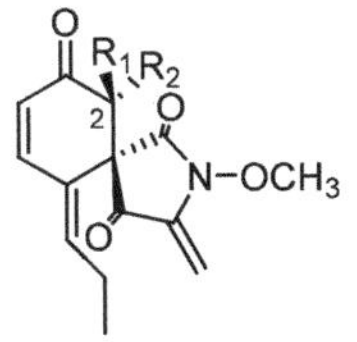

Triticone A, also spirostaphylotrichin C (**12**): R_1 = OH, R_2 = H
Triticone B, also spirostaphylotrichin D (**13**): R_1 = H, R_2 = OH

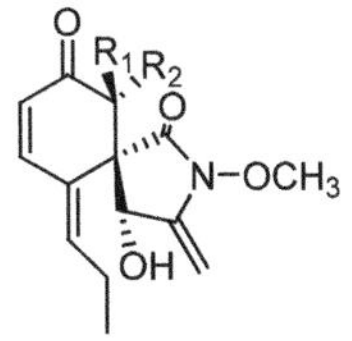

Triticone C, also spirostaphylotrichin A (**14**): R_1 = OH, R_2 = H
Triticone D (**15**): R_1 = H, R_2 = OH

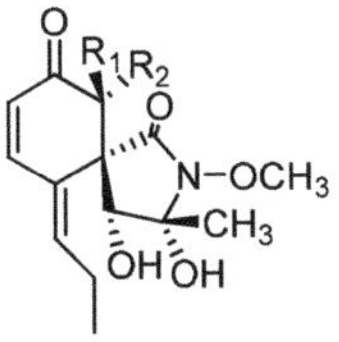

Triticone E (**16**): R_1 = OH, R_2 = H
Triticone F, also spirostaphylotrichin R (**17**): R_1 = H, R_2 = OH

Figure 2. Structures of triticones A-F, toxins produced by *P. tritici-repentis*.

The most studied toxins produced by *P. tritici-repentis* are the proteins known as Ptr ToxA and Ptr ToxB, obtained from cultures grown in Fries' medium. They are host-selective toxins reported as necrosis-inducing in the case of Ptr ToxA [57], and chlorosis-inducing in the case of Ptr ToxB [58]. Ptr ToxA causes quicker symptoms than Ptr ToxB, though the defense responses observed have multiple similarities [59]. It was also found that Ptr ToxB has a greater distribution than the common host-selective toxins [60]. Pandelova et al. [59] provided an excellent overview of the biochemical mechanisms and effects of both toxins.

Ptr ToxC was also reported as a chlorosis-inducing and low-molecular-weight compound, grown in a PDA medium [61,62]. This compound has a difficult isolation process and is not stable; its genetics are still under study. It has recently been suggested that it is not a protein [63].

As mentioned earlier, a family of spirocyclic lactams (**12**–**17**), named triticones or spirostaphylotrichins (Figure 2), has been described as toxins produced by *P. tritici-repentis* [64]. All of these were obtained from cultures grown in an M1D-modified liquid medium. Triticones A and B (**12** and **13**, Figure 2), epimeric compounds at C-2, were the first to be reported, isolated in 1988 as new chemotypes for which no closely related molecules had been described [65]. This study highlighted the instability of the active fractions to high temperatures and silica gel, making possible the isolation of the compounds by crystallization after the slow evaporation of the solvent. The ratio of production is approximately 1:1 [64]. Another relevant finding is that triticone A (**12**) undergoes racemization to form triticone B (**13**), and vice versa, which means that studies on the bioactivities of these compounds are commonly carried out on mixtures of both compounds.

Triticones A and B (**12** and **13**) showed remarked phytotoxicity in leaf assays [64], and also showed phytotoxic activity at 4.0 μM in a wheat protoplast assay [65]. The mixture of triticones A and B induces chlorosis and necrosis on a wide range of monocot and dicot plants [56,66] and also inhibits CO_2 fixation by 50% in wheat at 32 ± 13 μM [66]. Antibacterial activity against the Gram-positive species *Bacillus subtilis* and *Rhodococcus erythropolis* was reported, whereas no activity was observed against different Gram-negative bacteria or fungal species [56]. Triticone B (**13**) showed attributes of pharmacological interest, as it enhances plasmin activity of bovine aortic endothelial cells, causing direct and reversible inhibition of plasminogen activator inhibitor-1 [67].

As for triticones A and B (**12** and **13**), triticones C and D (**14** and **15**, Figure 2) were also described as epimers at C-2, and this is also the case for triticones E and F (**16** and **17**, Figure 2) [64,66]. Interestingly, triticones C and D (**14** and **15**) do not undergo the quick interconversion previously described for triticones A and B [64]. Unlike triticones A and B (**12** and **13**), which possess a marked phytotoxicity, triticones C and D (**14** and **15**) are weakly phytotoxic in leaf protoplast assays, whereas triticones E and F (**16** and **17**) are essentially inactive [64]. On the other hand, it is worth highlighting that these two latter compounds, in a mixture of 2:1, possess antibacterial activity against *Escherichia coli* (minimum inhibitory concentration = 62.5 μg/mL) [68].

Catenarin (**11**, Figure 1), a toxin produced by *P. teres* with phytotoxic and diverse pharmacological activities as previously described in Section 2.1.2, is also produced by *P. tritici-repentis* [46]. A study on *P. tritici-repentis* reported that the highest catenarin concentrations can be obtained in the Fries medium supplemented with starch. It was also shown that in specific conditions of incubation, a rapid accumulation of catenarin can occur during the first week, followed by a large decline after 14 days. This indicates that it may be bio-transformed to other anthraquinones or incorporated into melanin [50,69].

2.3. *Pyrenophora semeniperda*

2.3.1. Biology and Pathogenicity of *Pyrenophora semeniperda*

P. semeniperda (alternate spelling *P. seminiperda*) is a generalist seed pathogen that attacks seeds in field seed banks [70]. It is known almost entirely from its anamorph *Drechslera campanulata*, as the sexual state is very rarely observed in nature and nearly impossible to obtain in culture [71]. The fungus forms macroscopic fingerlike stromata that protrude from killed seeds, earning it the moniker 'black fingers of death'. Early studies on this pathogen in Australia addressed its potential as a biocontrol for annual grass weeds [72]. This has also been the motivating force behind extensive studies on the biology of this species in semiarid North America [8,9]. The Australian studies were initially based on the inoculation of non-dormant seeds, a treatment that resulted in very low seed mortality. These workers surmised that floral infection during seed development must account for the high natural mortality in soil seed banks of these weeds, and they demonstrated experimentally that this was at least possible [73]. Working with the host *Bromus tectorum* in the US, it was later discovered that the inoculation of mature seeds could cause very high mortality if seeds were inoculated when dormant [74]. Non-dormant seeds could escape mortality as in the Australian studies. Non-dormant *B. tectorum* seeds could also be killed in field seed banks under conditions of water stress that retarded seed germination but permitted pathogen activity [75].

In studies with multiple strains, it was discovered that slower-growing strains were better able to kill non-dormant *B. tectorum* seeds than fast-growing strains [76]. This was interpreted as a trade-off between the growth rate and production of cytochalasin B, a toxin produced in abundance by this pathogen [77]. This hypothesis was later confirmed experimentally [78].

Molecular genetic studies showed that *P. semeniperda* exhibits high levels of genetic diversity and regional genetic differentiation, even at the ITS locus, which is most often monomorphic at the species level [79]. It was later demonstrated that strains with different ITS haplotypes are strongly genetically differentiated and likely represent cryptic species [80].

Studies on the host range of this seed pathogen determined that it has a very wide host range, but that some hosts were more susceptible than others [81]. Reciprocal inoculation experiments with strains from different annual grass hosts demonstrated a complete lack of host specialization [82]. Strains varied in virulence and host species varied in resistance, but there was no pattern of increased virulence in the host of origin.

A provisional genome mining exercise (C. Coleman, Brigham Young University, unpublished data) using an annotated genome assembly [83] yielded 12 predicted PKS loci, 8 predicted NRPS loci, and 2 PKS-NRPS hybrid loci. The two hybrid loci were later determined to be responsible for the biosynthesis of cytochalasins and spirostaphylotrichins, both of which are known to be produced by this fungus in culture.

2.3.2. Phytotoxins Produced by *Pyrenophora semeniperda*

P. semeniperda is a species for which a higher diversity of compounds (Figure 3) has been found, in comparison to *P. teres* and *P. tritici-repentis*. They include cytochalasan, spirocyclic lactam, and sesquiterpenoid acid structures. Interestingly, some of the compounds produced by *P. semeniperda* have been also discovered in *P. tritici-repentis*, i.e., triticones A–C and E–F (**12–14, 16** and **17**, Figure 2), previously described in Section 2.2.2. These will be referred as spirostaphylotrichins in this section when possible, as they were designated as spirostaphylotrichins in subsequent publications on *P. semeniperda*. Cytochalasins B, F, T, and deoxaphomin (**18–21**, Figure 3), as well as the previously undescribed cytochalasins Z1, Z2, and Z3 (**22–24**, Figure 3), were isolated in 2002 by Evidente et al. as the first phytotoxins produced on solid wheat culture by an Australian strain of *P. semeniperda* [84]. They belong to the cytochalasan group of fungal polyketide-amino acid hybrid metabolites with several biological activities [85,86]. Cytochalasins Z1, Z2, and Z3 (**22–24**) were characterized as 24-oxa[14]cytochalasans by NMR and MS techniques. Compounds **18–24** were assayed on wheat and tomato seedlings, and the most active compounds proved to be cytochalasin B (**18**), F (**19**), Z3 (**24**), and deoxaphomin (**21**). These showed a remarkable ability to inhibit root elongation. In leaf-puncture assay, only deoxaphomin (**21**) showed the ability to produce small necrotic lesions, whereas no effects were observed in the immersion assay from any of the tested cytochalasins [84].

Preliminary in vitro experiments showed that the fungus was able to produce other low-molecular-weight lipophilic phytotoxins in liquid culture, but they were not characterized [84,87]. These metabolites were identified as spirocyclic γ-lactams by Masi et al. [88] working with the PDB liquid cultures of a *P. semeniperda* strain collected in the USA. In particular, this strain produced the known spirostaphylotrichins A, C, D, R (**12–14** and **17**, Figure 2) and V (**25**, Figure 3), as well as triticone E (**16**, Figure 2), and a previously undescribed related compound, which was named spirostaphylotrichin W (**26**, Figure 3). The structure of this latter compound, as well as its relative stereochemistry, was characterized by spectroscopic and chemical methods. All the isolated compounds were tested in a *B. tectorum* coleoptile bioassay at a concentration of 10^{-3} M. Spirostaphylotrichin A (**12**) proved to be the most active compound, followed by spirostaphylotrichins C and D (**13** and **14**). Furthermore, in a leaf puncture bioassay carried out on host and non-host plants, only spirostaphylotrichins A, C, and D (**12–14**) exhibited phytotoxicity [88]. When the same strain was grown in solid culture on wheat culture, cytochalasin B (**18**) was identified as the main metabolite. Its production by other strains was also evaluated using a high-pressure liquid chromatography method (HPLC). This study revealed that the production of cytochalasin B (**18**) is strongly dependent on cultural conditions and that it is produced in large quantities in solid wheat seed culture (with production varying from 535 to 2256 mg kg^{-1}). Furthermore, in a *B. tectorum* coleoptile bioassay, solid culture extracts of the strain studied showed higher toxicity than the cytochalasin B standard at the highest concentration tested. This suggested the possible presence of other phytotoxic metabolites in the organic extracts [77].

Thus, the organic extract of *P. semeniperda* strain WRR10-16, one of the most active strains in the *B. tectorum* coleoptile bioassay [89], was purified using different steps of column chromatography, also yielding the other known cytochalasins F and Z3 (**19** and **24**) and deoxaphomin (**21**), as well as a previously undescribed sesquiterpenoid penta-2,4-dienoic acid that was named pyrenophoric acid (**27**, Figure 3) [89]. Its relative stereochemistry was assigned by NMR studies while its absolute configuration was determined by applying the advanced Mosher's method [90]. Pyrenophoric acid (**27**) proved to be very phytotoxic in a cheatgrass coleoptile elongation test at 10^{-3} M and its negative effect on coleoptile elongation was additive with that of cytochalasin B when tested in a mixture at 10^{-4} M. This result demonstrated that the high toxicity shown by the organic extract was due to the combined action of multiple phytotoxic compounds [89].

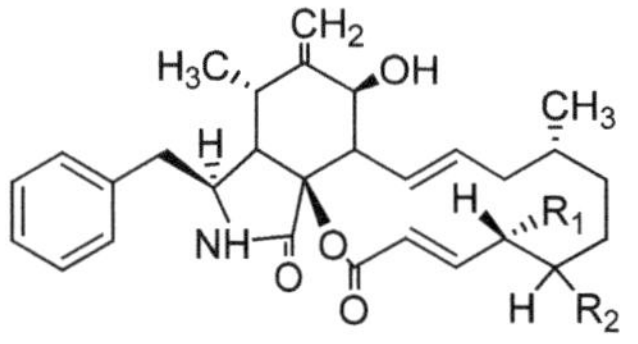

Cytochalasin B (**18**): R_1=OH, R_2=H
Cytochalasin Z_3 (**24**): R_1=H, R_2=OH

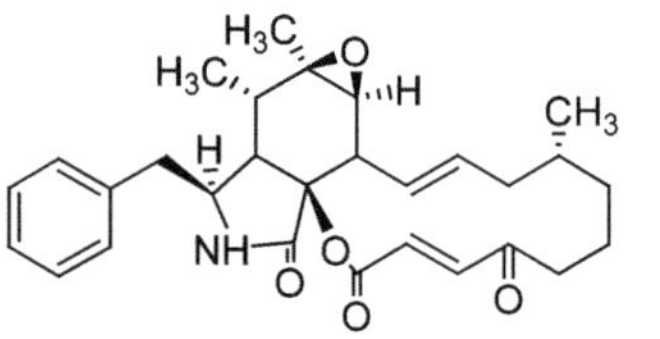

Cytochalasin F (**19**)

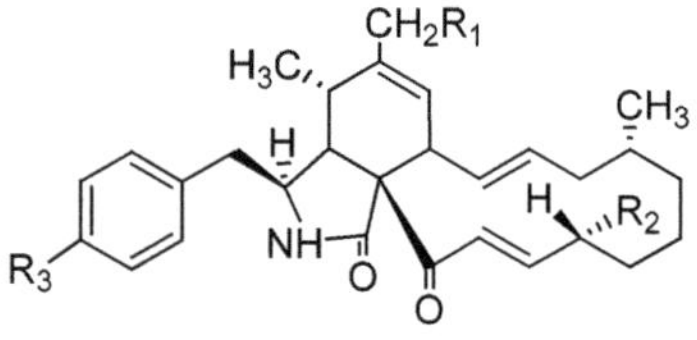

Cytochalasin T (**20**): R_1=R_3=H, R_2=OH
Cytochalasin Z_1 (**22**): R_1=R_2=H, R_3=OH
Cytochalasin Z_2 (**23**): R_1=R_2=OH, R_3=H

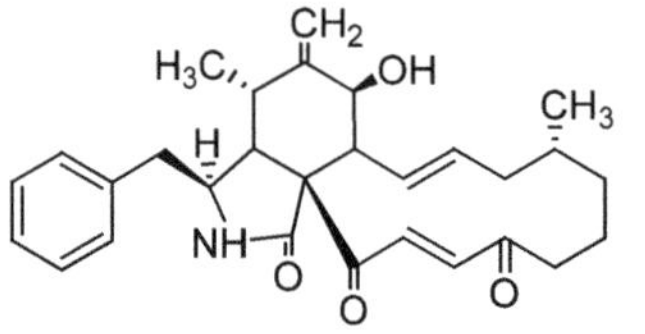

Deoxaphomin (**21**)

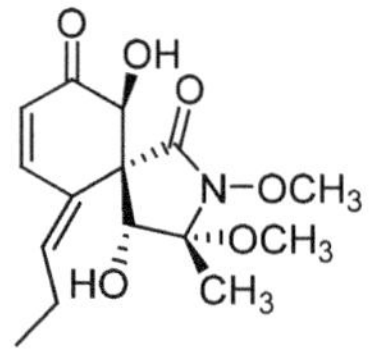

Spirostaphylotrichin V (**25**)

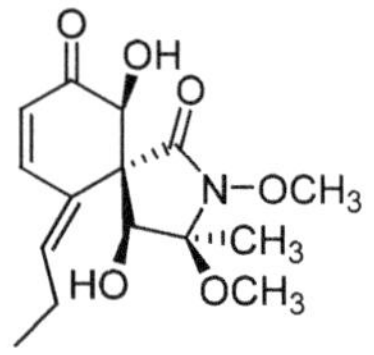

Spirostaphylotrichin W (**26**)

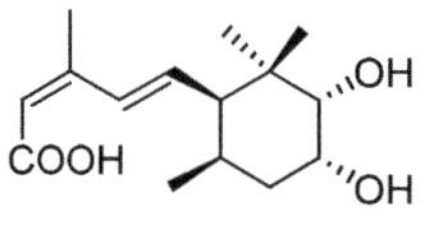

Pyrenophoric acid (**27**)

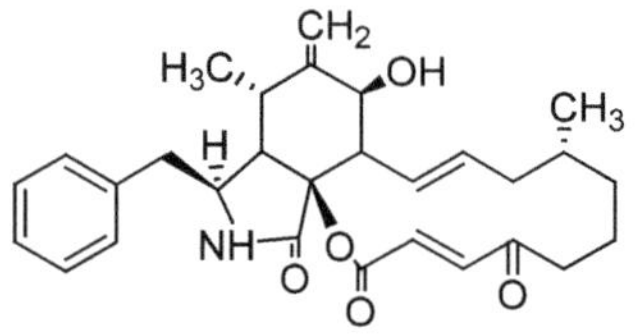

Cytochalasin A (**28**)

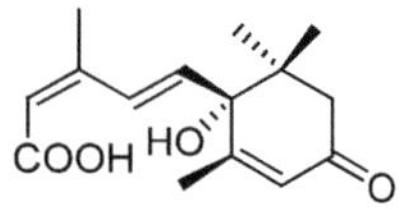

Abscisic acid (**29**)

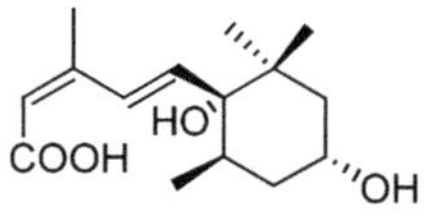

Pyrenophoric acid B (**30**)

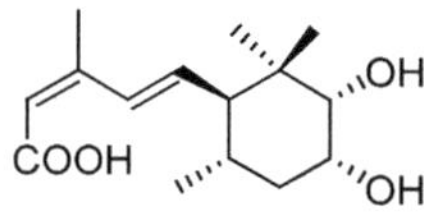

Pyrenophoric acid C (**31**)

Figure 3. Structures of the toxins produced by *Pyrenophora semeniperda*.

When the same fungus was grown in cheatgrass seed culture, two other previously undescribed compounds were isolated together with cytochalasins A, B, F, and Z3 (**28**, **18**, **19** and **24**, respectively, Figure 3), deoxaphomin, pyrenophoric acid, and abscisic acid (**21**, **27** and **29**, respectively, Figure 3). The two new compounds that were characterized by spectroscopic methods and, as they were related to pyrenophoric acid, were named pyrenophoric acids B and C (**30** and **31**, Figure 3). In a cheatgrass seedling bioassay at 10^{-3} M, pyrenophoric acid B (**30**) showed higher coleoptile toxicity than pyrenophoric acid, while pyrenophoric acid C (**31**) showed lower phytotoxicity [91].

Another study demonstrated that the production of cytochalasin B (**18**) could also be induced in liquid media only if they contained host seed constituents. This strongly suggests that the production of cytochalasin B is directly implicated in the pathogenesis of seeds [78]. Research on the mode of action of pyrenophoric acid B (**30**) using mutant lines of *Arabidopsis thaliana* demonstrated that this compound activates the abscisic acid (ABA) signaling pathway in order to inhibit seed germination. It was demonstrated that it uses the ABA biosynthesis pathway at the level of alcohol dehydrogenase ABA2 to achieve this inhibition. This result suggested that *P. semeniperda* may manipulate plant ABA biosynthesis in the seed as a strategy to reduce germination, increasing its ability to cause seed mortality and thereby increase its fitness through higher reproductive success [92].

2.4. Other *Pyrenophora* spp.

2.4.1. Biology and Pathogenicity of other *Pyrenophora* Species

Many other *Pyrenophora* species are foliar grass pathogens with life histories similar to *P. teres* and *P. tritici-repentis*, and this is especially true of those that have been studied in terms of secondary product chemistry. As these pathogens are less economically important, their biology and pathogenicity have received much less attention. Four species have been investigated to varying degrees for toxin production: *P. avenae* (syn. *P. chaetomioides*, anamorph *D. avenae*), *P. lolii* (anamorph *D. siccans*), *P. catenaria* (anamorph *D. catenaria*), and *P. biseptata* (anamorph *D. biseptata*). *Pyrenophora avenae* is primarily a disease of cultivated oats [93,94] while *P. lolii* infects cultivated and wild species of *Lolium* (ryegrass; [95,96]). Little information is available on the biology of the other two species. There is a report on secondary product chemistry for *D. dematioidea* as an endophyte in a species of marine algae [97], but as this identification was based only on morphology in a group where even the generic boundaries are not clear [98,99], we have chosen not to include this paper in our survey of toxin production in *Pyrenophora*.

2.4.2. Phytotoxins Produced by other *Pyrenophora* spp.

As reviewed in Sections 2.1–2.3, diverse families of toxins with different structures have been isolated from *P. teres*, *P. tritici-repentis*, and *P. semeniperda*. Nevertheless, markedly different toxins have been isolated from other *Pyrenophora* species (Figure 4). These toxins are reviewed in this section.

Pyrenophora avenae, a pathogen of oats, produces toxins with macrocyclic and anthraquinone structures. The toxins with a macrocyclic structure produced are pyrenophorin (**32**, Figure 4) [100] and the structurally related compounds dihydropyrenophorin and pyrenophorol (**33** and **34**, Figure 4) [101]. Pyrenophorin (**32**) inhibited radicle growth in oat and non-host plants [102]. This toxin has antifungal properties, as it is significantly active against the biotrophic pathogen *Microbotryum violaceum* and the yeast *Saccharomyces cerevisiae* at 5 μM [103]. Moreover, pyrenophorin (**32**) showed strong cytotoxicity against several cancer cell lines (IC_{50} values ranging from 0.07 to 7.8 μM) [104]. The stereoselective total synthesis of pyrenophorin has been published [105]. Dihydropyrenophorin (**33**) showed phytotoxic activity [101], as well as antibacterial, antifungal, and antialgal activities [106]. These last antimicrobial activities were also found for pyrenophorol (**34**) [101,106]. Compound **34** showed phytotoxicity (leaf necrosis) on *Avena sterilis* and, at a lower level, on *Avena fatua* L. On the other hand, the seed germination and seedling growth of *A. sterilis* were not affected [107]. The stereoselective total synthesis of pyrenophorol has been published [108].

In regard to the toxins with an anthraquinones structure produced by *P. avenae*, these compounds are helminthosporin and cynodontin (**35** and **36**, Figure 4), two metabolites produced by diverse fungal species. As for the previously described anthraquinone catenarin (**11**), the growth medium was PDA [45], while Czapek-Dox was also employed as a medium for obtaining compound **35 [109]**. Helminthosporin (**35**) is a toxin that showed herbicidal activity against different weed and crop plants, though species such as soybean, tomato, or cotton were resistant when tested at 500 μg/mL [110]. Compound **35** also showed positive results in pharmacological assays. It inhibited the growth of hepatic bile duct (TFK-1) and liver (HuH7) cancer cell lines [111] and also showed significant inhibition of electric eel acetylcholinesterase (IC_{50} = 2.53 μM) and brain permeable properties [112]. In the case of cynodontin (**36**), relevant antifungal activity was found against *Sclerotinia minor*, *Sclerotinia sclerotiorum*, and *Botrytis cinerea* [113]. It is worth highlighting the study by Đorović et al. [114], which examined the antioxidative mechanisms of action of cynodontin.

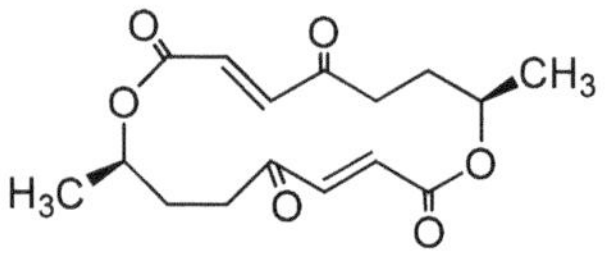

Pyrenophorin (**32**)

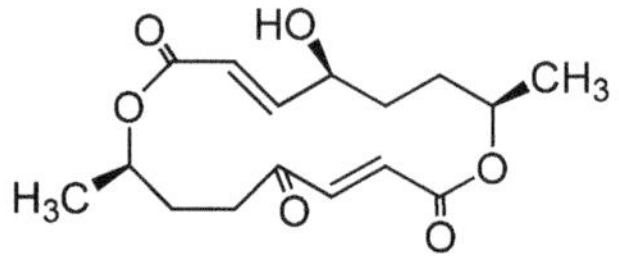

Dihydropyrenophorin (**33**)

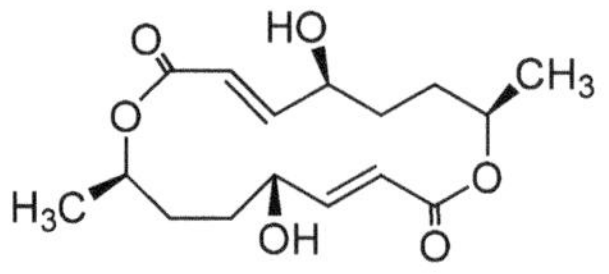

Pyrenophorol (**34**)

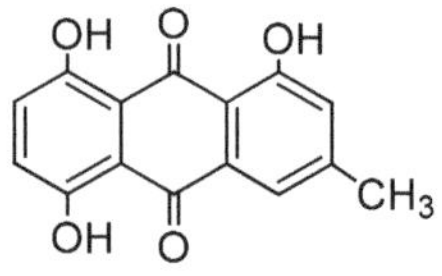

Helminthosporin (**35**)

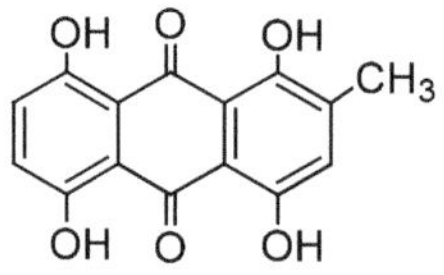

Cynodontin (**36**)

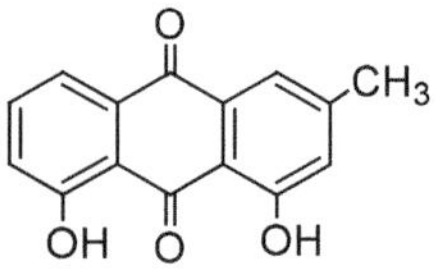

Crysophanol (**37**)

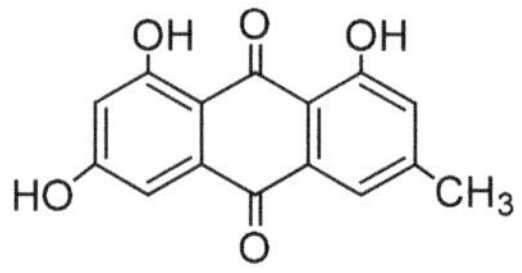

Emodin (**38**)

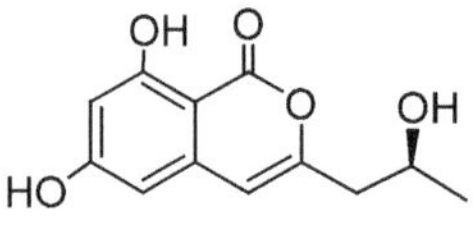

De-*O*-methyldiaporthin (**39**)

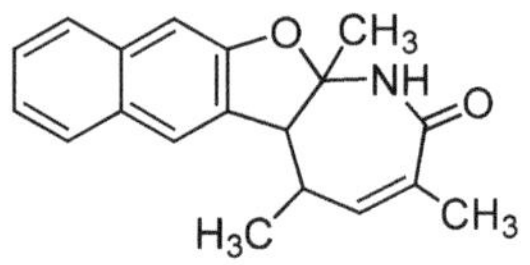

Drazepinone
(**40**, proposed structure)

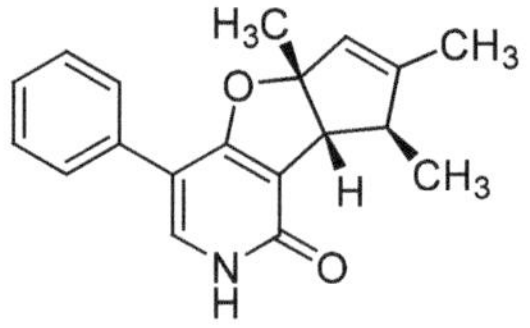

(±) Drazepinone
(**40**, revised structure)

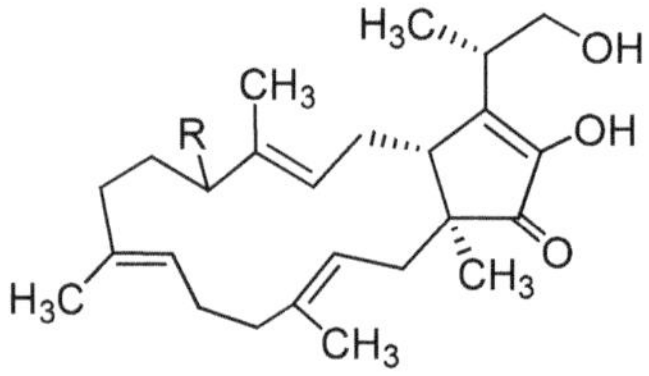

Siccanol, (**41**, proposed structure) R=β-OH
(-)-Terpestacin (**41**) R=α-OH

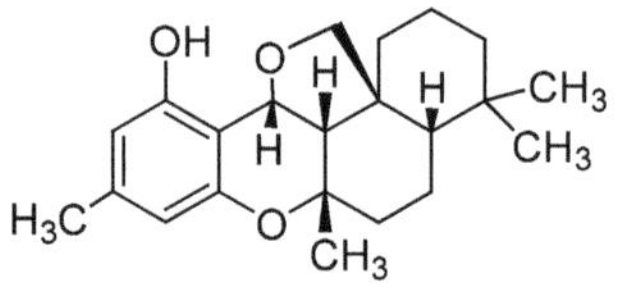

Siccanin (**42**)

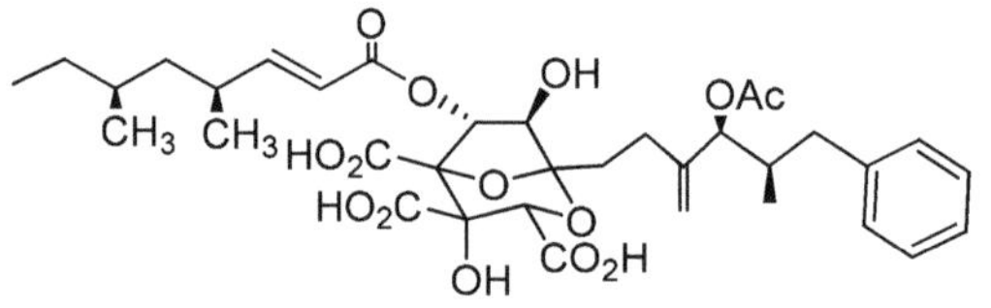

Zaragozic acid A (**43**)

Figure 4. Structures of toxins produced by other *Pyrenophora* species.

Three relevant anthraquinones were also isolated from the species *Drechslera catenaria* (grown in Czapek-Dox medium), named chrysophanol and emodin (**37** and **38**, Figure 4), as well as the already-described catenarin (**11**, Figure 1, Section 2.1.2) [115]. Chrysophanol (**37**) possessed poor phytotoxic activity, as tested on *Arabidopsis thaliana* [116], although it showed antifungal properties, including against plant pathogenic fungi [117]. Indeed, curative and protective activity against barley powdery mildew was demonstrated [118]. On the other hand, chrysophanol (**37**) has remarkable pharmacological potential, as recently reviewed by Yusuf et al. (2019) [118] and Su et al. (2020) [119]. Particularly, this compound showed anti-inflammatory, antiviral, anti-cancer, neuroprotective, anti-cardiovascular disease, and anti-ulcer activities. Research on the pharmacological bioactivities of chrysophanol (**37**) continues to be a topical issue. As examples of recent discoveries, the findings on its role in protecting against acute kidney injury [120], autologous blood-induced intracerebral hemorrhage [121], and in vivo hippocampal damage and mitochondrial autophagy [122] could be highlighted. Regarding emodin (**38**), it has been traditionally used in Chinese medicine, with a wide spectrum of later-proven pharmacological activities, but also adverse effects when used long-term at high doses [123]. This compound is the direct precursor of catenarin (**11**, Figure 1) [124] and is also a phytotoxin. It was found to have inhibitory activity on sunflowers (*Helianthus annuus*) [125] and the weeds *Amaranthus hypochondriacus* and *Echinochloa crus-galli* [126].

Toxins with diverse types of structures have been found for the pathogen *Drechslera siccans* (**39**–**42**, Figure 4) through the use of the liquid growth medium M1D modified, or glucose-potato broth-agar in the case of compound **42**. De-*O*-methyldiaporthin (**39**) is phytotoxic to barnyard grass, corn, and soybean, though poor or null activity was found for host plants of *D. siccans* [127]. Drazepinone (**40**) was isolated as a new phytotoxic trisubstituted naphthofuroazepinone, though its structure was recently revised (see **40**, Figure 4) [128,129]. This compound causes necrosis in a wide range of plant species, with *Urtica dioica* L. being the most affected tested species [128]. It also showed protein tyrosine phosphatase inhibitory activity [129] but low zootoxicity [128]. Siccanol (**41**), a bicyclic sesquiterpene that showed phytotoxicity on the root growth of Italian ryegrass (*Lolium multiflorum*, a *D. siccans* host plant), was also isolated from *D. siccans* [130]. Its structure was revised and assigned as (-)-terpestacin based on the total synthesis of this compound, which was isolated from other fungal species [131,132]. Siccanin (**42**), another toxin isolated from *D. siccans*, was active against *Trichophyton* [133]. Inhibitory activity to succinate dehydrogenase was also found (IC_{50} = 0.9 μM) [134]. Its total synthesis was reported [135].

Finally, it is worth highlighting zaragozic acid A (**43**), also known as squalestatin S1, a toxin produced by *Drechslera biseptata*. Although few references have been published on its activity, squalene synthase inhibitor activity was described [136,137]. The synthesis of this compound was also accomplished [138].

3. Classification of the Toxins Produced by *Pyrenophora* spp. according to Their Structures

In order to provide a clear overview in relation to the structures, origin, and biological activities described for the compounds under review (**1**–**43**), Table 1 compiles this information through a classification of the compounds according to their chemical classes.

This classification highlights how phytotoxic activity, whether detected for host plants or other species, has been shown by the vast majority of classes of compounds produced. This result, obtained after numerous studies carried out over decades, emphasizes the interest that exists in continuing with the study of the genomic aspects and modes of action involved in the phytopathogenic *Pyrenophora* species. Likewise, finding phytotoxic compounds could provide new herbicides based on natural products. A priori, they could present the advantages of reducing environmental impact, requiring lower doses of the active compound, or applying alternative modes of action to conventional herbicides, thus avoiding resistance problems. However, a significant difficulty is that the isolation of the toxins from natural sources often has excessively low yields. For this reason, throughout this review, the most outstanding publications on the synthesis of some of these toxins have been highlighted.

This discussion can be extrapolated to the pharmacological field, given the activity shown by some of the toxins in tests for antimicrobial or cytotoxic effects. In this regard, available references on pharmacological activities are provided for anthraquinones, cytochalasans, and macrocyclic or spirocyclic compounds. The anthraquinone chrysophanol (**37**) represents one of the most studied. It was noted in a recent review that relevant aspects of its mechanism of action and pharmacokinetics are still unknown [118].

Table 1. Classification of the toxins (**1–43**) according to their chemical classes.

Class	Compound	*Pyrenophora* species	Activity	References
Amino acid derivatives	Toxin A [*N*-(2-amino-2-carboxyethyl) aspartic acid] (**1**, Figure 1)	*P. teres*	Phytotoxic to barley	[14–16,26,27,139]
	Toxin B [1-(2-amino-2-carboxyethyl)-6-carboxy-3-carboxymethyl-2-piperazinone]; anhydroaspergillomarasmine A (**2**, Figure 1)	*P. teres*	Phytotoxic to barley	[14–16,26,27,139]
	Toxin C [*N*-[2-(2-amino-2-carboxy ethyl-amino)-2-carboxyethyl] aspartic acid]; aspergillomarasmine A (**3**, Figure 1)	*P. teres*	Phytotoxic to barley; reverse of resistance to Gram-negative pathogens	[15,16,24,26,27,139]
	Aspergillomarasmine B; lycomarasmic acid (**4**, Figure 1)	*P. teres*	Phytotoxic to barley	[27]
Anthraquinones	Catenarin (**11**, Figure 1)	*P. catenaria* *P. teres* *P. tritici-repentis*	Phytotoxic to wheat; antibacterial; antifungal; cytotoxic; antidiabetic	[45–47,50,51,109,115]
	Chrysophanol (**37**, Figure 4)	*P. catenaria*	Antifungal; anti-inflammatory; antiviral; anti-cancer; neuroprotective; anti-cardiovascular disease; antiulcer	[115,117–122]
	Cynodontin (**36**, Figure 4)	*P. avenae*	Antifungal; antioxidant	[45,109,113,114]
	Emodin (**38**, Figure 4)	*P. catenaria*	Phytotoxic to sunflower, *Amaranthus hypochondriacus* and *Echinochloa crus-galli*; antibacterial; anticancer; hepatoprotective; anti-inflammatory; antioxidant; antimicrobial	[115,123–126]
	Helminthosporin (**35**, Figure 4)	*P. avenae* *P. catenaria*	Herbicidal; cytotoxic; inhibition of cholinesterase	[45,109–112]
Bicyclic sesquiterpene	Siccanol; (-)-terpestacin (**41**, Figure 4)	*D. siccans*	Phytotoxic to *Lolium multiflorum*	[130]
Cytochalasans	Cytochalasin A (**28**, Figure 3)	*P. semeniperda*	Phytotoxic to *Bromus tectorum*, *Cirsium arvense* and *Sonchus arvensis*; anticancer; antibacterial; antifungal; antiviral	[85,86,91,140,141]
	Cytochalasin B (**18**, Figure 3)	*P. semeniperda*	Phytotoxic to wheat, tomato, *B. tectorum*, *Lilium longiflorum*, *C. arvense* and *S. arvensis*; algicidal; anticancer; cytotoxic; antiparasital; enzyme inhibition	[77,78,84–86,89,91,140–142]
	Cytochalasin F (**19**, Figure 3)	*P. semeniperda*	Phytotoxic to wheat, tomato, *B. tectorum*, *C. arvense* and *S. arvensis*; algicidal; anticancer	[84–86,89,91,140–142]
	Cytochalasin T (**20**, Figure 3)	*P. semeniperda*	Phytotoxic to *C. arvense* and *S. arvensis*	[84,141]
	Cytochalasin Z1 (**22**, Figure 3)	*P. semeniperda*	-	[84]
	Cytochalasin Z2 (**23**, Figure 3)	*P. semeniperda*	Phytotoxic to *C. arvense* and *S. arvensis*	[84,141,142]
	Cytochalasin Z3 (**24**, Figure 3)	*P. semeniperda*	Phytotoxic to wheat, tomato, *C. arvense* and *S. arvensis*; anticancer	[84,89,91,140–142]
	Deoxaphomin (**21**, Figure 3)	*P. semeniperda*	Phytotoxic to *B. tectorum*, s *C. arvense* and *S. arvensis*; anticancer	[84,89,91,140–142]

Table 1. *Cont.*

Class	Compound	*Pyrenophora* species	Activity	References
Isocoumarin	De-*O*-methyldiaporthin (**39**, Figure 4)	*D. siccans*	Phytotoxic to corn, soybean, *Amaranthus spinosus*, *Digitaria ischaemum* and *E. crus-galli*	[127]
Isoquinoline derivatives	Pyrenoline A (**9**, Figure 1)	*P. teres*	Phytotoxic to barley, *Festuca* spp., *Agropyron repens* and *Cynodon dactylon*	[43]
	Pyrenoline B (**10**, Figure 1)	*P. teres*	Phytotoxic to barley, oat, *Hibiscus sabdariffa* and *Euphorbia heterophylla*	[43]
Macrocyclic compounds	Pyrenophorin (**32**, Figure 4)	*P. avenae*	Inhibition of radical growth in oat and non-host plants; antifungal; cytotoxic	[100,102–104]
	Dihydropyrenophorin (**33**, Figure 4)	*P. avenae*	Phytotoxic to barley, soybean, wheat, maize, oat, *Sorghum halepense* and different weeds; antibacterial; antifungal; antialgal	[101,106]
	Pyrenophorol (**34**, Figure 4)	*P. avenae*	Phytotoxic to oat and tomato; antibacterial; antifungal; antialgal	[106,107,143]
Naphthofuroazepinone	Drazepinone (**40**, Figure 4)	*D. siccans*	Phytotoxic to durum wheat and diverse weed species; protein tyrosine phosphatase inhibitor	[128,129]
Nonenolides	Pyrenolide A (**5**, Figure 1)	*P. teres*	Antifungal	[30]
	Pyrenolide B (**6**, Figure 1)	*P. teres*	Antifungal	[29]
	Pyrenolide C (**7**, Figure 1)	*P. teres*	Antifungal	[29]
Phenolic compound	Siccanin (**42**, Figure 4)	*D. siccans*	Antifungal; succinate dehydrogenase inhibition	[133,134]
Proteins	Ptr ToxA	*P. tritici-repentis*	Phytotoxic to wheat	[57]
	Ptr ToxB	*P. tritici-repentis*	Phytotoxic to wheat	[58]
Sesquiterpenoids	Abscisic acid (**29**, Figure 3)	*P. semeniperda*	Phytotoxic to *B. tectorum*	[91,92]
	Pyrenophoric acid (**27**, Figure 3)	*P. semeniperda*	Phytotoxic to *B. tectorum*	[89,91,92]
	Pyrenophoric acid B (**30**, Figure 3)	*P. semeniperda*	Phytotoxic to *Arabidopsis thaliana* and *B. tectorum*	[91,92]
	Pyrenophoric acid C (**31**, Figure 3)	*P. semeniperda*	Phytotoxic to *B. tectorum*	[91,92]
Spirocyclic lactams	Triticone A; spirostaphylotrichin C (**12**, Figure 2)	*P. semeniperda* *P. tritici-repentis*	Phytotoxic to wheat, tomato, oat, and different weed species	[64–66,88]
	Triticone B; spirostaphylotrichin D (**13**, Figure 2)	*P. semeniperda* *P. tritici-repentis*	Phytotoxic to wheat, tomato and different weed species	[64,65,88]
	Triticone C; spirostaphylotrichin A (**14**, Figure 2)	*P. semeniperda* *P. tritici-repentis*	Phytotoxic to *B. tectorum* coleoptiles, weakly to wheat, tomato and different weed species	[64,66,88]
	Triticone D (**15**, Figure 2)	*P. tritici-repentis*	Weakly phytotoxic to wheat and different weed species	[64,66]
	Triticone E (**16**, Figure 2)	*P. semeniperda* *P. tritici-repentis*	Antibacterial	[64,68,88]
	Triticone F; spirostaphylotrichin R (**17**, Figure 2)	*P. semeniperda* *P. tritici-repentis*	Antibacterial	[64,68,88]
	Spirostaphylotrichin V (**25**, Figure 3)	*P. semeniperda*	Weakly phytotoxic to *B. tectorum* coleoptiles	[88]
	Spirostaphylotrichin W (**26**, Figure 3)	*P. semeniperda*	Weakly phytotoxic to tomato and *B. tectorum* coleoptiles	[88]

Table 1. *Cont.*

Class	Compound	*Pyrenophora* species	Activity	References
Spirocyclic lactone	Pyrenolide D (**8**, Figure 1)	*P. teres*	Cytotoxic	[37]
Squalestatin	Zaragozic acid A; squalestatin S1 (**43**, Figure 4)	*D. biseptata*	Squalene synthase inhibition	[136,137]
Unknown	Ptr ToxC	*P. tritici-repentis*	Phytotoxic to wheat	[61]

4. Conclusions

The research to date on toxin production in the genus *Pyrenophora* described here has likely only scratched the surface in terms of the potential of members of this genus to produce novel and interesting toxic compounds. First, very few species have been investigated, and there is remarkably little overlap among study species in the compounds produced. Of the several classes of compounds detected, only the spirocyclic lactams were common to both *P. tritici-repentis* and *P. semeniperda*, and the only other compound common to multiple species was the anthraquinone catenarin. The unusual compounds produced by economically unimportant *Pyrenophora* species were especially noteworthy. Another indication that many potential compounds have gone undetected is the large number of predicted biosynthesis genes from in silico analyses of the three well-studied species that have no known corresponding gene products. New molecular tools may make it possible to induce the production of some of these secondary metabolites in vitro so that they can be characterized and understood [144]. In the meantime, traditional approaches to the discovery of new secondary metabolites, in *Pyrenophora* and perhaps in general, are more likely to be successful if they are focused on understudied fungal pathogens from non-agronomic systems.

Author Contributions: Conceptualization, M.M. and S.M.; methodology, M.M., J.G.Z. and S.M.; software, M.M., J.G.Z. and S.M.; validation, M.M. and S.M.; resources, S.M.; data curation, M.M., J.G.Z. and S.M.; writing—original draft preparation, M.M., J.G.Z. and S.M.; writing—review and editing, M.M., J.G.Z. and S.M.; visualization, M.M. and J.G.Z.; supervision, M.M. and S.M.; project administration, S.M. All authors have read and agreed to the published version of the manuscript.

Funding: This research received no external funding.

Institutional Review Board Statement: Not applicable.

Informed Consent Statement: Not applicable.

Data Availability Statement: The data presented in this study are available in this article.

Acknowledgments: J.G.Z. thanks the University of Cadiz for the postdoctoral support with the Margarita Salas fellowship (2021-067/PN/MS-RECUAL/CD), funded by the NextGenerationEU program of the European Union.

Conflicts of Interest: The authors declare no conflict of interest.

References

1. Index Fungorum. Available online: http://www.indexfungorum.org (accessed on 16 July 2022).
2. Zhang, G.; Berbee, M.L. *Pyrenophora* phylogenetics inferred from ITS and glyceradehyde-3-phosphate dehydrogenase gene sequences. *Mycologia* **2001**, *93*, 1048–1063. [CrossRef]
3. Kodsueb, R.; Dhanasekaran, V.; Aptroot, A.; Lumyong, S.; McKenzie, E.H.; Hyde, K.D.; Jeewon, R. The family Pleosporaceae: Intergeneric relationships and phylogenetic perspectives based on sequence analyses of partial 28S rDNA. *Mycologia* **2006**, *98*, 571–583. [CrossRef]
4. Ariyawansa, H.A.; Thambugala, K.M.; Manamgoda, D.S.; Jayawardena, R.; Camporesi, E.; Boonmee, S.; Wanasinghe, D.N.; Phookamsak, R.; Hongsanan, S.; Singtripop, C.; et al. Towards a natural classification and backbone tree for Pleosporaceae. *Fungal Divers.* **2015**, *71*, 85–139. [CrossRef]
5. Ciuffetti, L.M.; Manning, V.A.; Pandelova, I.; Faris, J.D.; Friesen, T.L.; Strelkov, S.E.; Weber, G.L.; Goodwin, S.B.; Wolpert, T.J.; Figueroa, M. *Pyrenophora tritici-repentis*: A plant pathogenic fungus with global impact. In *Genomics of Plant-Associated Fungi: Monocot Pathogens*; Dean, R.A., Lichens-Park, A., Kole, C., Eds.; Springer: Berlin/Heidelberg, Germany, 2014; pp. 1–39.

6. Clare, S.J.; Wyatt, N.A.; Brueggeman, R.S.; Friesen, T.L. Research advances in the *Pyrenophora teres*–barley interaction. *Mol. Plant Pathol.* **2020**, *21*, 272–288. [CrossRef]
7. Backes, A.; Guerriero, G.; Ait Barka, E.; Jacquard, C. *Pyrenophora teres*: Taxonomy, morphology, interaction with barley, and mode of control. *Front. Plant Sci.* **2021**, *12*, 614951. [CrossRef]
8. Meyer, S.E.; Nelson, D.L.; Clement, S.; Beckstead, J. Cheatgrass (*Bromus tectorum*) biocontrol using indigenous fungal pathogens. In *Proceedings-Shrublands under Fire: Disturbance and Recovery in a Changing World, Cedar City, UT, USA, 6–8 June 2006*; Kitchen, S.G., Pendleton, R.L., Monaco, T.A., Vernon, J.C., Eds.; Proc. RMRS-P-52.; U.S. Department of Agriculture, Forest Service, Rocky Mountain Research Station: Fort Collins, CO, USA, 2008; pp. 61–67.
9. Meyer, S.E.; Beckstead, J.; Pearce, J. Community ecology of fungal pathogens on Bromus tectorum. In *Exotic Brome-Grasses in Arid and Semiarid Ecosystems of the Western US: Causes, Consequences, and Management Implications*; Germino, M.J., Chambers, J.C., Brown, C.S., Eds.; Series on Environmental Management; Springer: Berlin/Heidelberg, Germany, 2016; pp. 193–221.
10. Akhavan, A.; Turkington, T.; Askarian, H.; Tekauz, A.; Xi, K.; Tucker, J.R.; Kutcher, H.R.; Strelkov, S.E. Virulence of *Pyrenophora teres* populations in western Canada. *Can. J. Plant Pathol.* **2016**, *38*, 183–196. [CrossRef]
11. Tekauz, A. A numerical scale to classify reactions of barley to *Pyrenophora teres*. *Can. J. Plant Pathol.* **1985**, *7*, 181–183. [CrossRef]
12. Liu, Z.; Ellwood, S.R.; Oliver, R.P.; Friesen, T.L. *Pyrenophora teres*: Profile of an increasingly damaging barley pathogen. *Mol. Plant Pathol.* **2011**, *12*, 1–19. [CrossRef]
13. Moolhuijzen, P.M.; Muria-Gonzalez, M.J.; Syme, R.; Rawlinson, C.; See, P.T.; Moffat, C.S.; Ellwood, S.R. Expansion and conservation of biosynthetic gene clusters in pathogenic *Pyrenophora* spp. *Toxins* **2020**, *12*, 242. [CrossRef]
14. Smedegård-Petersen, V. Isolation of two toxins produced by *Pyrenophora teres* and their significance in disease development of net-spot blotch of barley. *Physiol. Plant Pathol.* **1977**, *10*, 203–211. [CrossRef]
15. Bach, E.; Christensen, S.; Dalgaard, L.; Larsen, P.O.; Olsen, C.E.; Smedegård-Petersen, V. Structures, properties and relationship to the aspergillomarasmines of toxins produced by *Pyrenophora teres*. *Physiol. Plant Pathol.* **1979**, *14*, 41–46. [CrossRef]
16. Friis, P.; Olsen, C.E.; Møller, B.L. Toxin production in *Pyrenophora teres*, the ascomycete causing the net-spot blotch disease of barley (*Hordeum vulgare* L.). *J. Biol. Chem.* **1991**, *266*, 13329–13335. [CrossRef]
17. Haenni, A.L.; Robert, M.; Vetter, W.; Roux, L.; Barbier, M.; Lederer, E. Structure chimique des aspergillomarasmines A et B. *Helv. Chim. Acta* **1965**, *48*, 729–750. [CrossRef]
18. Arai, K.; Ashikawa, N.; Nakakita, Y.; Matsuura, A.; Ashizawa, N.; Munekata, M. Aspergillomarasmine A and B, potent microbial inhibitors of endothelin-converting enzyme. *Biosci. Biotechnol. Biochem* **1993**, *57*, 1944–1945. [CrossRef]
19. Liao, D.; Yang, S.; Wang, J.; Zhang, J.; Hong, B.; Wu, F.; Lei, X. Total synthesis and structural reassignment of aspergillomarasmine A. *Angew. Chem.* **2016**, *128*, 4363–4367. [CrossRef]
20. Albu, S.A.; Koteva, K.; King, A.M.; Al-Karmi, S.; Wright, G.D.; Capretta, A. Total synthesis of aspergillomarasmine A and related compounds: A sulfamidate approach enables exploration of structure–activity relationships. *Angew. Chem.* **2016**, *128*, 13453–13456. [CrossRef]
21. Koteva, K.; King, A.M.; Capretta, A.; Wright, G.D. Total synthesis and activity of the metallo-β-lactamase inhibitor aspergillomarasmine A. *Angew. Chem. Int. Ed.* **2016**, *55*, 2210–2212. [CrossRef]
22. Zhang, J.; Wang, S.; Bai, Y.; Guo, Q.; Zhou, J.; Lei, X. Total syntheses of natural metallophores staphylopine and aspergillomarasmine A. *J. Org. Chem.* **2017**, *82*, 13643–13648. [CrossRef]
23. Fu, H.; Zhang, J.; Saifuddin, M.; Cruiming, G.; Tepper, P.G.; Poelarends, G.J. Chemoenzymatic asymmetric synthesis of the metallo-β-lactamase inhibitor aspergillomarasmine A and related aminocarboxylic acids. *Nat. Catal.* **2018**, *1*, 186–191. [CrossRef]
24. King, A.M.; Reid-Yu, S.A.; Wang, W.; King, D.T.; De Pascale, G.; Strynadka, N.C.; Walsh, T.R.; Coombes, B.K.; Wright, G.D. Aspergillomarasmine A overcomes metallo-β-lactamase antibiotic resistance. *Nature* **2014**, *510*, 503–506. [CrossRef]
25. Sychantha, D.; Rotondo, C.M.; Tehrani, K.H.; Martin, N.I.; Wright, G.D. Aspergillomarasmine A inhibits metallo-β-lactamases by selectively sequestering Zn^{2+}. *J. Biol. Chem.* **2021**, *297*, 100918. [CrossRef] [PubMed]
26. Weiergang, I.; Jørgensen, H.L.; Møller, I.M.; Friis, P.; Smedegaard-Petersen, V. Correlation between sensitivity of barley to *Pyrenophora teres* toxins and susceptibility to the fungus. *Physiol. Mol. Plant Pathol.* **2002**, *60*, 121–129. [CrossRef]
27. Sarpeleh, A.; Tate, M.E.; Wallwork, H.; Catcheside, D.; Able, A.J. Characterisation of low molecular weight phytotoxins isolated from *Pyrenophora teres*. *Physiol. Mol. Plant Pathol.* **2008**, *73*, 154–162. [CrossRef]
28. Ballio, A.; Bottalico, A.; Buonocore, V.; Carilli, A.; Di Vittorio, V.; Graniti, A. Production and isolation of aspergillomarasmin B (lycomarasmic acid) from cultures of *Colletotrichum gloeosporioides* Penz. (*Gloeosporium olivarum* Aim.). *Phytopathol. Mediterr.* **1969**, *8*, 187–196.
29. Nukina, M.; Ikeda, M.; Sassa, T. Two new pyrenolides, fungal morphogenic substances produced by *Pyrenophora teres* (Diedicke) Drechsler. *Agric. Biol. Chem.* **1980**, *44*, 2761–2762. [CrossRef]
30. Nukina, M.; Sassa, T.; Ikeda, M. A new fungal morphogenic substance, pyrenolide A from *Pyrenophora teres*. *Tetrahedron Lett.* **1980**, *21*, 301–302. [CrossRef]
31. Venkatasubbaiah, P.; Chilton, W.S. Phytotoxins of *Ascochyta hyalospora*, causal agent of lambsquarters leaf spot. *J. Nat. Prod.* **1992**, *55*, 461–467. [CrossRef]
32. Greve, H.; Schupp, P.J.; Eguereva, E.; Kehraus, S.; König, G.M. Ten-membered lactones from the marine-derived fungus *Curvularia* sp. *J. Nat. Prod.* **2008**, *71*, 1651–1653. [CrossRef]
33. Asaoka, M.; Naito, S.; Takei, H. Total synthesis of (±)-pyrenolide B. *Tetrahedron Lett.* **1985**, *26*, 2103–2106. [CrossRef]

34. Suzuki, S.; Tanaka, A.; Yamashita, K. Synthesis and biological activity of (+)-pyrenolide B. *Agric. Biol. Chem.* **1987**, *51*, 3095–3098.
35. Moricz, A.; Gassmann, E.; Bienz, S.; Hesse, M. Synthesis of (±)-pyrenolide B. *Helv. Chim. Acta* **1995**, *78*, 663–669. [CrossRef]
36. Wasserman, H.H.; Prowse, K.S. The singlet oxygen conversion of oxazoles to triamides. Application in the synthesis of (±)-pyrenolide C. Assignment of stereochemistry. *Tetrahedron* **1992**, *48*, 8199–8212. [CrossRef]
37. Nukina, M.; Hirota, H. Pyrenolide D, a new cytotoxic fungal metabolite from *Pyrenophora teres*. *Biosci. Biotechnol. Biochem.* **1992**, *56*, 1158–1159. [CrossRef]
38. Engstrom, K.M.; Mendoza, M.R.; Navarro-Villalobos, M.; Gin, D.Y. Total synthesis of (+)-pyrenolide D. *Angew. Chem. Int. Ed.* **2001**, *40*, 1128–1130. [CrossRef]
39. Thirupathi, B.; Reddy, P.P.; Mohapatra, D.K. A carbohydrate-based total syntheses of (+)-pyrenolide D and (−)-4-*epi*-pyrenolide D. *J. Org. Chem.* **2011**, *76*, 9835–9840. [CrossRef] [PubMed]
40. Zhang, C.; Liu, J.; Du, Y. A concise total synthesis of (+)-pyrenolide D. *Tetrahedron Lett.* **2013**, *54*, 3278–3280. [CrossRef]
41. Markovič, M.; Lopatka, P.; Koóš, P.; Gracza, T. Asymmetric formal synthesis of (+)-pyrenolide D. *Synthesis* **2014**, *46*, 817–821.
42. Ogawa, Y.; Kato, M.; Sasaki, I.; Sugimura, H. Total synthesis of (+)-pyrenolide D. *J. Org. Chem.* **2018**, *83*, 12315–12319. [CrossRef]
43. Coval, S.J.; Hradil, C.M.; Lu, H.S.; Clardy, J.; Satouri, S.; Strobel, G.A. Pyrenoline-A and-B, two new phytotoxins from *Pyrenophora teres*. *Tetrahedron Lett.* **1990**, *31*, 2117–2120. [CrossRef]
44. Benali, D.; Lyamani, A.; Zaid, A.; Samih, M.; Haloui, N. Cinétique de production de toxines de type pyrenoline A et pyrenoline B par des isolats marocains de *Pyrenophora teres*. *Phytopathol. Mediterr.* **1995**, *34*, 120–125.
45. Engström, K.; Brishammar, S.; Svensson, C.; Bengtsson, M.; Andersson, R. Anthraquinones from some *Drechslera* species and *Bipolaris sorokiniana*. *Mycol. Res.* **1993**, *97*, 381–384. [CrossRef]
46. Wakuliński, W.; Kachlicki, P.; Sobiczewski, P.; Schollenberger, M.; Zamorski, C.; Łotocka, B.; Sarova, J. Catenarin production by isolates of *Pyrenophora tritici-repentis* (Died.) Drechsler and its antimicrobial activity. *J. Phytopathol.* **2003**, *151*, 74–79. [CrossRef]
47. Sadorn, K.; Saepua, S.; Boonyuen, N.; Komwijit, S.; Rachtawee, P.; Pittayakhajonwut, P. Phenolic glucosides and chromane analogs from the insect fungus *Conoideocrella krungchingensis* BCC53666. *Tetrahedron* **2019**, *75*, 3463–3471. [CrossRef]
48. Anslow, W.K.; Raistrick, H. Synthesis of catenarin (1:4:5:7-tetrahydroxy-2-methylanthraquinone), a metabolic product of species of *Helminthosporium*. *Biochem.* **1941**, *35*, 1006–1010.
49. Chandrasenan, K.; Neelakantan, S.; Seshadri, T.R. A new synthesis of catenarin and erythroglaucin. *Proc. Indian Natl. Sci. Acad.* **1960**, *51*, 296–300. [CrossRef]
50. Bouras, N.; Strelkov, S.E. The anthraquinone catenarin is phytotoxic and produced in leaves and kernels of wheat infected by *Pyrenophora tritici-repentis*. *Physiol. Mol. Plant Pathol.* **2008**, *72*, 87–95. [CrossRef]
51. Martorell, M.; Castro, N.; Victoriano, M.; Capó, X.; Tejada, S.; Vitalini, S.; Pezzani, R.; Sureda, A. An update of anthraquinone derivatives emodin, diacerein, and catenarin in diabetes. *Evid. Based Complementary Altern. Med.* **2021**, *2021*, 3313419. [CrossRef]
52. Mehrabi, R.; Bahkali, A.H.; Abd-Elsalam, K.A.; Moslem, M.; M'Barek, S.B.; Gohari, A.M.; Jashni, M.K.; Stergiopoulos, I.; Kema, G.H.J.; de Wit, P.J.G.M. Horizontal gene and chromosome transfer in plant pathogenic fungi affecting host range. *FEMS Microbiol. Rev.* **2011**, *35*, 542–554. [CrossRef]
53. Friesen, T.L.; Stukenbrock, E.H.; Liu, Z.H.; Meinhardt, S.; Ling, H.; Faris, J.D.; Rasmussen, J.B.; Solomon, P.S.; McDonald, B.A.; Oliver, R.P. Emergence of a new disease as a result of interspecific virulence gene transfer. *Nat. Genet.* **2006**, *38*, 953–956. [CrossRef]
54. Antoni, E.A.; Rybak, K.; Tucker, M.P.; Hane, J.K.; Solomon, P.S.; Drenth, A.; Shankar, M.; Oliver, R.P. Ubiquity of ToxA and absence of ToxB in Australian populations of *Pyrenophora tritici-repentis*. *Australas. Plant Pathol.* **2010**, *39*, 63–68. [CrossRef]
55. Leisova-Syobodova, L.; Hanzalova, A.; Kucera, L. Expansion and variability of the Ptr Tox A gene in populations of *Pyrenophora tritici-repentis* and *Pyrenophora teres*. *J. Plant Pathol.* **2010**, *92*, 729–735.
56. Rawlinson, C.; See, P.T.; Moolhuijzen, P.; Li, H.; Moffat, C.S.; Chooi, Y.H.; Oliver, R.P. The identification and deletion of the polyketide synthase-nonribosomal peptide synthase gene responsible for the production of the phytotoxic triticone A/B in the wheat fungal pathogen *Pyrenophora tritici-repentis*. *Environ. Microbiol.* **2019**, *21*, 4875–4886. [PubMed]
57. Ballance, G.M.; Lamari, L.; Bernier, C.C. Purification and characterization of a host-selective necrosis toxin from *Pyrenophora tritici-repentis*. *Physiol. Mol. Plant Pathol.* **1989**, *35*, 203–213. [CrossRef]
58. Strelkov, S.E.; Lamari, L.; Ballance, G.M. Characterization of a host-specific protein toxin (Ptr ToxB) from *Pyrenophora tritici-repentis*. *Mol. Plant-Microbe Interact.* **1999**, *12*, 728–732. [CrossRef]
59. Pandelova, I.; Figueroa, M.; Wilhelm, L.J.; Manning, V.A.; Mankaney, A.N.; Mockler, T.C.; Ciuffetti, L.M. Host-selective toxins of *Pyrenophora tritici-repentis* induce common responses associated with host susceptibility. *PLoS ONE* **2012**, *7*, e40240.
60. Andrie, R.M.; Schoch, C.L.; Hedges, R.; Spatafora, J.W.; Ciuffetti, L.M. Homologs of ToxB, a host-selective toxin gene from *Pyrenophora tritici-repentis*, are present in the genome of sister-species *Pyrenophora bromi* and other members of the Ascomycota. *Fungal Genet. Biol.* **2008**, *45*, 363–377.
61. Effertz, R.J.; Meinhardt, S.W.; Anderson, J.A.; Jordahl, J.G.; Francl, L.J. Identification of a chlorosis-inducing toxin from *Pyrenophora tritici-repentis* and the chromosomal location of an insensitivity locus in wheat. *Phytopathology* **2002**, *92*, 527–533.
62. Betts, M.F.; Manning, V.A.; Cardwell, K.B.; Pandelova, I.; Ciuffetti, L.M. The importance of the N-terminus for activity of Ptr ToxB, a chlorosis-inducing host-selective toxin produced by *Pyrenophora tritici-repentis*. *Physiol. Mol. Plant Pathol.* **2011**, *75*, 138–145.
63. Shi, G.; Kariyawasam, G.; Liu, S.; Leng, Y.; Zhong, S.; Ali, S.; Moolhuijzen, P.; Moffat, C.S.; Rasmussen, J.B.; Friesen, T.L.; et al. A conserved hypothetical gene is required but not sufficient for Ptr ToxC production in *Pyrenophora tritici-repentis*. *Mol. Plant-Microbe Interact.* **2022**, *35*, 336–348. [CrossRef]

64. Hallock, Y.F.; Lu, H.S.; Clardy, J.; Strobel, G.A.; Sugawara, F.; Samsoedin, R.; Yoshida, S. Triticones, spirocyclic lactams from the fungal plant pathogen *Drechslera tritici-repentis*. *J. Nat. Prod.* **1993**, *56*, 747–754. [CrossRef]
65. Sugawara, F.; Takahashi, N.; Strobel, G.A.; Strobel, S.A.; Lu, H.S.; Clardy, J. Triticones A and B, novel phytotoxins from the plant pathogenic fungus *Drechslera tritici-repentis*. *J. Am. Chem. Soc.* **1988**, *110*, 4086–4087. [CrossRef]
66. Kenfield, D.; Strobel, S.; Sugawara, F.; Berglund, D.; Strobel, G. Triticone A: A novel bioactive lactam with potential as a molecular probe. *Biochem. Biophys. Res. Commun.* **1988**, *157*, 174–182. [CrossRef]
67. Shinohara, C.; Chikanishi, T.; Nakashima, S.; Hashimoto, A.; Hamanaka, A.; Endo, A.; Hasumi, K. Enhancement of fibrinolytic activity of vascular endothelial cells by chaetoglobosin A, crinipellin B, geodin and triticone B. *J. Antibiot.* **2000**, *53*, 262–268. [CrossRef] [PubMed]
68. Hilario, F.; Polinário, G.; de Amorim, M.R.; de Sousa Batista, V.; do Nascimento, N.M., Jr.; Araújo, A.R.; Baubab, T.M.; Dos Santos, L.C. Spirocyclic lactams and curvulinic acid derivatives from the endophytic fungus *Curvularia lunata* and their antibacterial and antifungal activities. *Fitoterapia* **2020**, *141*, 104466. [CrossRef] [PubMed]
69. Bouras, N.; Strelkov, S.E. Influence of carbon source on growth and mycotoxin production by isolates of *Pyrenophora tritici-repentis* from wheat. *Can. J. Microbiol.* **2010**, *56*, 874–882. [CrossRef] [PubMed]
70. Meyer, S.E.; Quinney, D.; Nelson, D.L.; Weaver, J. Impact of the pathogen *Pyrenophora semeniperda* on *Bromus tectorum* seedbank dynamics in North American cold deserts. *Weed Res.* **2007**, *47*, 54–62. [CrossRef]
71. Paul, A.R. The production of *Pyrenophora semeniperda* in culture. *Trans. Br. Mycol. Soc.* **1969**, *52*, 373–379. [CrossRef]
72. Medd, R.W.; Murray, G.M.; Pickering, D.I. Review of the epidemiology and economic importance of *Pyrenophora semeniperda*. *Australas. Plant Pathol.* **2003**, *32*, 539–550. [CrossRef]
73. Medd, R.W.; Campbell, M.A. Grass seed infection following inundation with *Pyrenophora semeniperda*. *Biocontrol. Sci. Technol.* **2005**, *15*, 21–36. [CrossRef]
74. Beckstead, J.; Meyer, S.E.; Molder, C.J.; Smith, C. A race for survival: Can *Bromus tectorum* seeds escape *Pyrenophora semeniperda*-caused mortality by germinating quickly? *Ann. Bot.* **2007**, *99*, 907–914. [CrossRef]
75. Allen, P.S.; Finch-Boekweg, H.; Meyer, S.E. A proposed mechanism for high pathogen-caused mortality in the seed bank of an invasive annual grass. *Fungal Ecol.* **2018**, *35*, 108–115. [CrossRef]
76. Meyer, S.E.; Stewart, T.E.; Clement, S. The quick and the deadly: Growth vs virulence in a seed bank pathogen. *New Phytol.* **2010**, *187*, 209–216. [CrossRef] [PubMed]
77. Masi, M.; Evidente, A.; Meyer, S.; Nicholson, J.; Muñoz, A. Effect of strain and cultural conditions on the production of cytochalasin B by the potential mycoherbicide *Pyrenophora semeniperda* (Pleosporaceae, Pleosporales). *Biocontrol. Sci. Technol.* **2014**, *24*, 53–64. [CrossRef]
78. Meyer, S.E.; Masi, M.; Clement, S.; Davis, T.L.; Beckstead, J. Mycelial growth rate and toxin production in the seed pathogen *Pyrenophora semeniperda*: Resource trade-offs and temporally varying selection. *Plant Pathol.* **2015**, *64*, 1450–1460. [CrossRef]
79. Boose, D.; Harrison, S.; Clement, S.; Meyer, S. Population genetic structure of the seed pathogen *Pyrenophora semeniperda* on *Bromus tectorum* in western North America. *Mycologia* **2011**, *103*, 85–93. [CrossRef]
80. Coleman, C.E.; Meyer, S.E.; Ricks, N. Mating system complexity and cryptic speciation in the seed bank pathogen *Pyrenophora semeniperda*. *Plant Pathol.* **2019**, *68*, 369–382. [CrossRef]
81. Beckstead, J.; Meyer, S.E.; Reinhart, K.O.; Bergen, K.M.; Holden, S.R.; Boekweg, H.F. Factors affecting host range in a generalist seed pathogen of semi-arid shrublands. *Plant Ecol.* **2014**, *15*, 427–440. [CrossRef]
82. Beckstead, J.; Meyer, S.E.; Ishizuka, T.S.; McEvoy, K.M.; Coleman, C.E. Lack of host specialization on winter annual grasses in the fungal seed bank pathogen *Pyrenophora semeniperda*. *PLoS ONE* **2016**, *11*, e0151058. [CrossRef]
83. Soliai, M.M.; Meyer, S.E.; Udall, J.A.; Elzinga, D.E.; Hermansen, R.A.; Bodily, P.M.; Hart, A.A.; Coleman, C.E. De novo genome assembly of the fungal plant pathogen *Pyrenophora semeniperda*. *PLoS ONE* **2014**, *9*, e87045. [CrossRef] [PubMed]
84. Evidente, A.; Andolfi, A.; Vurro, M.; Zonno, M.C.; Motta, A. Cytochalasins Z1, Z2 and Z3, three 24-oxa[14]cytochalasans produced by *Pyrenophora semeniperda*. *Phytochemistry* **2002**, *60*, 45–53. [CrossRef]
85. Aldridge, D.C.; Armstrong, J.J.; Speake, R.N.; Turner, W.B. The cytochalasins, a new class of biologically active mould metabolites. *Chem. Comm.* **1967**, 26–27. [CrossRef]
86. Scherlach, K.; Boettger, D.; Remme, N.; Hertweck, C. The chemistry and biology of cytochalasans. *Nat. Prod. Rep.* **2010**, *27*, 869–886. [CrossRef]
87. Campbell, M.A.; Medd, R.W.; Brown, J.B. Optimizing conditions for growth and sporulation of *Pyrenophora semeniperda*. *Plant Pathol.* **2003**, *52*, 448–454. [CrossRef]
88. Masi, M.; Meyer, S.; Clement, S.; Andolfi, A.; Cimmino, A.; Evidente, A. Spirostaphylotrichin W, a spirocyclic γ-lactam isolated from liquid culture of *Pyrenophora semeniperda*, a potential mycoherbicide for cheatgrass (*Bromus tectorum*) biocontrol. *Tetrahedron* **2014**, *70*, 1497–1501. [CrossRef]
89. Masi, M.; Meyer, S.; Cimmino, A.; Andolfi, A.; Evidente, A. Pyrenophoric acid, a phytotoxic sesquiterpenoid penta-2,4-dienoic acid produced by a potential mycoherbicide, *Pyrenophora semeniperda*. *J. Nat. Prod.* **2014**, *77*, 925–930. [CrossRef] [PubMed]
90. Cimmino, A.; Masi, M.; Evidente, M.; Superchi, S.; Evidente, A. Application of Mosher's method for absolute configuration assignment to bioactive plants and fungi metabolites. *J. Pharm. Biomed. Anal.* **2017**, *144*, 59–89. [CrossRef]
91. Masi, M.; Meyer, S.; Cimmino, A.; Clement, S.; Black, B.; Evidente, A. Pyrenophoric acids B and C, two new phytotoxic sesquiterpenoids produced by *Pyrenophora semeniperda*. *J. Agric. Food Chem.* **2014**, *62*, 10304–10311. [CrossRef]

92. Lozano-Juste, J.; Masi, M.; Cimmino, A.; Clement, S.; Fernández, M.A.; Antoni, R.; Meyer, S.; Rodriguez, P.L.; Evidente, A. The fungal sesquiterpenoid pyrenophoric acid B uses the plant ABA biosynthetic pathway to inhibit seed germination. *J. Exp. Bot.* **2019**, *70*, 5487–5494. [CrossRef]
93. da Rosa, C.R.; Martinelli, J.A.; Federizzi, L.C.; Bocchese, C.A. Quantification of conidia produced by *Pyrenophora chaetomioides* on dead leaves of *Avena sativa* under field condition. *Fitopatol. Bras.* **2003**, *28*, 319–322.
94. Chen, H.; Xue, L.; White, J.F.; Kamran, M.; Li, C. Identification and characterization of *Pyrenophora* species causing leaf spot on oat (*Avena sativa*) in western China. *Plant Pathol.* **2022**, *71*, 566–577. [CrossRef]
95. Lam, A. *Drechslera siccans* from ryegrass fields in England and Wales. *Trans. Br. Mycol. Soc.* **1984**, *83*, 305–311. [CrossRef]
96. Wiewióra, B.; Żurek, G.; Żurek, M. Endophyte-mediated disease resistance in wild populations of perennial ryegrass (*Lolium perenne*). *Fungal Ecol.* **2015**, *15*, 1–8. [CrossRef]
97. Osterhage, C.; König, G.M.; Höller, U.; Wright, A.D. Rare sesquiterpenes from the algicolous fungus *Drechslera dematioidea*. *J. Nat. Prod.* **2002**, *65*, 306–313. [CrossRef] [PubMed]
98. Shoemaker, R.A. *Marielliottia*, a new genus of cereal and grass parasites segregated from *Drechslera*. *Can. J. Bot.* **1998**, *76*, 1558–1569.
99. Jones, E.B.G.; Sakayaroj, J.; Suetrong, S.; Somrithipol, S.; Pang, K.L. Classification of marine Ascomycota, anamorphic taxa and Basidiomycota. *Fungal Divers.* **2009**, *35*, 187.
100. Nozoe, S.; Hirai, K.; Tsuda, K.; Ishibashi, K.; Shirasaka, M.; Grove, J.F. The structure of pyrenophorin. *Tetrahedron Lett.* **1965**, *6*, 4675–4677. [CrossRef]
101. Sugawara, F.; Strobel, G.A. (−)-Dihydropyrenophorin, a novel and selective phytotoxin produced by *Drechslera avenae*. *Plant Sci.* **1986**, *43*, 1–5. [CrossRef]
102. Lerario, P.; Graniti, A. Attività fitotossica della pirenoforina e sua produzione nelle colture di *Pyrenophora avenae* Ito *et* Kurib. *Phytopathol. Mediterr.* **1985**, *24*, 280–283.
103. McMullin, D.R.; Green, B.D.; Miller, J.D. Antifungal sesquiterpenoids and macrolides from an endophytic *Lophodermium* species of *Pinus strobus*. *Phytochemistry Lett.* **2015**, *14*, 148–152. [CrossRef]
104. Yu, H.; Sperlich, J.; Höfert, S.P.; Janiak, C.; Teusch, N.; Stuhldreier, F.; Wesselborg, S.; Wang, C.; Kassack, M.U.; Dai, H.; et al. Azaphilone pigments and macrodiolides from the coprophilous fungus *Coniella fragariae*. *Fitoterapia* **2019**, *137*, 104249. [CrossRef]
105. Ramakrishna, K.; Sreenivasulu, R.; Vidavalur, S.; Jagan Mohan Reddy, B. Stereoselective total synthesis of (-)-pyrenophorin. *Lett. Org. Chem.* **2016**, *13*, 693–697. [CrossRef]
106. Zhang, W.; Krohn, K.; Egold, H.; Draeger, S.; Schulz, B. Diversity of antimicrobial pyrenophorol derivatives from an endophytic fungus, *Phoma* sp. *Eur. J. Org. Chem.* **2008**, *2008*, 4320–4328. [CrossRef]
107. Kastanias, M.A.; Chrysayi-Tokousbalides, M. Herbicidal potential of pyrenophorol isolated from a *Drechslera avenae* pathotype. *Pest Manag. Sci.* **2000**, *56*, 227–232. [CrossRef]
108. Yadav, J.S.; Reddy, U.S.; Reddy, B.S. Stereoselective total synthesis of (−)-pyrenophorol. *Tetrahedron Lett.* **2009**, *50*, 5984–5986. [CrossRef]
109. Raistrick, H.; Robinson, R.; Todd, A.R. Studies in the biochemistry of micro-organisms: (a) On the production of hydroxyanthraquinones by species of *Helminthosporium*. (b) Isolation of tritisporin, a new metabolic product of *Helminthosporium tritici-vulgaris* Nisikado. (c) The molecular constitution of catenarin. *Biochem. J.* **1934**, *28*, 559–572. [PubMed]
110. Shujun, J.; Sheng, Q.; Yunzhi, Z. Isolation, purification, identification, and bioassay of helminthosporin with herbicidal activity from *Curvularia eragrostidis*. *Acta Phytophylacica Sin.* **2006**, *33*, 313–318.
111. Fozia, A.A. Phytochemical Investigation of *Aloe turkanensis* for Anticancer Activity. Doctoral Dissertation, University of Nairobi, Nairobi, Kenya, 2014.
112. Augustin, N.; Nuthakki, V.K.; Abdullaha, M.; Hassan, Q.P.; Gandhi, S.G.; Bharate, S.B. Discovery of helminthosporin, an anthraquinone isolated from *Rumex abyssinicus* Jacq as a dual cholinesterase inhibitor. *ACS Omega* **2020**, *5*, 1616–1624. [CrossRef] [PubMed]
113. Chrysayi-Tokousbalides, M.; Kastanias, M.A. Cynodontin: A fungal metabolite with antifungal properties. *J. Agric. Food Chem.* **2003**, *51*, 4920–4923. [CrossRef] [PubMed]
114. Đorović, J.; Antonijević, M.; Marković, Z. Antioxidative and inhibition potency of cynodontin. *J. Serb. Soc. Comput. Mech.* **2020**, *2020*. [CrossRef]
115. van Eijk, G.W. Chrysophanol and emodin from *Drechslera catenaria*. *Phytochemistry* **1974**, *13*, 650. [CrossRef]
116. Dussart, F.; Jakubczyk, D. Biosynthesis of rubellins in *Ramularia collo-cygni*—Genetic basis and pathway proposition. *Int. J. Mol. Sci.* **2022**, *23*, 3475. [CrossRef] [PubMed]
117. Choi, G.J.; Lee, S.W.; Jang, K.S.; Kim, J.S.; Cho, K.Y.; Kim, J.C. Effects of chrysophanol, parietin, and nepodin of *Rumex crispus* on barley and cucumber powdery mildews. *Crop Prot.* **2004**, *23*, 1215–1221. [CrossRef]
118. Yusuf, M.A.; Singh, B.N.; Sudheer, S.; Kharwar, R.N.; Siddiqui, S.; Abdel-Azeem, A.M.; Fraceto, L.F.; Dashora, K.; Gupta, V.K. Chrysophanol: A natural anthraquinone with multifaceted biotherapeutic potential. *Biomolecules* **2019**, *9*, 68.
119. Su, S.; Wu, J.; Gao, Y.; Luo, Y.; Yang, D.; Wang, P. The pharmacological properties of chrysophanol, the recent advances. *Biomed. Pharmacother.* **2020**, *125*, 110002. [CrossRef]
120. Lin, C.H.; Tseng, H.F.; Hsieh, P.C.; Chiu, V.; Lin, T.Y.; Lan, C.C.; Tzeng, I.S.; Chao, H.N.; Hsu, C.C.; Kuo, C.Y. Nephroprotective role of chrysophanol in hypoxia/reoxygenation-induced renal cell damage via apoptosis, ER stress, and ferroptosis. *Biomedicines* **2021**, *9*, 1283. [CrossRef] [PubMed]

121. Jadaun, K.S.; Mehan, S.; Sharma, A.; Siddiqui, E.M.; Kumar, S.; Alsuhaymi, N. Neuroprotective effect of chrysophanol as a PI3K/AKT/mTOR signaling inhibitor in an experimental model of autologous blood-induced intracerebral hemorrhage. *Curr. Med. Sci.* **2022**, *2022*, 1–18. [CrossRef]
122. Cui, W.H.; Zhang, H.H.; Qu, Z.M.; Wang, Z.; Zhang, D.J.; Wang, S. Effects of chrysophanol on hippocampal damage and mitochondrial autophagy in mice with cerebral ischemia reperfusion. *Int. J. Neurosci.* **2022**, *132*, 613–620. [CrossRef]
123. Dong, X.; Fu, J.; Yin, X.; Cao, S.; Li, X.; Lin, L.; Huyiligeqi; Ni, J. Emodin: A review of its pharmacology, toxicity and pharmacokinetics. *Phytother. Res.* **2016**, *30*, 1207–1218. [CrossRef]
124. Anke, H.; Kolthoum, I.; Laatsch, H. Metabolic products of microorganisms. 192. The anthraquinones of the *Aspergillus glaucus* group. II. Biological activity. *Arch. Microbiol.* **1980**, *126*, 231–236. [CrossRef]
125. Hasan, H.A.H. Studies on toxigenic fungi in roasted foodstuff (salted seed) and halotolerant activity of emodin-producing *Aspergillus wentii*. *Folia Microbiol.* **1998**, *43*, 383–391. [CrossRef]
126. Macías, M.; Ulloa, M.; Gamboa, A.; Mata, R. Phytotoxic compounds from the new coprophilous fungus *Guanomyces polythrix*. *J. Nat. Prod.* **2000**, *63*, 757–761. [CrossRef] [PubMed]
127. Hallock, Y.F.; Clardy, J.; Kenfield, D.S.; Strobel, G. De-*O*-methyldiaporthin, a phytotoxin from *Drechslera siccans*. *Phytochemistry* **1988**, *27*, 3123–3125. [CrossRef]
128. Evidente, A.; Andolfi, A.; Vurro, M.; Fracchiolla, M.; Zonno, M.C.; Motta, A. Drazepinone, a trisubstituted tetrahydronaphthofuroazepinone with herbicidal activity produced by *Drechslera siccans*. *Phytochemistry* **2005**, *66*, 715–721. [CrossRef]
129. Cao, F.; Pan, L.; Gao, W.; Liu, Y.; Zheng, C.; Zhang, Y. Structure revision and protein tyrosine phosphatase inhibitory activity of drazepinone. *Mar. Drugs* **2021**, *19*, 714. [CrossRef] [PubMed]
130. Lim, C.H.; Miyagawa, H.; Ueno, T.; Takenaka, H.; Sung, N.D. Siccanol: Sesterterpene isolated from pathogenic fungus *Drechslera siccans*. *Appl. Biol. Chem.* **1996**, *39*, 241–244.
131. Chan, J.; Jamison, T.F. Enantioselective synthesis of (−)-terpestacin and structural revision of siccanol using catalytic stereoselective fragment couplings and macrocyclizations. *J. Am. Chem. Soc.* **2004**, *126*, 10682–10691. [CrossRef]
132. Masi, M.; Zonno, M.C.; Boari, A.; Vurro, M.; Evidente, A. Terpestacin, a toxin produced by *Phoma exigua* var. *heteromorpha*, the causal agent of a severe foliar disease of oleander (*Nerium oleander* L.). *Nat. Prod. Res.* **2022**, *36*, 1253–1259. [CrossRef] [PubMed]
133. Ishibashi, K. Studies on antibiotics from *Helminthosporium* sp. fungi. VII Siccanin, a new antifungal antibiotic produced by *Helminthosporium siccans*. *J. Antibiot.* **1962**, *15*, 161–167.
134. Mogi, T.; Kawakami, T.; Arai, H.; Igarashi, Y.; Matsushita, K.; Mori, M.; Shiomi, K.; Ōmura, S.; Harada, S.; Kita, K. Siccanin rediscovered as a species-selective succinate dehydrogenase inhibitor. *J. Biochem.* **2009**, *146*, 383–387. [CrossRef]
135. Trost, B.M.; Shen, H.C.; Surivet, J.P. An enantioselective biomimetic total synthesis of (−)-siccanin. *Angew. Chem.* **2003**, *115*, 4073–4077. [CrossRef]
136. Bills, G.F.; Peláez, F.; Polishook, J.D.; Diez-Matas, M.T.; Harris, G.H.; Clapp, W.H.; Dufresne, C.; Byrne, K.M.; Nallin-Omstead, M.; Jenkins, R.G.; et al. Distribution of zaragozic acids (squalestatins) among filamentous ascomycetes. *Mycol. Res.* **1994**, *98*, 733–739. [CrossRef]
137. Huang, L.; Lingham, R.B.; Harris, G.H.; Singh, S.B.; Dufresne, C.; Nallin-Omstead, M.; Bills, G.F.; Mojena, M.; Sanchez, M.; Karkas, J.D.; et al. New fungal metabolites as potential antihypercholesterolemics and anticancer agents. *Can. J. Bot.* **1995**, *73*, 898–906. [CrossRef]
138. Nicolaou, K.C.; Yue, E.W.; La Greca, S.; Nadin, A.; Yang, Z.; Leresche, J.E.; Tsuri, T.; Naniwa, Y.; de Riccardis, F. Synthesis of zaragozic acid A/squalestatin S1. *Eur. J. Chem.* **1995**, *1*, 467–494. [CrossRef]
139. Sarpeleh, A.; Wallwork, H.; Catcheside, D.E.; Tate, M.E.; Able, A.J. Proteinaceous metabolites from *Pyrenophora teres* contribute to symptom development of barley net blotch. *Phytopathology* **2007**, *97*, 907–915. [CrossRef] [PubMed]
140. Van Goietsenoven, G.; Mathieu, V.; Andolfi, A.; Cimmino, A.; Lefranc, F.; Kiss, R.; Evidente, A. In vitro growth inhibitory effects of cytochalasins and derivatives in cancer cells. *Planta Med.* **2011**, *77*, 711–717. [CrossRef]
141. Berestetskiy, A.; Dmitriev, A.; Mitina, G.; Lisker, I.; Andolfi, A.; Evidente, A. Nonenolides and cytochalasins with phytotoxic activity against *Cirsium arvense* and *Sonchus arvensis*: A structure–activity relationships study. *Phytochemistry* **2008**, *69*, 953–960. [CrossRef] [PubMed]
142. Cimmino, A.; Andolfi, A.; Berestetskiy, A.; Evidente, A. Production of phytotoxins by *Phoma exigua* var. exigua, a potential mycoherbicide against perennial thistles. *J. Agric. Food Chem.* **2008**, *56*, 6304–6309. [CrossRef]
143. Sumarah, M.W.; Kesting, J.R.; Sørensen, D.; Miller, J.D. Antifungal metabolites from fungal endophytes of *Pinus strobus*. *Phytochemistry* **2011**, *72*, 1833–1837. [CrossRef]
144. Chooi, Y.H.; Solomon, P.S. A chemical ecogenomics approach to understand the roles of secondary metabolites in fungal cereal pathogens. *Front. Microbiol.* **2014**, *5*, 640. [CrossRef]

toxins

MDPI

Review

Defensive Molecules Momilactones A and B: Function, Biosynthesis, Induction and Occurrence

Hisashi Kato-Noguchi

Department of Applied Biological Science, Faculty of Agriculture, Kagawa University, Miki, Kagawa 761-0795, Japan; kato.hisashi@kagawa-u.ac.jp

Abstract: Labdane-related diterpenoids, momilactones A and B were isolated and identified in rice husks in 1973 and later found in rice leaves, straws, roots, root exudate, other several Poaceae species and the moss species *Calohypnum plumiforme*. The functions of momilactones in rice are well documented. Momilactones in rice plants suppressed the growth of fungal pathogens, indicating the defense function against pathogen attacks. Rice plants also inhibited the growth of adjacent competitive plants through the root secretion of momilactones into their rhizosphere due to the potent growth-inhibitory activity of momilactones, indicating a function in allelopathy. Momilactone-deficient mutants of rice lost their tolerance to pathogens and allelopathic activity, which verifies the involvement of momilactones in both functions. Momilactones also showed pharmacological functions such as anti-leukemia and anti-diabetic activities. Momilactones are synthesized from geranylgeranyl diphosphate through cyclization steps, and the biosynthetic gene cluster is located on chromosome 4 of the rice genome. Pathogen attacks, biotic elicitors such as chitosan and cantharidin, and abiotic elicitors such as UV irradiation and $CuCl_2$ elevated momilactone production through jasmonic acid-dependent and independent signaling pathways. Rice allelopathy was also elevated by jasmonic acid, UV irradiation and nutrient deficiency due to nutrient competition with neighboring plants with the increased production and secretion of momilactones. Rice allelopathic activity and the secretion of momilactones into the rice rhizosphere were also induced by either nearby *Echinochloa crus-galli* plants or their root exudates. Certain compounds from *Echinochloa crus-galli* may stimulate the production and secretion of momilactones. This article focuses on the functions, biosynthesis and induction of momilactones and their occurrence in plant species.

Keywords: allelopathy; biosynthesis; diterpenoid; *Echinochloa crus-galli*; elicitation; momilactone; *Oryza sativa*; pathogen; rice blast

Key Contribution: The allelopathic and defense functions of momilactones may play important ecological roles in rice evolution because of the existence of a dedicated biosynthetic gene cluster in the rice genome. The potential of momilactones to serve as natural fungicides and herbicides provides significant benefits when applied to other important crops.

Citation: Kato-Noguchi, H. Defensive Molecules Momilactones A and B: Function, Biosynthesis, Induction and Occurrence. *Toxins* **2023**, *15*, 241. https://doi.org/10.3390/toxins15040241

Received: 24 February 2023
Revised: 22 March 2023
Accepted: 24 March 2023
Published: 25 March 2023

1. Introduction

Labdane-related diterpenoids, momilactones A and B (Figure 1) were first isolated and identified in rice husks as potent germination and growth-inhibitory substances in 1973 [1]. Momilactones were later isolated from rice leaves as phytoalexins against fungal pathogens such as the rice blast fungus *Magnaporthe oryzae* [2,3]. The concentrations of momilactones increased 2 days after infection with *Magnaporthe oryzae*, and momilactones suppressed the further growth of the fungus [4,5]. The fungal elicitors chitosan and cholic acid also induced the accumulation of momilactone A in rice leaves and suspension-cultured rice cells [6,7].

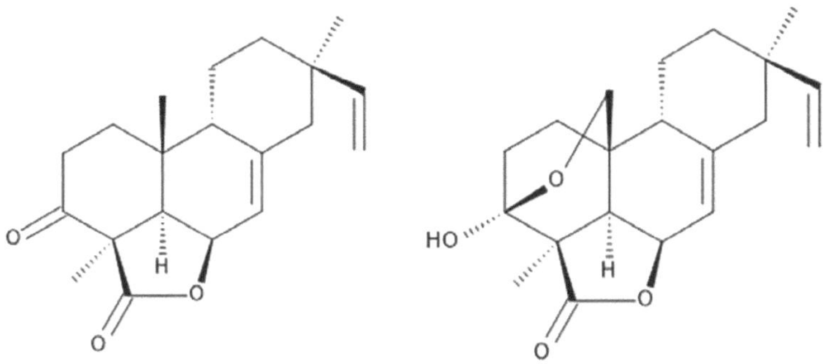

Figure 1. Momilactones.

The function of momilactones, especially momilactone A, as phytoalexins has been extensively studied, and the evidence suggests that momilactones may play a role in the rice defense function against fungal pathogens [8–10].

The first finding of rice allelopathy was made in field examinations in Arkansas, U.S.A., where 191 of over 5000 rice accessions suppressed the growth of the aquatic weed *Heteranthera limosa* [11]. Allelopathy is defined as the chemical interactions among various plant species [12]. Certain plants release some secondary metabolites, termed allelochemicals, into their immediate environment, and these allelochemicals affect the growth and development of other plant species nearby [13–17]. The observation of rice allelopathy led to large field screening programs. Among over 16,000 rice germplasm collections of the USDA-ARS from 99 countries, 412 rice accessions suppressed the growth of *Heteranthera limosa*, and 145 rice accessions suppressed the growth of *Ammannia coccinea* [18,19]. More than 40 rice cultivars among 1000 rice collections inhibited the growth of *Echinochloa crus-galli* and *Cyperus difformis* [20]. Screening programs in the field and/or laboratories have also been carried out in several other countries, and it was found that certain rice cultivars released allelochemicals from their root systems into their immediate environments, such as rhizosphere soil, cultural solutions and other incubation media [21–24]. Thereafter, momilactones A and B were again isolated and identified in rice root exudates as rice allelochemicals [25,26]. It was also found that rice plants released momilactones throughout their life cycles with sufficient amounts of momilactones for allelopathy [27,28].

Momilactones are synthesized in rice plants from geranylgeranyl diphosphate, which is also a precursor of other phytoalexins and a plant hormone, gibberellic acid [29]. Momilactones are synthesized and accumulated in rice leaves as phytoalexins and secreted into their root zones as allelochemicals [30,31]. A gene cluster related to momilactone synthesis was found on chromosome 4 of the rice genome. Momilactones were later found in some other Gramineae plant species and the moss species *Calohypnum plumiforme* (syn. *Hypnum plumaeform*) as allelochemicals [32–35]. This review provides an overview of the functions, biosynthesis, induction and occurrence of momilactones in plant species and highlights the importance of momilactones.

2. Defense Function against Pathogens, Microbes and Insects

2.1. Rice Blast Fungal Pathogen

Infection with the rice blast pathogen *Magnaporthe oryzae* (syn. *Pyricularia oryzae*; renamed from *Magnaporthe grisea*) induced momilactone A accumulation in rice leaves. The accumulation was abundant at the edges of necrotic lesions, which are symptoms of the infection of leaves [36]. Blast fungus susceptibility diffed among rice cultivars, and tolerance to the fungus correlated positively with momilactone A accumulation in rice leaves [37]. Blast-fungus-resistant rice mutants accumulated momilactone A 2 days after fungus inoculation, and the concentration of momilactone A was 100–400-fold greater than that in wild-type rice and suppressed the further growth of the fungus [4,5]. Exogenously applied momilactone A also suppressed the growth of the fungus on agar media [5]. In addition, the susceptibility of momilactone-deficient rice mutants to the blast fungus was high compared to wild-type rice [38]. These observations suggest that momilactone A may prevent the subsequent spread of the fungus infection through the increased production of momilactone A after pathogen infection.

2.2. Other Fungal Pathogens

Momilactones A and B inhibited the growth of the pathogenic fungi *Rhizoctonia solani*, *Blumeria graminis*, *Fusarium oxysporum*, *Fusarium solani*, *Botrytis cinereal* and the *Colletrichum gloesporides* complex [39,40]. Infection with *Xanthomonas oryzae* pv. *oryzae*, which causes bacterial blight, increased jasmonic acid and momilactone A concentrations in rice leaves [41]. Jasmonic acid is a plant defense signaling hormone and induces several defense responses for protection [42–44].

2.3. Anti-Microbe Activity

Momilactone A inhibited the mycelia growth of the mushroom *Coprinus cinereus* [45] and the cyanobacteria *Microcystis aeruginosa* [46]. Momilactones A and B inhibited the growth of the bacteria *Escherichia coli*, *Pseudomonas putida* (former name, *Pseudomonas ovalis*), *Bacillus cereus* and *Bacillus pumilus* [39].

2.4. Insect Attack

An insect attack by the white-back planthopper (*Sogatella furcifera*) induced the accumulation of momilactone A in rice leaves through a jasmonic acid-mediated pathway [47]. The jasmonic acid-mediated pathway is described in Section 7. The digestive waste of the rice brown planthopper (*Nilaparvata lugens*) induced momilactone A and B accumulation in rice leaves. Filtration and heat treatments of digestive wastes reduced their accumulation. A symbiont of the insect, *Serratia marcescens*, in the digestive waste also induced the accumulation of momilactones A and B [48]. The function of momilactones A and B against insect attacks is not clear.

3. Function in Allelopathy

A considerable number of rice accessions or cultivars have been found to suppress the growth of several other plant species, including weed species, when these rice and other plants were grown together under field and/or laboratory conditions [11,21–24,49]. These observations suggest that rice is allelopathic and contains allelochemicals. A compound causing the growth-inhibitory effect of rice was later isolated from its root exudates and identified as momilactone B [25]. Momilactone A was also identified in rice secretory fluid [26]. These investigations suggest that momilactones A and B may function as rice allelochemicals.

3.1. Activities of Momilactones A and B as Allelochemicals

Momilactones A and B inhibited the growth of several plant species, including weed species such as *Echinochloa crus-galli* and *Echinochloa colonum*. Both *Echinochloa* species are known as the most noxious weeds in rice fields because of their potential to significantly disturb rice production [50,51]. Momilactones A and B inhibited the root and shoot growth of *Echinochloa crus-galli* at concentrations greater than 3 μM and 1 μM, respectively, and the root and shoot growth of *Echinochloa colonum* at concentrations greater than 10 μM and 1 μM, respectively [52]. Table 1 shows the concentrations of momilactones A and B required for 50% growth inhibition (defined as IC_{50}) of target plant species. Smaller values of IC_{50} indicate the higher susceptibly of the target plants to momilactones. On the basis of IC_{50} values, monocotyledonous weed plant species (*Echinochloa crus-galli*, *Echinochloa colonum*, *Phleum pretense*, *Digitaria sanguinalis* and *Lolium multiflorum*) showed higher susceptibly compared to dicotyledonous plant species (*Arabidopsis thaliana*, *Lepidium sativum*, *Lactuca sativa* and *Medicago sativa*) [52–55]. In addition, momilactone B showed much higher growth-inhibitory activity than momilactone A, which has also been confirmed by other bioassay systems [55–59].

Table 1. The concentrations (μM) required for 50% growth inhibition (IC_{50}) of various plant species.

Target Plant Species	Momilactone A Roots	Momilactone A Shoots	Momilactone B Roots	Momilactone B Shoots	Reference
Echinochola crus-gall	28.7	46.4	6.1	6.3	[53]
Echinochloa colonum	65.4	240	5.04	12.5	[52]
Phleum pratense	76.5	157	5.6	7.9	[55]
Digitaria sanguinalis	98.5	275	9.5	12.4	[55]
Lolium multiflorum	91.9	138	6.9	6.5	[55]
Arabidopsis thiliana	203	84.4	12	6.5	[54]
Lepidium sativum	425	285	6.3	4.6	[35]
Lactuca sativa	472	395	54.3	77.9	[55]
Medicago sativa	379	315	67.8	82.4	[55]

On the other hand, momilactones A and B showed relatively weak inhibitory activity on rice growth compared to *Echinochloa crus-galli*. The rice roots and shoots were suppressed by momilactones A and B at concentrations greater than 300 μM and 100 μM, respectively [52,53]. Thus, the effect of momilactones on rice was only 1% of that on *Echinochloa crus-galli*, which was inhibited at concentrations greater than 3 μM and 1 μM for roots and shoots, respectively, as described above [52,53]. In addition, momilactones A and B did not cause any visible damage to rice plants at concentrations that were phytotoxic to other plant species [52–55]. These observations suggest that the toxicity of momilactones A and B to rice plants is much less than that to other plant species. The resistance mechanism of rice to momilactones is unknown. This tolerance may possibly involve either rapid secretion, the insensitivity of the molecular target and/or the degradation of momilactones.

3.2. Concentration and Secretion of Momilactones

The endogenous concentrations of momilactones A and B, respectively, in rice were 4.5 μg/g and 3.0 μg/g of rice straw [60] and 4.9 μg/g and 2.9 μg/g of rice husks [61]. Momilactone B was found in rice seedlings 7 days after germination, and the concentrations of momilactones A and B increased until day 80 after germination, which is when flowering is initiated [52,62–64]. The 80-day-old rice plants contained momilactones A and B at 140 μg/g and 95 μg/g in rice plants, respectively [52,64]. Considering their reported concentrations, the ratio of momilactone A to momilactone B is 1.5–1.6.

The secretion of momilactone B from rice roots was observed 3 days after germination [62]. The levels of momilactone A and B secretion increased up to day 80 after germination and decreased thereafter [52,63]. The secretion levels of momilactones A and B at day 80 were 1.1 and 2.3 μg per plant per day, respectively [52,63], which indicates that the secretion ratio of momilactone B to momilactone A is 2.1. The observation suggests that rice secretes momilactones A and B into its rhizosphere throughout its entire life cycle, and the secretion increases until flowering initiation. Thus, it may be possible that rice allelopathy increases over this time frame. In addition, momilactone B was secreted at a higher rate than momilactone A, even though the concentration of momilactone A is higher than that of momilactone B in rice plants, which suggests that momilactone B may be preferentially secreted into the rhizosphere over momilactone A. Plants are reported to secrete a wide range of compounds from their roots through their cell membranes, for example, by proton-pumping mechanisms, plasmalemma-derived exudation and endoplasmic-derived exudation [65–67]. However, the mechanism of the exudation of momilactones from rice roots is unknown.

3.3. Contribution of Momilactones to Rice Allelopathy

When eight cultivars of rice seedlings (7 days old) were incubated for four days with *Echinochloa crus-galli* seedlings (4 days old) in a buffered bioassay medium, all rice cultivars suppressed the growth of *Echinochloa crus-galli* with different suppression levels. All rice cultivars produced and secreted momilactones A and B into the media, and the concentrations of momilactones A and B in the media were 0.21–1.45 μM and 0.66–3.84 μM, respectively [53]. Based on the growth-inhibitory activity and secreted amounts of momilactones A and B in the media, momilactone A may only account for 1.0–4.9% of the observed growth inhibition of *Echinochloa crus-galli* by the respective rice cultivars. By contrast, momilactone B may account for 58.8–81.9% of the observed growth inhibition. In addition, the momilactone B concentration in the media was significantly ($p < 0.01$) correlated with the extent of the growth suppression of *Echinochloa crus-galli* by these eight rice cultivars [53]. A similar correlation was also found between the level of momilactone B secretion and the extent of the growth suppression of *Lactuca sativa* by these rice cultivars [68,69]. The observations suggest that momilactone B may be a major contributor to the allelopathic activity of rice, and the secretion levels of momilactone B reflect the variation in allelopathic activity observed rice cultivars. The leaf, straw and husk extracts of 41 rice cultivars differed in their growth-inhibitory activity against *Alisma plantago-aquatica*. The concentration of momilactone B in the extracts was also correlated with the inhibitory activity of the extracts [70].

3.4. Genetic Evidence for Momilactones in Rice Allelopathy

Momilactone-biosynthesis-deficient mutants (*cps4* and *ksl4*) were obtained through insertion gene knockouts for OsCPS4 and OsKSL4 [71,72], which is described in Section 5. Allelopathic activity after removing all *syn*-copalyl diphosphate-derived labdane-related diterpenoids (*cps4* mutant) or, more selectively, only momilactones (*ksl4* mutant) was compared to the respective wild-type rice. The wild types showed allelopathic activity, whereas both mutants lost this activity [73]. The investigation suggests that the loss of allelopathic activity may be attributed to the specific loss of momilactones, which verifies the involvement of momilactones in rice allelopathy.

3.5. Inhibitory Mechanism

Molecular targets of momilactone B were investigated through SDS-PAGE and two-dimensional gel electrophoresis with MALDI-TOF-MS. Momilactone B suppressed the germination of *Arabidopsis thaliana* and inhibited the breakdown of the storage proteins cruciferina, cruciferin 2 and cruciferin 3 during germination [74]. The breakdown of these proteins is essential to construct cell structures for germination and seedling growth [75–77]. The application of momilactone B to *Arabidopsis thaliana* seedlings inhibited the accumulation of amyrin synthase LUP2, subtilisin-like serine protease, β-glucosidase and malate synthase [78]. Those proteins are involved in the production of intermediates and metabolic turnover for cell structures [79–82]. On the contrary, momilactone B induced the accumulation of translationally controlled tumor protein, 1-cysteine peroxiredoxin 1 and glutathione-*S*-transferase [75]. These proteins elevate the tolerance to drought and oxidative stress conditions [83–85]. In addition, glutathione-*S*-transferase showed herbicide detoxification activity [86], and 1-cysteine peroxiredoxin 1 showed germination-inhibitory activity under unfavorable conditions [87]. These observations suggest that momilactone B may cause growth inhibition through the suppression of metabolic turnover and the production of intermediates and induce tolerance to stress conditions.

3.6. Induction of Rice Allelopathy and Momilactone

The allelopathic activity of rice was increased by nutrient deficiency, which is often caused by competition with neighboring plants [88–90]. The nutrient-deficient condition also increased the production and secretion of momilactone B from rice [91]. In addition, the allelopathic activity of rice was also elevated by either nearby *Echinochloa crus-galli* plants or their root exudates [91–94]. This elevation was not only owing to nutrient competition between rice and *Echinochloa crus-galli* [95,96]. The momilactone B concentration in rice and its secretion level from rice were also increased by either *Echinochloa crus-galli* or its root exudates. Rice may recognize certain components of the root exudation of *Echinochloa crus-galli*, and the compounds trigger the increased production and secretion of momilactone B [91,95,96]. Other weed species, namely, *Eclipta prostate* and *Leptochola chinensis*, also increased the secretion of momilactone B [97].

Rice allelopathic activity was also elevated by jasmonic acid [98]. The application of jasmonic acid and cantharidin with UV irradiation also increased the concentration of momilactone B in rice and the secretion levels of momilactones from rice roots into its rhizosphere [99]. As momilactones, especially momilactone B, have strong allelopathic activity, as described previously, such increasing secretion levels of momilactones may provide a competitive advantage for rice through the suppression of the growth of nearby competing plant species.

4. Pharmacological Activity

4.1. Anticancer Activity

Momilactones A and B showed growth suppression activity in the murine leukemia P399 cell line [100]. Momilactones A and B induced apoptosis in acute promyelocytic leukemia HL-60 and multiple myeloma U266 cell lines through the activation of apoptosis-inducing factors such as caspase-3 [101]. Momilactone B also induced G_1 arrest in the cell cycle and apoptosis in the human leukemia U937 cell line through the suppression of pRB phosphorylation and the induction of the kinase inhibitor p21 [102], and it induced apoptosis in human leukemia T cells through the activation of caspase [103] and in human breast cancer cells through signal transducer and activator of transcription 5 and a caspase-3-dependent pathway [104]. Momilactone B showed cytotoxic activity in the human colon cancer HT-29 and SW620 cell lines [105].

4.2. Anti-Inflammatory Activity

Momilactone A suppressed the inflammatory response in mouse macrophage RAW264.7 cells through a reduction in NO production and iNOS mRNA expression [106].

4.3. Anti-Diabetic Activity

Momilactones A and B suppressed pancreatic α-amylase, α-glucosidase and trypsin activity in vitro, which indicates that momilactones A and B may work as diabetes inhibitors [107,108].

4.4. Anti-Ketosis Activity

Momilactone B inhibited ketosis in vitro through the suppression of the mitochondrial enzyme 3-hydroxy-3-methylglutaryl-CoA synthase-2, which converts acetyl-CoA to ketone bodies [109].

4.5. Anti-Melanogenic Activity

Momilactone B inhibited the accumulation of melanin in B16 melanocytes through the suppression of protein kinase A signaling and tyrosinase-related proteins [110].

5. Biosynthesis and Related Genes

Geranylgeranyl diphosphate (GGDP) is the precursor of the plant hormone gibberellin and rice diterpenoid phytoalexins such as oryzalexins and phytocassanes, including momilactones [29]. GGDP is synthesized by GGDP synthase (GGPS) from two five-carbon isoprenoids, isopentyl diphosphate or dimethylallyl diphosphate, which are synthesized through the methylerythritol phosphate pathway from pyruvate and glyceraldehyde-3-phosphate [111] (Figure 2).

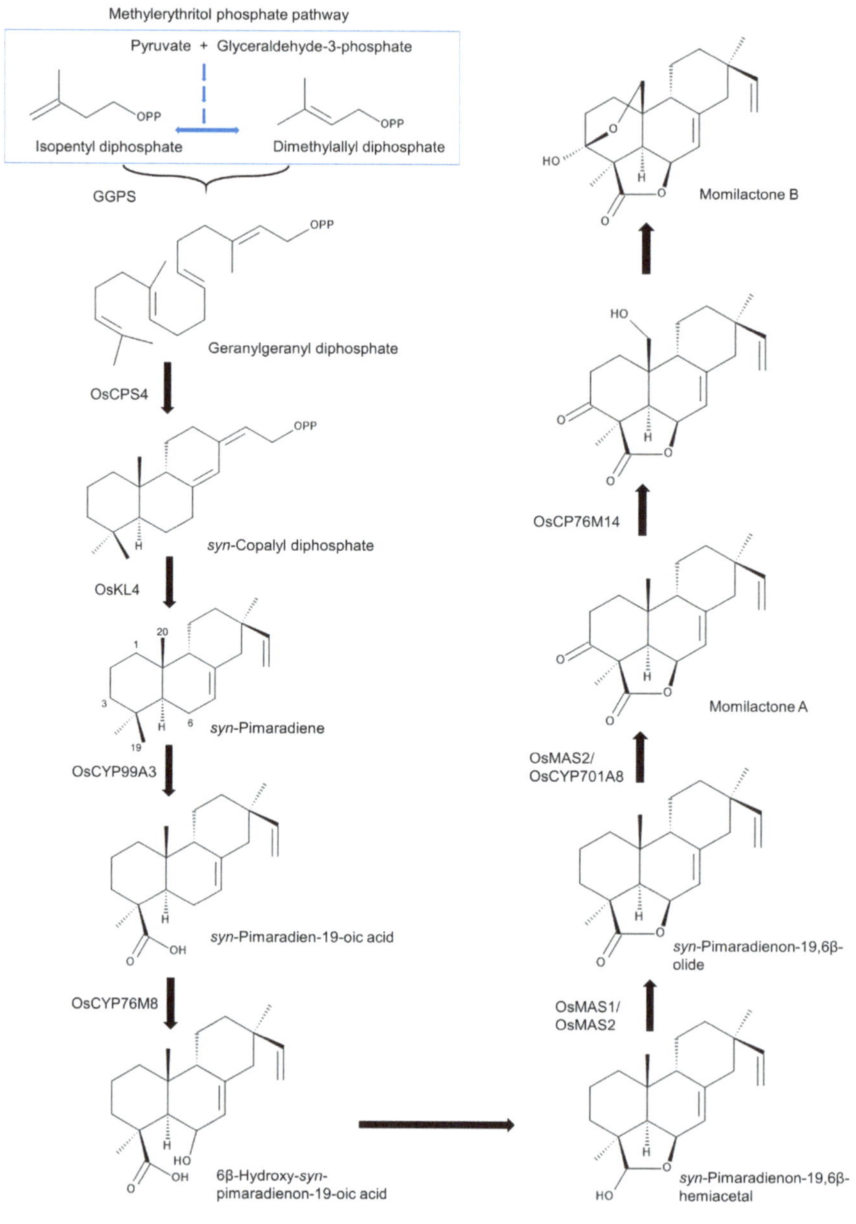

Figure 2. Biosynthetic pathway of momilactones in rice.

GGDP is cyclized into *syn*-copalyl diphosphate (*syn*-CDP) by CDP synthases (OsCPS4). *syn*-CDP is further cyclized into *syn*-pimaradiene by *ent*-kaurene synthase-like 4 (OsKSL4) [112–114]. cDNA encoding OsCPS4 was obtained from UV-irradiated rice leaves [115]. *OsCOS4* and *OsKSL4* are located close to each other on chromosome 4 and were demonstrated to have sequential activity producing *syn*-CDP and *syn*-pimaradiene [116,117].

Cytochrome P450 enzymes (CYPs) are involved in the further metabolism of *syn*-pimaradiene. OsCYP99A3 oxidizes the C19 methyl of *syn*-pimaradiene into *syn*-pimaradien-19-oic acid [118,119], and OsCPY76M8 then hydroxylates its C6 position into 6β-hydroxy-*syn*-pimaradienon-19-oic acid, followed by the spontaneous closure of the ring between

C19 and C6, which forms *syn*-pimaradienon-19,6β-hemiacetal [120]. Momilactone synthase (OsMS1 or OsMS2) converts the C19 hydroxyl group into a ketone to form *syn*-pimaradienon-19,6β-olide [120]. OsMS2 (or OsCPY701A8) then catalyzes C3 hydroxy into a ketone, forming momilactone A [120]. C20 hydroxylation of momilactone A by OsCP76M14 leads to the spontaneous closure of the hemiacetal ring and forms momilactone B [120,121]. The momilactone-synthesis-related genes *OsCPS4, OsKSL4, CYP99A2, CYP99A3, OsMS1* and *OsMS2* were reported to be located on chromosome 4 in plastids of rice cells [32,122] (Figure 3), which indicates that momilactones may play an important ecological role in rice evolution because of the presence of a dedicated biosynthetic gene cluster in the rice genome.

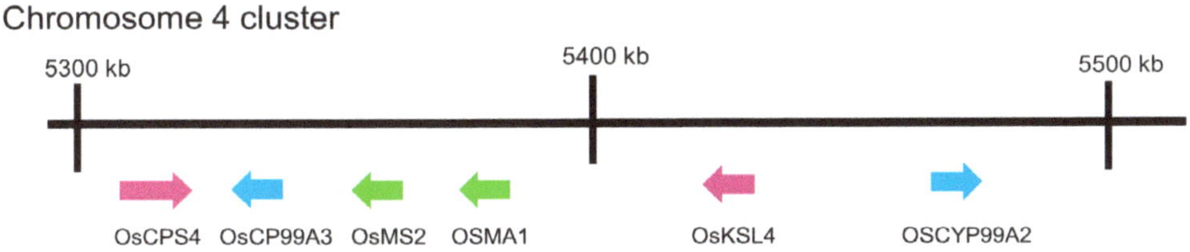

Figure 3. Gene cluster on chromosome 4 of rice genome for momilactone biosynthesis.

6. Momilactone Induction

Plants often respond by increasing their production of certain phytoalexins when they are attacked by pathogens and insects. The reaction involves the induction of active oxygen species, lignification, protease inhibitors and some enzymes, such as chitinase and β-glucanase. Plant defense reactions are also induced by a variety of biological, chemical and physical elicitors, such as oligosaccharides, cantharidin and UV irradiation [123–125]. Momilactone A and B production and accumulation were also induced by these elicitors.

6.1. Biotic Elicitors

Chitosan (oligosaccharide) is a deacetylated derivative of chitin, which is a long-chain polymer of *N*-acetylglucosamine and a primary component of fungal cell walls, arthropod exoskeletons and insect exuviae [126,127]. Chitosan increased the accumulation of momilactone A in rice leaves and suspension-cultured rice cells [6,7] and increased the tolerance of rice to the rice blight pathogen *Fusarium oxysporum* [128]. *N*-Acetylchitooligosaccharides, which are released from the cell walls of pathogenic fungi, also induced the accumulation of momilactones A and B in suspension-cultured rice cells, and their accumulation was 100–500 g/g of cultured cells, which is a sufficient concentration to prevent the growth of pathogenic fungi [129].

Tetraglucosyl glucitol [β-(1,3/1,6)-derived glucan] increased momilactone A production in rice cells [130]. Cantharidin, a protein serine/threonine phosphatase inhibitor contained in some insects, has been shown to mimic elicitor action in plants and to activate defense responses [131,132], and it increased the concentrations of momilactones A and B in rice [132,133] and the secretion level of momilactone B [134]. Cerebrosides (monoglycosylceramides), which are important components of animal cell membranes, induced β-glucanase, chitinase and peroxidase-encoding transcripts and enhanced the production of momilactone A [36,135]. The application of methionine also increased the momilactone A concentration in rice leaves. A free radical scavenger, Tiron (disodium 4,5-dihydroxy-1,3-benzenedisulfonate), increased the momilactone A concentration, which suggests that active oxygen species may stimulate methionine-induced momilactone A production [136].

6.2. Abiotic Elicitors

UV irradiation (254 nm, 20 min) increased momilactone A and B concentrations in rice leaves, and the maximum accumulation was found 3 days after UV irradiation [3,137]. The increase in the levels of momilactone A differed among rice varieties, and blast-resistant rice varieties accumulated more momilactone A than susceptible rice varieties [37].

The application of $CuCl_2$ to rice leaves also induced momilactone A accumulation. The accumulation was detected 12 h after application and reached maximum accumulation at 72 h. $FeCl_2$ and $HgCl_2$ also increased momilactone A accumulation by 37% and 20% compared to $CuCl_2$ application, respectively [138]. The application of $CuCl_2$ to rice leaves induced jasmonic acid and momilactone A. Jasmonic acid biosynthesis inhibitors, quinacrine, nordihydroguaiaretic acid and salicylhydroxamic acid, suppressed momilactone A accumulation after the application of $CuCl_2$. However, additional jasmonic acid application induced momilactone A accumulation after the application of $CuCl_2$ and jasmonic acid biosynthesis inhibitors [139]. These observations suggest that $CuCl_2$ increased the concentration of jasmonic acid in the leaves, and jasmonic acid then stimulated the biosynthesis of momilactone A. In addition, the application of $CuCl_2$ and $FeCl_2$ increased the production and secretion levels of momilactone B in rice and its allelopathic activity [133].

Other metal ions, such as silver, potassium, calcium, sodium zinc and magnesium, also increased the accumulation of momilactone A in suspension-cultured rice cells [140]. The air pollutant sulfur dioxide (SO_2) induced reddish-brown necrotic spots on rice leaves and increased the momilactone A concentration in the leaves [141]. A fungicide, 2,2-dichloro-3,3-dimethyl cyclopropane carboxylic acid, also induced the accumulation of momilactones A and B in rice leaves [2]. Protein synthesis inhibitor herbicides, pretilachlor and butachlor, increased momilactone A accumulation in rice leaves [142].

7. Induction Signaling

The generation of elicitor fragments after pathogen and insect attacks may occur through the induction of chitinase and β-1,3-glucanase [143,144]. Elicitor fragments such as *N*-acetylchitooligosaccharide induced the formation of hetero-oligomer complexes of OsCEBiP (chitin elicitor binding protein) and OsCERK1 (chitin elicitor receptor kinase) [145]. OsCERK1 is part of the defensome complex at the plasma membrane (Figure 4). The defensome contains OsHsp70 (heat shock protein 70), OsHps90, OsHop/Sti1 (Hsp70/Hsp90 organizing protein/stress-induced protein 1), OsSGT1 (suppressor of G/two allele of *Skp*1) and OsRAR1 (required for *Mla12* resistance) as molecular chaperone proteins and co-chaperon-like proteins [146–148]. OsRac1 (small-specific Rho-type GTPase), which is another important component, may cause mitogen-activated protein kinase (MAPK) signal cascades [149]. The earliest MAPK signaling step is OsACDR1 (accelerated cell death and resistance 1), followed by OsMKK4 and then OsMK3 and/or OsMK6 [150,151]. OsTGAP1 (TGA factor for phytoalexin production 1) may then induce the methylerythritol phosphate pathway and the expression of momilactone biosynthetic genes, including OsKSL4 [152,153].

OsRac1 may interact with OsRbohB (respiratory burst oxidase homolog B) in a Ca^{2+}-dependent manner [154]. The constitutive expression of OsRac1 causes an increase in H_2O_2 production, *OsCP2* transcripts and momilactone A accumulation in rice [155].

Tricoderma viride-derived xylanase (TvX) requires specific receptors [156] and increased cytosolic Ca^{2+} within minutes [157,158]. Cytosolic Ca^{2+} induction by TvX is partly mediated by the plasma membrane putative voltage-gated cation channel OsTPC1 [158]. TvX-induced signaling targets Ca^{2+}-sensing calcineurin B-like proteins (OsCBL) and CBL-interacting protein kinases (CIPK14 and 15), which may act as Ca^{2+} sensors [157]. Increased momilactone production was found 24 h after TvX application [157,158].

Exogenous jasmonic acid (JA) induced the accumulation of momilactones [159]. Jasmonic acid production in plants after exposure to stress factors is initiated by the peroxidation of linolenic acid, followed by allene oxide cyclase-mediated epoxide formation, cyclization by allene oxide cyclase (OsAOC) and β-oxidation [159,160]. The produced jasmonic acid is then conjugated with isoleucine by OsJAR1 (Jasmonate Resistant 1), resulting in the formation of JA-isoleucine (JA-Il). JA-Il may then stimulate momilactone synthesis [159]. The exogenous application of salicylic acid also induced momilactone accumulation in rice. However, the mechanism of salicylic acid induction of momilactones remains unclear [161].

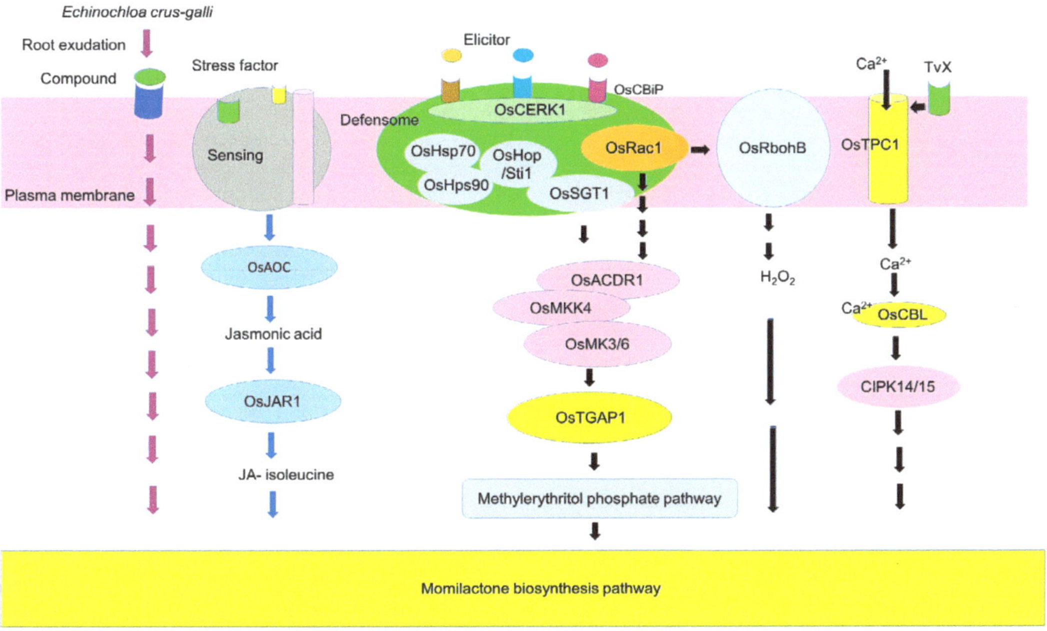

Figure 4. Signaling pathway for the elicitation of rice momilactone biosynthesis.

8. Occurrence of Momilactone

Momilactones A and B were first isolated from seed husks of *Oryza sativa* cv. Koshihikari [1] and then found in the leaves of *Oryza sativa* [2], but these studies did not clearly mention the cultivar or accession of the rice. Momilactones A and B were found in whole plants of rice, including their roots [60,64], and in multiple rice cultivars [53,68–70,162]. The concentrations of momilactones A and B were determined in the leaves of 69 rice cultivars from World Rice Core Collections, and in 64 and 31 cultivars, the presence of momilactones A and B were detected, respectively. The concentrations of momilactones A and B varied among these cultivars. The maximum amount of momilactone A was recorded in the cultivar Urasan at 495 nmol/g leaf, but the exact value for momilactone B was not reported. The concentrations of momilactones A and B in the leaves were greater in Japonica-type cultivars than in Indica-type cultivars [162].

Wild rice species such as *Oryza rufipogon*, *O. burthii*, *O. glaberrima*, *O. glumaepatula*, *O. meridionalis*, *O. punctatas* and *O. brachyatha* also contained momilactones A and B. The concentrations of momilactone A were 0.97–667 nmol/g leaf [162]. Momilactone biosynthesis genes of *O. punctatas* (*OpCPS4*, *OpCYP99A*, *OpMS1*, *OpMS2*, *OpKSL4* and *OpCYP99A*) form a gene cluster on the same chromosome [163]. These genes are equivalent to rice *OsCPS4*, *OsCYP99A*, *OsMS1*, *OsMS2*, *OsKSL4* and *OsCYP99A* genes, respectively. A gene cluster for momilactone biosynthesis was also found in *Echinochloa crus-galli*. The gene cluster contains only single copies of *EcCY99A* and *EcMS*, and its gene sequence on the chromosome is different from that in rice [164]. However, the endogenous concentration of momilactones in *Echinochloa crus-galli* has not yet been reported.

Momilactones A and B were also found in the moss species *Calohypnum plumiforme* (syn. *Hypnum plumaeform*), which is quite taxonomically distinct from rice [33–35]. *Calohypnum plumiforme* belongs to the Hypnaceae family of the Bryophyta division, often dominates in plant communities and forms large pure colonies in sunny places in lowland to upland areas, including marshy places in eastern Asia [165,166]. Momilactones are also synthesized from GGDP in the moss. GGDP is cyclized to *syn*-pimaradiene by diterpene cyclase (CpDTC1/HpDTC1) [167]. *syn*-Pimaradiene is catalyzed into 3β-hydroxy-*syn*-pimaradienon-19,6β-olide by CpCYP770A14 and CpCYP964A1. 3β-Hydroxy-*syn*-pimaradienon-19,6β-olide is then metabolized to momilactone A by momilactone synthase (CpMS) [168]. Those genes also form a gene cluster in the order *CpMS, CpCYP970A14, CpDTC1/HpDTC1* and *CpCYP964A1* on the same chromosome [168].

Momilactone A and B concentrations in the moss were 58.7 μg/g and 23.4 μg/g dry weight of the moss, respectively. The moss also secretes momilactones A and B into the rhizosphere at ratios of 4.0 μg/g and 6.3 μg/g dry weight of the moss, respectively, which were 7.3% and 27% of the endogenous concentrations of momilactones A and B in the moss [35]. The observations suggest that the moss selectively secretes momilactone B into the rhizosphere rather than momilactone A. UV irradiation, jasmonic acid and cantharidin also increased the production and secretion levels of momilactones A and B [169]. These observations suggest that elicitors and/or pathogen attacks may increase the production and secretion levels of momilactones A and B in the moss. Momilactones A and B secreted from moss are also able to suppress the growth of neighboring plant species. Therefore, momilactones in the moss may function in the defense against pathogen attacks and allelopathy.

9. Conclusions

The literature reviewed here demonstrates an important role for momilactones in the defense function and allelopathic function. Momilactones in rice plants may provide resistance to fungal pathogen attacks, and momilactones in rice root exudate may provide rice with the ability to compete with neighboring plant species, which was confirmed with momilactone-deficient mutants. The momilactone biosynthesis pathway and related genes have been investigated by many researchers. The elicitation of momilactone production and secretion and the endogenous signaling cascades involved in the elicitation are also well documented. These findings suggest that the allelopathic and defense functions of momilactones may play important ecological roles in rice evolution because of the existence of a dedicated biosynthetic gene cluster in the genome. However, the mechanism and molecular targets of momilactone functions remain unknown. Momilactones A and B did not cause growth suppression or any visible damage to rice plants at concentrations that were phytotoxic to other plant species. The resistance mechanism of rice to momilactones is also unknown. It is worth investigating the mechanism underlying this tolerance for developing resistant crop plants. The potential of momilactones to serve as endogenous natural fungicides and herbicides provides significant benefits when applied to other important crops. The identification of momilactones may provide a molecular marker for breeding and engineering directed at increasing defense and allelopathic abilities. In addition, momilactones have shown anti-leukemia and anti-diabetic activities. Further investigations are necessary to develop their medical applications.

Funding: This work was supported by JSPS Grants-in-Aid for Scientific Research, Grant Number JP21K05598.

Institutional Review Board Statement: Not applicable.

Informed Consent Statement: Not applicable.

Conflicts of Interest: The authors declare no conflict of interest.

References

1. Kato, T.; Kabuto, C.; Sasaki, N.; Tsunagawa, M.; Aizawa, H.; Fujita, K.; Kato, Y.; Takahashi, N. Momilactones, growth inhibitors from rice, *Oryza sativa* L. *Tetrahedron Lett.* **1973**, *39*, 3861–3864. [CrossRef]
2. Cartwright, D.; Langcake, P.; Pryce, R.J.; Leworthy, D.P.; Ride, J.P. Chemical activation of host defense mechanisms as a basis for crop protection. *Nature* **1977**, *267*, 511–513. [CrossRef]
3. Cartwright, D.W.; Langcake, P.; Pryce, R.J.; Leworthy, D.P.; Ride, J.P. Isolation and characterization of two phytoalexins from rice as momilactones A and B. *Phytochemistry* **1981**, *20*, 535–537. [CrossRef]

4. Takahashi, A.; Kawasaki, T.; Henmi, K.; Shii, K.; Kodama, O.; Satoh, H.; Shimamoto, K. Lesion mimic mutants of rice with alterations in early signaling events of defense. *Plant J.* **1999**, *17*, 535–545. [CrossRef] [PubMed]
5. Hasegawa, M.; Mitsuhara, I.; Seo, S.; Imai, T.; Koga, J.; Okada, K.; Yamane, H.; Ohashi, Y. Phytoalexin accumulation in the interaction between rice and the blast fungus. *Mol. Plant-Micro. Intrac.* **2010**, *23*, 1000–1011. [CrossRef] [PubMed]
6. Agrawal, G.K.; Rakwal, R.; Tamogami, S.; Yonekura, M.; Kubo, A.; Saji, H. Chitosan activates defense/stress response(s) in the leaves of *Oryza sativa* seedlings. *Plant Physiol. Biochem.* **2002**, *40*, 1061–1069. [CrossRef]
7. Shimizu, T.; Jikumaru, Y.; Okada, A.; Okada, K.; Koga, J.; Umemura, K.; Minami, E.; Shibuya, N.; Hasegawa, M.; Kodama, O.; et al. Effects of a bile acid elicitor, cholic acid, on the biosynthesis of diterpenoid phytoalexins in suspension-cultured rice cells. *Phytochemistry* **2008**, *69*, 973–981. [CrossRef]
8. Tamogami, S.; Kodama, O. Coronatine elicits phytoalexin production in rice leaves (*Oryza sativa* L.) in the same manner as jasmonic acid. *Phytochemistry* **2000**, *54*, 689–694.
9. Jung, Y.H.; Lee, J.H.; Agrawal, G.K.; Rakwal, R.; Kim, J.A.; Shim, J.K.; Lee, S.K.; Jeon, J.S.; Koh, H.J.; Lee, Y.H.; et al. The rice (*Oryza sativa*) blast lesion mimic mutant, blm, may confer resistance to blast pathogens by triggering multiple defense-associated signaling pathways. *Plant Physiol. Biochem.* **2005**, *43*, 397–406. [CrossRef]
10. Okada, A.; Shimizu, T.; Okada, K.; Kuzuyama, T.; Koga, J.; Shibuya, N.; Nojiri, H.; Yamane, H. Elicitor induced activation of the methylerythritol phosphate pathway toward phytoalexins biosynthesis in rice. *Plant Mol. Biol.* **2007**, *65*, 177–187. [CrossRef]
11. Dilday, R.H.; Nastasi, P.; Smith, R.J., Jr. Allelopathic observations in rice (*Oryza sativa* L.) to ducksalad (*Heteranthera limosa*). *Proc. Arkansas. Acad. Sci.* **1989**, *43*, 21–22.
12. Rice, E.L. *Allelopathy*, 2nd ed.; Academic Press: Orlando, FL, USA, 1984; pp. 1–422.
13. Putnam, A.R.; Tang, C.S. Allelopathy: State of the science. In *The Science of Allelopathy*; Putnam, A.R., Tang, C.S., Eds.; John Wiley and Sons: Ithaca, NY, USA, 1986; pp. 1–19.
14. Inderjit. Plant phenolics in allelopathy. *Bot. Rev.* **1996**, *62*, 186–202. [CrossRef]
15. Bais, H.P.; Weir, T.L.; Perry, L.G.; Gilroy, S.; Vivanco, J.M. The role of root exudates in rhizosphere interactions with plants and other organisms. *Annu. Rev. Plant Biol.* **2006**, *57*, 233–266. [CrossRef] [PubMed]
16. Bonanomi, G.; Sicurezza, M.G.; Caporaso, S.; Esposito, A.; Mazzoleni, S. Phytotoxicity dynamics of decaying plant materials. *New Phytol.* **2006**, *169*, 571–578. [CrossRef] [PubMed]
17. Belz, R.G. Allelopathy in crop/weed interactions—An update. *Pest Manag. Sci.* **2007**, *63*, 308–326. [CrossRef] [PubMed]
18. Dilday, R.H.; Lin, J.; Yan, W. Identification of allelopathy in the USDA-ARS rice germplasm collection. *Aust. J. Exp. Agric.* **1994**, *34*, 907–910. [CrossRef]
19. Dilday, R.H.; Yan, W.G.; Moldenhauer, K.A.K.; Gravois, K.A. Allelopathic activity in rice for controlling major aquatic weeds. In *Allelopathy in Rice*; Olofsdotter, M., Ed.; International Rice Research Institute: Manila, Philippines, 1998; pp. 7–26.
20. Hassan, S.M.; Aidy, I.R.; Bastawisi, A.O.; Draz, A.E. Weed management using allelopathic rice varieties in Egypt. In *Allelopathy in Rice*; Olofsdotter, M., Ed.; International Rice Research Institute: Manila, Philippines, 1998; pp. 27–37.
21. Kim, K.U.; Shin, D.H. Rice allelopathy research in Korea. In *Allelopathy in Rice*; Olofsdotter, M., Ed.; International Rice Research Institute: Manila, Philippines, 1998; pp. 39–43.
22. Olofsdotter, M.; Navarez, D.; Rebulanan, M.; Streibig, J.C. Weed-suppressing rice cultivars: Does allelopathy play a role? *Weed Res.* **1999**, *39*, 441–454. [CrossRef]
23. Pheng, S.; Adkins, S.; Olofsdotter, M.; Jahn, G. Allelopathic effects of rice (*Oryza sativa* L.) on the growth of awnless barnyardgrass (*Echinochloa colona* (L.) Link): A new form for weed management. *Cambodian J. Agri.* **1999**, *2*, 42–49.
24. Kato-Noguchi, H.; Ino, T. Assessment of allelopathic potential of root exudate of rice seedlings. *Biol. Plant.* **2001**, *44*, 635–638. [CrossRef]
25. Kato-Noguchi, H.; Ino, T.; Sata, N.; Yamamura, S. Isolation and identification of a potent allelopathic substance in rice root exudates. *Physiol. Plant.* **2002**, *115*, 401–405. [CrossRef] [PubMed]
26. Kato-Noguchi, H.; Ino, T.; Ota, K. Secretion of momilactone A from rice roots to the rhizosphere. *J. Plant Physiol.* **2008**, *165*, 691–696. [CrossRef] [PubMed]
27. Kato-Noguchi, H. Allelopathic substance in rice root exudates: Rediscovery of momilactone B as an allelochemical. *J. Plant Physiol.* **2004**, *161*, 271–276. [CrossRef]
28. Kato-Noguchi, H.; Peters, R.J. The role of momilactones in rice allelopathy. *J. Chem. Ecol.* **2013**, *39*, 175–185. [CrossRef]
29. Schmelz, E.A.; Huffaker, A.; Sims, J.W.; Christensen, S.A.; Lu, X.; Okada, K.; Peters, R.J. Biosynthesis, elicitation and roles of monocot terpenoid phytoalexins. *Plant J.* **2014**, *79*, 659–678. [CrossRef]
30. Kato-Noguchi, H. Convergent or parallel molecular evolution of momilactone A and B: Potent allelochemicals, momilactones have been found only in rice and the moss *Hypnum plumaeforme*. *J. Plant Physiol.* **2011**, *168*, 1511–1516. [CrossRef]
31. Serra, N.S.; Shanmuganathan, R.; Becker, C. Allelopathy in rice: A story of momilactones, kin recognition, and weed management. *J. Exp. Bot.* **2021**, *72*, 4022–4037. [CrossRef] [PubMed]
32. Zhang, J.; Peters, R.J. Why are momilactones always associated with biosynthetic gene clusters in plants? *Proc. Natl. Acad. Sci. USA* **2020**, *117*, 13867–13869. [CrossRef] [PubMed]
33. Kobayashi, K.; Shigemori, H.; Kato-Noguch, H. Allelopathic potential of *Hypnum plumaeforme* L. and its allelopathic substances. In Proceedings of the 4th Asia-Pacific Conference on Chemical Ecology, from Biomolecules to Ecosystems an Interactive Chemical Message for our Future, Tsukuba, Japan, 10–14 September 2007; p. 77.

34. Nozaki, H.; Hayashi, K.I.; Nishimura, N.; Kawaide, H.; Matsuo, A.; Takaoka, D. Momilactone A and B as allelochemicals from moss *Hypnum plumaeforme*: First occurrence in bryophytes. *Biosci. Biotech. Biochem.* **2007**, *71*, 3127–3130. [CrossRef]
35. Kato-Noguchi, H.; Kobayashi, K.; Shigemori, H. Allelopathy of the moss *Hypnum plumaeforme* by the production of momilactone A and B. *Weed Res.* **2009**, *49*, 621–627. [CrossRef]
36. Umemura, K.; Ogawa, N.; Shimura, M.; Koga, J.; Usami, H.; Kono, T. Possible role of phytocassane, rice phytoalexin, in disease resistance of rice against the blast fungus *Magnaporthe grisea*. *Biosci. Biotech. Biochem.* **2003**, *67*, 899–902. [CrossRef]
37. Dillon, V.M.; Overton, J.; Grayer, R.J.; Harborne, J.B. Differences in phytoalexin response among rice cultivars of different resistance to blast. *Phytochemistry* **1997**, *44*, 599–603. [CrossRef]
38. Toyomasu, T.; Usui, M.; Sugawara, C.; Otomo, K.; Hirose, Y.; Miyao, A.; Hirochik, H.; Okad, K.; Shimizu, T.; Koga, J.; et al. Reverse-genetic approach to verify physiological roles of rice phytoalexins: Characterization of a knockdown mutant of OsCPS4 phytoalexin biosynthetic gene in rice. *Physiol. Plant.* **2014**, *150*, 55–62. [CrossRef] [PubMed]
39. Fukuta, M.; Xuan, T.D.; Deba, F.; Tawata, S.; Dang Khanh, T.; Chung, M.I. Comparative efficacies in vitro of antibacterial, fungicidal, antioxidant, and herbicidal activities of momilatones A and B. *J. Plant Interac.* **2007**, *2*, 245–251. [CrossRef]
40. Gu, C.Z.; Xia, X.M.; Lv, J.; Tan, J.W.; Baerson, S.R.; Pan, Z.Q.; Song, Y.Y.; Zeng, R.S. Diterpenoids with herbicidal and antifungal activities from hulls of rice (*Oryza sativa*). *Fitoterapia* **2019**, *136*, 104183. [CrossRef] [PubMed]
41. Liu, H.; Li, X.; Xiao, J.; Wang, S. A convenient method for simultaneous quantification of multiple phytohormones and metabolites: Application in study of rice-bacterium interaction. *Plant Methods* **2012**, *8*, 1–12. [CrossRef]
42. Howe, G.A.; Major, I.T.; Koo, A.J. Modularity in jasmonate signaling for multistress resilience. *Ann. Rev. Plant Biol.* **2018**, *69*, 387–415. [CrossRef] [PubMed]
43. Mostafa, S.; Wang, Y.; Zeng, W.; Jin, B. Plant responses to herbivory, wounding, and infection. *Int. J. Mol. Sci.* **2022**, *23*, 7031. [CrossRef] [PubMed]
44. Nguyen, T.H.; Goossens, A.; Lacchini, E. Jasmonate: A hormone of primary importance for plant metabolism. *Curr. Opin. Plant Biol.* **2022**, *67*, 102197. [CrossRef] [PubMed]
45. Hanai, H.; Ishida, S.; Saito, C.; Maita, T.; Kusano, M.; Tamogami, S.; Noma, M. Stimulation of mycelia growth in several mushroom species by rice husks. *Biosci. Biotech. Biochem.* **2005**, *69*, 123–127. [CrossRef]
46. Chung, I.M.; Ali, M.; Ahmad, A.; Chun, S.C.; Kim, J.T.; Sultana, S.; Kim, J.S.; Seo, B.R. Steroidal constituents of rice (*Oryza sativa*) hulls with Algicidal and Herbicidal activity against blue-green algae and duckweed. *Phytochem. Anal.* **2007**, *18*, 133–145. [CrossRef]
47. Kanno, H.; Hasegawa, M.; Kodama, O. Accumulation of salicylic acid, jasmonic acid and phytoalexins in rice, *Oryza sativa*, infested by the white-backed planthopper, *Sogatella furcifera* (Hemiptera: Delphacidae). *Appl. Entomol. Zool.* **2012**, *47*, 27–34. [CrossRef]
48. Wari, D.; Alamgir, K.M.; Mujiono, K.; Hojo, Y.; Tani, A.; Shinya, T.; Nakatania, H.; Galis, I. Brown planthopper honeydew-associated symbiotic microbes elicit momilactones in rice. *Plant Signal. Behav.* **2019**, *14*, 1655335. [CrossRef] [PubMed]
49. Azmi, M.; Abdullah, M.Z.; Fujii, Y. Exploratory study on allelopathic effect of selected Malaysian rice varieties and rice field weed species. *J. Trop. Agric. Food Sci.* **2000**, *28*, 39–54.
50. Rao, A.N.; Johnson, D.E.; Sivaprasad, B.; Ladaha, J.K.; Mortimer, A.M. Weed management in direct-seeded rice. *Adv. Agron.* **2007**, *93*, 153–255.
51. Kong, C.H. Rice allelopathy. *Allelopathy J.* **2008**, *22*, 261–278.
52. Kato-Noguchi, H.; Ota, K.; Ino, T. Release of momilactone A and B from rice plants into the rhizosphere and its bioactivities. *Allelopathy J.* **2008**, *22*, 321–328.
53. Kato-Noguchi, H.; Hasegawa, M.; Ino, T.; Ota, K.; Kujime, H. Contribution of momilactone A and B to rice allelopathy. *J. Plant Physiol.* **2010**, *167*, 787–791. [CrossRef] [PubMed]
54. Kato-Noguchi, H.; Ota, K.; Kujime, H. Absorption of momilactone A and B by *Arabidopsis thaliana* L. and the growth inhibitory effects. *J. Plant Physiol.* **2012**, *169*, 1471–1476. [CrossRef]
55. Kato-Noguchi, H.; Ota, K. Biological activities of rice allelochemicals momilactone A and B. *Rice Res.* **2013**, *1*, 2. [CrossRef]
56. Takahashi, N.; Kato, T.; Tsunagawa, M.; Sasaki, N.; Kitahara, Y. Mechanisms of dormancy in rice seeds. II. New growth inhibitors, momilactone-A and -B isolated from the hulls of rice seeds. *Jpn. J. Breed.* **1976**, *26*, 91–98. [CrossRef]
57. Kato, T.; Tsunakawa, M.; Sasaki, N.; Aizawa, H.; Fujita, K.; Kitahara, Y.; Takahashi, N. Growth and germination inhibitors in rice husks. *Phytochemistry* **1977**, *16*, 45–48. [CrossRef]
58. Chung, I.M.; Hahh, S.J.; Ahmad, A. Confirmation of potential herbicidal agents in hulls of rice, *Oryza sativa*. *J. Chem. Ecol.* **2005**, *31*, 1339–1352. [CrossRef] [PubMed]
59. Toyomasu, T.; Kagahara, T.; Okada, K.; Koga, J.; Hasegawa, M.; Mitsuhashi, W.; Sassa, T.; Yamane, H. Diterpene phytoalexins are biosynthesized in and exuded from the roots of rice seedlings. *Biosci. Biotechnol. Biochem.* **2008**, *72*, 562–567. [CrossRef] [PubMed]
60. Lee, C.W.; Yoneyama, K.; Takeuchi, Y.; Konnai, M.; Tamogami, S.; Kodama, O. Momilactones A and B in rice straw harvested at different growth stages. *Biosci. Biotechnol. Biochem.* **1999**, *63*, 1318–1320. [CrossRef] [PubMed]
61. Chung, I.-M.; Kim, T.K.; Kim, S.H. Evaluation of allelopathic potential and quantification of momilactone A, B from rice hull extracts and assessment of inhibitory bioactivity on paddy field weeds. *J. Agric. Food. Chem.* **2006**, *54*, 2527–2536. [CrossRef] [PubMed]
62. Kato-Noguchi, H.; Ino, T. Rice seedlings release momilactone B into the environment. *Phytochemistry* **2003**, *63*, 551–554. [CrossRef]

63. Kato-Noguchi, H.; Ino, T.; Ichii, M. Changes in release level of momilactone B into the environment from rice throughout its life cycle. *Func. Plant Biol.* **2003**, *30*, 995–997. [CrossRef]
64. Kato-Noguchi, H.; Ino, T. Possible involvement of momilactone B in rice allelopathy. *J. Plant Physiol.* **2005**, *162*, 718–721. [CrossRef]
65. Hawes, M.C.; Gunawardena, U.; Miyasaka, S.; Zhao, X. The role of root border cells in plant defense. *Trends Plant Sci.* **2000**, *5*, 128–133. [CrossRef]
66. Bais, H.P.; Park, S.W.; Weir, T.L.; Callaway, R.M.; Vivanco, J.M. How plants communicate using the underground information superhighway. *Trends Plant Sci.* **2004**, *9*, 26–32. [CrossRef]
67. Badri, D.V.; Vivanco, J.M. Regulation and function of root exudates. *Plant Cell Environ.* **2009**, *32*, 666–681. [CrossRef] [PubMed]
68. Kato-Noguchi, H.; Ino, T. Concentration and release level of momilactone B in the seedlings of eight rice cultivars. *J. Plant Physiol.* **2005**, *162*, 965–969. [CrossRef]
69. Kato-Noguchi, H.; Ino, T.; Kujime, H. The relation between growth inhibition and secretion level of momilactone B from rice root. *J. Plant Interact.* **2010**, *5*, 87–90. [CrossRef]
70. Mennan, H.; Ngouajio, M.; Sahin, M.; Isik, D.; Altop, E.K. Quantification of momilactone B in rice hulls and the phytotoxic potential of rice extracts on the seed germination of *Alisma plantago*-aquatica. *Weed Biol. Manag.* **2012**, *12*, 29–39. [CrossRef]
71. Zhang, J.; Li, C.; Wu, C.; Xiong, L.; Chen, G.; Zhang, Q.; Wang, S. RMD: A rice mutant database for functional analysis of the rice genome. *Nucleic Acids Res.* **2006**, *34*, D745–D748. [CrossRef] [PubMed]
72. Jeon, J.S.; Lee, S.; Jung, K.H.; Jun, S.H.; Jeong, D.H.; Lee, J.; Kim, C.; Jang, S.; Yang, K.; Nam, J.; et al. T-DNA insertional mutagenesis for functional genomics in rice. *Plant J.* **2000**, *22*, 561–570. [CrossRef] [PubMed]
73. Xu, M.; Galhano, R.; Wiemann, P.; Bueno, E.; Tiernan, M.; Wu, W.; Chung, I.M.; Gershenzon, J.; Sesma, A.T.; Peters, R.J. Genetic evidence for natural product-mediated plant-plant allelopathy in rice (Oryza sativa). *New Phytol.* **2012**, *193*, 570–575. [CrossRef]
74. Kato-Noguchi, H.; Ota, K.; Kujime, H.; Ogawa, M. Effects of momilactone on the protein expression in Arabidopsis germination: Arabidopsis and momilactone. *Weed Biol. Manag.* **2013**, *13*, 19–23. [CrossRef]
75. Finkelstein, R.R.; Tenbarge, K.M.; Shumway, J.E.; Crouch, M.L. Role of ABA in maturation of rapeseed embryos. *Plant Physiol.* **1985**, *78*, 630–636. [CrossRef]
76. Bewley, J.D.; Bradford, K.J.; Hilhorst, H.W.M.; Nonogaki, H. *Seeds: Physiology of Development, Germination and Dormancy, 3rd ed*; Springer: New York, NY, USA, 2012; pp. 1–408.
77. Job, C.; Rajjou, L.; Lovigny, Y.; Belghazi, M.; Job, D. Patterns of protein oxidation in *Arabidopsis* seeds and during germination. *Plant Physiol.* **2005**, *138*, 790–802. [CrossRef]
78. Kato-Noguchi, H.; Kitajima, S. Momilactone sensitive proteins in *Arabidopsis thaliana*. *Nat. Prod. Commun.* **2015**, *10*, 729–732. [CrossRef] [PubMed]
79. Ohyama, K.; Suzuki, M.; Kikuchi, J.; Saito, K.; Muranaka, T. Dual biosynthetic pathways to phytosterol via cycloartenol and lanosterol in *Arabidopsis*. *Proc. Natl. Acad. Sci. USA* **2009**, *106*, 725–730. [CrossRef]
80. Kuroha, T.; Okuda, A.; Arai, M.; Komatsu, Y.; Sato, S.; Kato, T.; Tabata, S.; Satoh, S. Identification of *Arabidopsis* subtilisin-like serine protease specifically expressed in root stele by gene trapping. *Physiol. Plant.* **2009**, *137*, 281–288. [CrossRef] [PubMed]
81. Gallardo, K.; Job, C.; Groot, S.P.C.; Puype, M.; Demol, H.; Vandekerckhove, J.; Job, D. Proteomics of *Arabidopsis* seed germination. A comparative study of wild-type and gibberellin-deficient seeds. *Plant Physiol.* **2002**, *129*, 823–837. [CrossRef]
82. Eastmond, P.J.; Graham, I.A. Re-examining the role of the glyoxylate cycle in oilseeds. *Trends Plant Sci.* **2001**, *6*, 72–77. [CrossRef]
83. Stacy, R.A.P.; Nordeng, T.W.; Culianez-Macia, F.A.; Reidunn, B.; Aalen, R.B. The dormancy-related peroxiredoxin anti-oxidant, PER1, is localized to the nucleus of barley embryo and aleurone cells. *Plant J.* **1999**, *19*, 1–8. [CrossRef]
84. Kim, S.Y.; Paeng, S.K.; Nawkar, G.M.; Maibam, P.; Lee, E.S.; Kim, K.S.; Lee, D.H.; Park, D.J.; Kang, S.B.; Kim, M.R.; et al. The 1-cys peroxiredoxin, a regulator of seed dormancy, functions as a molecular chaperone under oxidative stress conditions. *Plant Sci.* **2011**, *181*, 119–124. [CrossRef]
85. Fanucchi, F.; Alpi, E.; Olivieri, S.; Cannistraci, C.V.; Bachi, A.; Alpi, A.; Alessio, M. Acclimation increases freezing stress response of *Arabidopsis thaliana* at proteome level. *Biochim. Biophys. Acta* **2012**, *1824*, 813–825. [CrossRef] [PubMed]
86. Neuefeind, T.; Reinemer, P.; Bieseler, B. Plant glutathione S-transferases and herbicide detoxification (Review). *Biol. Chem.* **1997**, *378*, 199–205. [PubMed]
87. Haslekås, C.; Viken, M.K.; Grini, P.E.; Nygaard, V.; Nordgard, S.H.; Meza, T.J.; Aalen, R.B. Seed 1-cysteine peroxiredoxin antioxidants are not involved in dormancy, but contribute to inhibition of germination during stress. *Plant Physiol.* **2003**, *133*, 1148–1157. [CrossRef]
88. Kim, K.U.; Shin, D.H.; Lee, I.J.; Kim, H.Y.; Kim, K.U.; Shin, D.H. Rice allelopathy in Korea. In *Rice Allelopathy*; Kim, K.U., Shin, D.H., Eds.; Kyungpook National University: Taegu, Korea, 2000; pp. 57–82.
89. Song, B.; Xiong, J.; Fang, C.; Qiu, L.; Lin, R.; Liang, Y.; Lin, W. Allelopathic enhancement and differential gene expression in rice under low nitrogen treatment. *J. Chem. Ecol.* **2008**, *34*, 688–695. [CrossRef]
90. Shen, L.; Lin, W. Effects of phosphorus levels on allelopathic potential of rice co-cultured with barnyardgrass. *Allelopathy J.* **2007**, *19*, 393–402.
91. Kato-Noguchi, H. Barnyard grass-induced rice allelopathy and momilactone B. *J. Plant Physiol.* **2011**, *168*, 1016–1020. [CrossRef] [PubMed]
92. Zhao, H.; Li, H.; Kong, C.; Xu, X.; Liang, W. Chemical response of allelopathic rice seedlings under varying environmental conditions. *Allelopathy J.* **2005**, *15*, 105–110.

93. Kong, C.H.; Li, H.B.; Hu, F.; Xu, X.H.; Wang, P. Allelochemicals released by rice roots and residues in soil. *Plant Soil* **2006**, *288*, 47–56. [CrossRef]
94. Li, L.L.; Zhao, H.H.; Kong, C.H. (−)-Loliolide, the most ubiquitous lactone, is involved in barnyardgrass-induced rice allelopathy. *J. Exp. Bot.* **2020**, *71*, 1540–1550. [CrossRef]
95. Kato-Noguchi, H. The chemical cross talk between rice and barnyardgrass. *Plant Signal. Behav.* **2011**, *6*, 1207–1209. [CrossRef] [PubMed]
96. Kato-Noguchi, H.; Ino, T. The chemical-mediated allelopathic interaction between rice and barnyard grass. *Plant Soil* **2013**, *370*, 267–275. [CrossRef]
97. Yang, X.F.; Kong, C.H. Interference of allelopathic rice with paddy weeds at the root level. *Plant Biol.* **2017**, *19*, 584–591. [CrossRef]
98. Bi, H.H.; Zeng, R.Z.; Su, L.M.; An, M.; Luo, S.H. Rice allelopathy induced by methyl jasmonate and methyl salicylate. *J. Chem. Ecol.* **2007**, *33*, 1089–1103. [CrossRef]
99. Kato-Noguchi, H.; Kujime, H.; Ino, T. UV-induced momilactone B accumulation in rice rhizosphere. *J. Plant Physiol.* **2007**, *164*, 1548–1551. [CrossRef]
100. Chung, I.M.; Ali, M.; Hahn, S.J.; Siddiqui, N.A.; Lim, Y.H.; Ahmad, A. Chemical constituents from the hulls of *Oryza sativa* with cytotoxic activity. *Chem. Nat. Compd.* **2005**, *41*, 182–189. [CrossRef]
101. Anh, L.H.; Lam, V.Q.; Takami, A.; Khanh, T.D.; Quan, N.V.; Xuan, T.D. Cytotoxic mechanism of momilactones A and B against acute promyelocytic leukemia and multiple myeloma cell Lines. *Cancers* **2022**, *14*, 4848. [CrossRef]
102. Park, C.; Jeong, N.Y.; Kim, G.Y.; Han, M.H.; Chung, I.M.; Kim, W.J.; Yoo, Y.Y.; Choi, Y.H. Momilactone B induces apoptosis and G1 arrest of the cell cycle in human monocytic leukemia U937 cells through downregulation of pRB phosphorylation and induction of the cyclin-dependent kinase inhibitor $p21^{Waf1/Cip1}$. *Oncol. Rep.* **2014**, *31*, 1653–1660. [CrossRef]
103. Lee, S.C.; Chung, I.M.; Jin, Y.J.; Song, Y.S.; Seo, S.Y.; Park, B.S.; Vho, K.H.; Yoo, K.S.; Yee, S.B.; Yoo, Y.H. Momilactone B, an allelochemical of rice hulls, induces apoptosis on human lymphoma cells (Jurkat) in a micromolar concentration. *Nutr. Cancer* **2008**, *60*, 542–551. [CrossRef] [PubMed]
104. Joung, Y.H.; Lim, E.J.; Kim, M.S.; Lim, S.D.; Yoon, S.Y.; Lim, Y.C.; Yoo, Y.B.; Ye, S.K.; Park, T.; Chung, I.M.; et al. Enhancement of hypoxia-induced apoptosis of human breast cancer cells via STAT5b by momilactone B. *Int. J. Oncol.* **2008**, *33*, 477–484. [CrossRef]
105. Kim, S.J.; Park, H.R.; Park, E.; Lee, S.C. Cytotoxic and antitumor activity of momilactone B from rice hulls. *J. Agric. Food Chem.* **2007**, *55*, 1702–1706. [CrossRef] [PubMed]
106. Cho, J.G.; Cha, B.J.; Lee, S.M.; Shrestha, S.; Jeong, R.H.; Lee, D.S.; Kim, Y.C.; Lee, D.G.; Kang, H.C.; Jiyoung Kima, J.; et al. Diterpenes from the roots of Oryza sativa L. and their inhibition activity on NO production in LPS-stimulated RAW264. 7 macrophages. *Chem. Biodivers.* **2015**, *12*, 1356–1364. [CrossRef] [PubMed]
107. Quan, N.V.; Tran, H.D.; Xuan, T.D.; Ahmad, A.; Dat, T.D.; Khanh, T.D.; Teschke, R. Momilactones A and B are α-amylase and α-glucosidase inhibitors. *Molecules* **2019**, *24*, 482. [CrossRef]
108. Quan, N.; Xuan, T.D.; Tran, H.D.; Ahmad, A.; Khanh, T.D.; Dat, T.D. Contribution of momilactones A and B to diabetes inhibitory potential of rice bran: Evidence from in vitro assays. *Saudi Pharm. J.* **2019**, *27*, 643–649. [CrossRef]
109. Kang, D.Y.; SP, N.; Darvin, P.; Joung, Y.H.; Byun, H.J.; Do, C.H.; Park, K.D.; Cho, K.H.; Yang, Y.M. Momilactone B inhibits ketosis in vitro by regulating the ANGPTL3-LPL pathway and inhibiting HMGCS2. *Anim. Biotechnol.* **2017**, *28*, 189–197. [CrossRef]
110. Lee, J.H.; Cho, B.; Jun, H.J.; Seo, W.D.; Kim, D.W.; Cho, K.J.; Lee, S.J. Momilactione B inhibits protein kinase A signaling and reduces tyrosinase-related proteins 1 and 2 expression in melanocytes. *Biotechnol. Let.* **2012**, *4*, 805–812. [CrossRef]
111. Vranova, E.; Coman, D.; Gruissem, W. Network analysis of the VA and MEP pathways for isoprenoid synthesis. *Annu. Rev. Plant Biol.* **2013**, *4*, 665–700. [CrossRef]
112. Nemoto, T.; Cho, E.M.; Okada, A.; Okada, K.; Otomo, K.; Kanno, Y.; Toyomasu, T.; Mitsuhashi, W.; Sassa, T.; Minami, E.; et al. Stemar-13-ene synthase, a diterpene cyclase involved in the biosynthesis of the phytoalexin oryzalexin S in rice. *FEBS Lett.* **2004**, *571*, 182–186. [CrossRef]
113. Otomo, K.; Kanno, Y.; Motegi, A.; Kenmoku, H.; Yamane, H.; Mitsuhashi, W.; Okikawa, H.; Toshima, H.; Itoh, H.; Matsuoka, M.; et al. Diterpene cyclases responsible or the biosynthesis of phytoalexins, momilactones A, B, and oryzalexins A-F in rice. *Biosci. Biotechnol. Biochem.* **2004**, *68*, 2001–2006. [CrossRef] [PubMed]
114. Xu, M.; Hillwig, M.L.; Prisic, S.; Coates, R.M.; Peters, R.J. Functional identification of rice *syn*-copalyl diphosphate synthase and its role in initiating biosynthesis of diterpenoid phytoalexin/allelopathic natural products. *Plant J.* **2004**, *39*, 309–318. [CrossRef] [PubMed]
115. Otomo, K.; Kenmoku, H.; Oikawa, H.; Konig, W.A.; Toshima, H.; Mitsuhashi, W.; Yamane, H.; Sassa, T.; Toyomasu, T. Biological functions of *ent*- and *syn*-copalyl diphosphate synthases in rice: Key enzymes for the branch point of gibberellin and phytoalexin biosynthesis. *Plant J.* **2004**, *39*, 886–893. [CrossRef]
116. Sakamoto, T.; Miura, K.; Itoh, H.; Tatsumi, T.; Ueguchi-Tanaka, M.; Ishiyama, K.; Kobayashi, M.; Agrawal, G.K.; Takeda, S.; Abe, K.; et al. An overview of gibberellin metabolism enzyme genes and their related mutants in rice. *Plant Physiol.* **2004**, *134*, 1642–1653. [CrossRef]
117. Wilderman, P.R.; Xu, M.; Jin, Y.; Coates, R.M.; Peters, R.J. Identification of syn-pimara-7,15-diene synthase reveals functional clustering of terpene synthases involved in rice phytoalexin/allelochemical biosynthesis. *Plant Physiol.* **2004**, *135*, 2098–2105. [CrossRef]

118. Shimura, K.; Okada, A.; Okada, K.; Jikumaru, Y.; Ko, K.W.; Toyomasu, T.; Sassa, T.; Hasegawa, M.; Kodama, O.; Shibuya, N.; et al. Identification of a biosynthetic gene cluster in rice for momilactones. *J. Biol. Chem.* **2007**, *282*, 34013–34018. [CrossRef] [PubMed]
119. Wang, Q.; Hillwig, M.L.; Peters, R.J. CYP99A3: Functional identification of a diterpene oxidase from the momilactone biosynthetic gene cluster in rice. *Plant J.* **2011**, *65*, 87–95. [CrossRef]
120. Kitaoka, N.; Zhang, J.; Oyagbenro, R.K.; Brown, B.; Wu, Y.; Yang, B.; Li, Z.; Peters, R.J. Interdependent evolution of biosynthetic gene clusters for momilactone production in rice. *Plant Cell* **2021**, *33*, 290–305. [CrossRef] [PubMed]
121. De La Peña, R.; Sattely, E.S. Rerouting plant terpene biosynthesis enables momilactone pathway elucidation. *Nat. Chem. Biol.* **2020**, *17*, 205–212. [CrossRef] [PubMed]
122. Li, R.; Zhang, J.; Li, Z.; Peters, R.J.; Yang, B. Dissecting the labdane-related diterpenoid biosynthetic gene clusters in rice reveals directional cross-cluster phytotoxicity. *New Phytologist.* **2022**, *233*, 878–889. [CrossRef]
123. Walters, D.; Walsh, D.; Newton, A.; Lyon, G. Induced resistance for plant disease control: Maximizing the effcacy of resistance elicitors. *Phytopathology* **2005**, *95*, 1368–1373. [CrossRef] [PubMed]
124. Langner, T.; Kamoun, S.; Belhaj, K. CRISPR crops: Plant genome editing toward disease resistance. *Annu. Rev. Phytopathol.* **2018**, *56*, 479–512. [CrossRef]
125. Van, D.E.; Koornneef, A.; Ton, J.; Pieterse, C.M. Induced resistance-orchestrating defence mechanisms through crosstalk and priming. *Annu. Plant Rev.* **2018**, *34*, 334–370.
126. Merzendorfer, H.; Zimoch, L. Chitin metabolism in insects: Structure, function and regulation of chitin synthases and chitinases. *J. Exp. Biol.* **2003**, *206*, 4393–4412. [CrossRef]
127. Bowman, S.M.; Free, S.J. The structure and synthesis of the fungal cell wall. *BioEssays* **2006**, *28*, 799–808. [CrossRef]
128. Ma, B.; Wang, J.; Liu, C.; Hu, J.; Tan, K.; Zhao, F.; Yuan, M.; Zhang, J.; Gai, Z. Preventive effects of fluoro-substituted benzothiadiazole derivatives and chitosan oligosaccharide against the rice seedling blight induced by *Fusarium oxysporum*. *Plants* **2019**, *8*, 538. [CrossRef]
129. Yamada, A.; Shibuya, N.; Kodama, O.; Akatsuka, T. Induction of phytoalexin formation in suspension-cultured rice cells by *N*-acetylchitooligosaccharides. *Biosci. Biotech. Biochem.* **1993**, *57*, 405–409. [CrossRef]
130. Yamaguchi, T.; Yamada, A.; Hong, N.; Ogawa, T.; Ishii, T.; Shibuya, N. Differences in the recognition of glucan elicitor signals between rice and soybean: B-glucan fragments from the rice blast disease fungus *Pyricularia oryzae* that elicit phytoalexin biosynthesis in suspension-cultured rice cells. *Plant Cell* **2000**, *12*, 817–826. [PubMed]
131. MacKintosh, C.; Lyon, G.D.; MacKintosh, R.W. Protein phosphatase inhibitors activate anti-fungal defense responses of soybean cotyledons and cell cultures. *Plant J.* **1994**, *5*, 137–147. [CrossRef]
132. Rakwal, R.; Shii, K.; Agrawal, G.K.; Yonekura, M. Protein phosphatase inhibitors activate defense responses in rice (*Oryza sativa*) leaves. *Physiol. Plant.* **2001**, *111*, 151–157. [CrossRef]
133. Kato-Noguchi, H.; Kobayashi, K. Jasmonic acid, protein phosphatase inhibitor, metals and UV-irradiation increased momilactone A and B concentrations in the moss *Hypnum plumaeforme*. *J. Plant Physiol.* **2009**, *166*, 1118–1122. [CrossRef]
134. Kato-Noguchi, H. Stress-induced allelopathic activity and momilactone B in rice. *Plant Growth Regul.* **2009**, *59*, 153–158. [CrossRef]
135. Koga, J.; Yamauchi, T.; Shimura, M.; Ogawa, N.; Oshima, K.; Umemura, K.; Kikuchi, M.; Ogasawara, N. Cerebrosides A and C, sphingolipid elicitors of hypersensitive cell death and phytoalexin accumulation in rice plants. *J. Biol. Chem.* **1998**, *273*, 31985–31991. [CrossRef]
136. Nakazato, Y.; Tamogami, S.; Kawai, H.; Hasegawa, M.; Kodama, O. Methionine-induced phytoalexin production in rice leaves. *Biosci. Biotech. Biochem.* **2000**, *64*, 577–583. [CrossRef]
137. Kodama, O.; Suzuki, T.; Miyakawa, J.; Akatsuka, T. Ultraviolet-induced accumulation of phytoalexins in rice leaves. *Agric. Biol. Chem.* **1988**, *52*, 2469–2473.
138. Kodama, O.; Yamada, A.; Yamamoto, A.; Takemoto, T.; Akatsuka, T. Induction of phytoalexins with heavy metal ions in rice leaves. *J. Pesticide Sci.* **1988**, *13*, 615–617. [CrossRef]
139. Rakwal, R.; Tamogami, S.; Kodama, O. Role of jasmonic acid as a signaling molecule in copper chloride-elicited rice phytoalexin production. *Biosci. Biotech. Biochem.* **1996**, *60*, 1046–1048. [CrossRef]
140. Qin, J.; Wand, Y.; He, G. Induction of phytoalexins (PA) formation in suspension-cultured rice cells by metal and nonmetal Ions. *Chin. J. Appl. Environ. Biol.* **2006**, *12*, 322.
141. Rakwal, R.; Agrawal, G.K.; Kubo, A.; Yonekura, M.; Tamogami, S.; Saji, H.; Iwahashi, H. Defense/stress responses elicited in rice seedlings exposed to the gaseous air pollutant sulfur dioxide. *Environ. Exp. Bot.* **2003**, *49*, 223–235. [CrossRef]
142. Tamogami, S.; Kodama, O.; Hirose, K.; Akatsuka, T. Pretilachlor [2-chloro-N-(2, 6-diethylphenyl)-N-(2-propoxyethyl) acetamide]- and butachlor [N-(butoxymethyl)-2-chloro-N-(2, 6-diethylphenyl) acetamide]-induced accumulation of phytoalexin in rice (*Oryza sativa*) plants. *J. Agric. Food Chem.* **1995**, *43*, 1695–1697. [CrossRef]
143. Ji, C.; Norton, R.A.; Wicklow, D.T.; Dowd, P.F. Isoform patterns of chitinase and b-1,3-glucanase in maturing corn kernels (*Zea mays* L.) associated with *Aspergillus flavus* milk stage infection. *J. Agric. Food Chem.* **2000**, *48*, 507–511. [CrossRef]
144. Rodriguez, V.M.; Santiago, R.; Malvar, R.A.; Butron, A. Inducible maize defense mechanisms against the corn borer *Sesamia nonagrioides*: A transcriptome and biochemical approach. *Mol. Plant-Microbe Interact.* **2012**, *25*, 61–68. [CrossRef]
145. Shimizu, T.; Nakano, T.; Takamizawa, D.; Desaki, Y.; Ishii-Minami, N.; Nishizawa, Y.; Minami, E.; Okada, K.; Yamane, H.; Kaku, H.; et al. Two LysM receptor molecules, CEBiP and OsCERK1, cooperatively regulate chitin elicitor signaling in rice. *Plant J.* **2010**, *64*, 204–214. [CrossRef]

146. Thao, N.P.; Chen, L.; Nakashima, A.; Hara, S.I.; Umemura, K.; Takahashi, A.; Shirasu, K.; Kawasaki, T.; Shimamoto, K. RAR1 and HSP90 form a complex with Rac/Rop GTPase and function in innate-immune responses in rice. *Plant Cell* **2007**, *19*, 4035–4045. [CrossRef]
147. Seo, N.S.; Lee, S.K.; Song, M.Y.; Suh, J.P.; Hahn, T.R.; Ronald, P.; Jeon, J.S. The HSP90–SGT1–RAR1 molecular chaperone complex: A core modulator in plant immunity. *J. Plant Biol.* **2008**, *51*, 1–10. [CrossRef]
148. Chen, L.; Hamada, S.; Fujiwara, M.; Zhu, T.; Thao, N.P.; Wong, H.L.; Krishna, P.; Ueda, T.; Kaku, H.; Naoto Shibuya, N.; et al. The Hop/Sti1–Hsp90 chaperone complex facilitates the maturation and transport of a PAMP receptor in rice innate immunity. *Cell Host Microbe* **2010**, *7*, 185–196. [CrossRef]
149. Lieberherr, D.; Thao, N.P.; Nakashima, A.; Umemura, K.; Kawasaki, T.; Shimamoto, K. A sphingolipid elicitor-inducible mitogen-activated protein kinase is regulated by the small GTPase OsRac1 and heterotrimeric G-protein in rice. *Plant Physiol.* **2005**, *138*, 1644–1652. [CrossRef]
150. Kim, J.A.; Cho, K.; Singh, R.; Jung, Y.H.; Jeong, S.H.; Kim, S.H.; Kim, S.H.; Lee, J.E.; Cho, Y.S.; Agrawal, G.K.; et al. Rice OsACDR1 (*Oryza sativa* accelerated cell death and resistance 1) is a potential positive regulator of fungal disease resistance. *Mol. Cells* **2009**, *28*, 431–439. [CrossRef]
151. Kishi-Kaboshi, M.; Okada, K.; Kurimoto, L.; Murakami, S.; Umezawa, T.; Shibuya, N.; Yamane, H.; Miyao, A.; Takatsuji, H.; Takahashi, A.; et al. A rice fungal MAMP-responsive MAPK cascade regulates metabolic flow to antimicrobial metabolite synthesis. *Plant J.* **2010**, *63*, 599–612. [CrossRef] [PubMed]
152. Okada, A.; Okada, K.; Miyamoto, K.; Koga, J.; Shibuya, N.; Nojiri, H.; Yamane, H. OsTGAP1, a bZIP transcription factor, coordinately regulates the inductive production of diterpenoid phytoalexins in rice. *J. Biol. Chem.* **2009**, *284*, 26510–26518. [CrossRef] [PubMed]
153. Yokotani, N.; Sato, Y.; Tanabe, S.; Chujo, T.; Shimizu, T.; Okada, K.; Yamane, H.; Shimono, M.; Sugano, S.; Takatsuji, H.; et al. OsWRKY76 is a rice transcriptional repressor playing opposite roles in blast disease resistance and cold stress tolerance. *J. Exp. Bot.* **2013**, *64*, 5085–5097. [CrossRef]
154. Wong, H.L.; Pinontoan, R.; Hayashi, K.; Tabata, R.; Yaeno, T.; Hasegawa, K.; Kojima, C.; Yoshioka, H.; Iba, L.; Kawasaki, T.; et al. Regulation of rice NADPH oxidase by binding of Rac GTPase to its N-terminal extension. *Plant Cell* **2007**, *19*, 4022–4034. [CrossRef] [PubMed]
155. Ono, E.; Wong, H.L.; Kawasaki, T.; Hasegawa, M.; Kodama, O.; Shimamoto, K. Essential role of the small GTPase Rac in disease resistance of rice. *Proc. Natl Acad. Sci. USA* **2001**, *98*, 759–764. [CrossRef] [PubMed]
156. Ron, M.; Avni, A. The receptor for the fungal elicitor ethylene-inducing xylanase is a member of a resistance-like gene family in tomato. *Plant Cell* **2004**, *16*, 1604–1615. [CrossRef] [PubMed]
157. Kurusu, T.; Hamada, J.; Nokajima, H.; Kitagawa, Y.; Kiyoduka, M.; Takahashi, A.; Hanamata, S.; Ohno, R.; Hayashi, T.; Okada, K.; et al. Regulation of microbe-associated molecular pattern-induced hypersensitive cell death, phytoalexin production, and defense gene expression by calcineurin B-like protein-interacting protein kinases, OsCIPK14/15, in rice cultured cells. *Plant Physiol.* **2010**, *153*, 678–692. [CrossRef]
158. Hamada, H.; Kurusu, T.; Okuma, E.; Nokajima, H.; Kiyoduka, M.; Koyano, T.; Sugiyama, Y.; Okada, K.; Koga, J.; Saji, H.; et al. Regulation of a proteinaceous elicitor-induced Ca^{2+} influx and production of phytoalexins by a putative voltage-gated cation channel, OsTPC1, in cultured rice cells. *J. Biol. Chem.* **2012**, *287*, 9931–9939. [CrossRef]
159. Riemann, M.; Haga, K.; Shimizu, T.; Okada, K.; Ando, S.; Mochizuki, S.; Nishizawa, Y.; Yamanouchi, U.; Nick, P.; Yano, M.; et al. Identification of rice allene oxide cyclase mutants and the function of jasmonate for defense against *Magnaporthe oryzae*. *Plant J.* **2013**, *74*, 226–238. [CrossRef] [PubMed]
160. Wasternack, C.; Hause, B. Jasmonates: Biosynthesis, perception, signal transduction and action in plant stress response, growth and development. An update to the 2007. *Ann. Bot.* **2013**, *111*, 1021–1058. [CrossRef]
161. Daw, B.D.; Zhang, L.H.; Wang, Z.Z. Salicylic acid enhances antifungal resistance to *Magnaporthe grisea* in rice plants. *Aust. Plant Pathol.* **2008**, *37*, 637–644. [CrossRef]
162. Kariya, K.; Ube, N.; Ueno, M.; Teraishi, M.; Okumoto, Y.; Mori, N.; Ueno, L.; Ishihara, A. Natural variation of diterpenoid phytoalexins in cultivated and wild rice species. *Phytochemistry* **2020**, *180*, 112518. [CrossRef]
163. Miyamoto, K.; Fujita, M.; Shenton, M.R.; Akashi, S.; Sugawara, C.; Sakai, A.; Horie, K.; Hasegawa, M.; Kawaide, H.; Mitsuhashi, W.; et al. Evolutionary trajectory of phytoalexin biosynthetic gene clusters in rice. *Plant J.* **2016**, *87*, 293–304. [CrossRef] [PubMed]
164. Guo, L.; Qiu, J.; Ye, C.; Jin, G.; Mao, L.; Zhang, H.; Yang, X.; Peng, Q.; Wang, Y.; Jia, L.; et al. *Echinochloa crus-galli* genome analysis provides insight into its adaptation and invasiveness as a weed. *Nat. Commun.* **2017**, *8*, 1031. [CrossRef]
165. Ando, H.; Matsuo, A. Applied bryology. In *Advance in Bryology, vol. 2.*; W. Schultze-Motel, W., Ed.; International Association of Bryologists: Vaduz, Liechtenstein, 1984; pp. 133–224.
166. Tsubota, H.; Kuroda, A.; Masuzaki, H.; Nakahara, M.; Deguchi, H. Preliminary study on allelopathic activity of bryophytes under laboratory conditions using the sandwich method. *J. Hattori Bot. Lab.* **2006**, *100*, 517–525.
167. Okada, K.; Kawaide, H.; Miyamoto, K.; Miyazaki, S.; Kainuma, R.; Kimura, H.; Fujiwara, K.; Natsume, M.; Nojiri, H.; Nakajima, M.; et al. HpDTC1, a stress-inducible bifunctional diterpene cyclase involved in momilactone biosynthesis, functions in chemical defense in the moss *Hypnum plumaeforme*. *Sci. Rep.* **2006**, *6*, 1–12.

168. Mao, L.; Kawaide, H.; Higuchi, T.; Chen, M.; Miyamoto, K.; Hirata, Y.; Kimura, H.; Miyazaki, S.; Teruya, M.; Fujiwara, K.; et al. Genomic evidence for convergent evolution of gene clusters for momilactone biosynthesis in land plants. *Proc. Natl Acad. Sci. USA* **2020**, *117*, 12472–12480. [CrossRef] [PubMed]
169. Kato-Noguchi, H. Secretion of momilactone A and B by the moss *Hypnum plumaeforme*. *Plant Signal. Behav.* **2009**, *4*, 737–739. [CrossRef]

toxins

Review

Piperine: Chemistry and Biology

Jin Han [1], Shaoyong Zhang [2], Jun He [3] and Tianze Li [3,*]

[1] School of Public Administration, Xi'an University of Finance and Economics, Xi'an 710061, China; hanjin202012@126.com
[2] Key Laboratory of Vector Biology and Pathogen Control of Zhejiang Province, College of Life Science, Huzhou University, Huzhou 313000, China; 1zhangshaoyong@163.com
[3] College of Plant Protection, Northwest A&F University, Xianyang 712100, China; hejun6206@126.com
* Correspondence: litianze0408@163.com

Abstract: Piperine is a plant-derived promising piperamide candidate isolated from the black pepper (*Piper nigrum* L.). In the last few years, this natural botanical product and its derivatives have aroused much attention for their comprehensive biological activities, including not only medical but also agricultural bioactivities. In order to achieve sustainable development and improve survival conditions, looking for environmentally friendly pesticides with low toxicity and residue is an extremely urgent challenge. Fortunately, plant-derived pesticides are rising like a shining star, guiding us in the direction of development in pesticidal research. In the present review, the recent progress in the biological activities, mechanisms of action, and structural modifications of piperine and its derivatives from 2020 to 2023 are summarized. The structure-activity relationships were analyzed in order to pave the way for future development and utilization of piperine and its derivatives as potent drugs and pesticides for improving the local economic development.

Keywords: piperine; piperine derivatives; biological activity; mechanism of action; structural modification; structure-activity relationship

Key Contribution: This review presents an overview on the biological activities, mechanisms of action, structural modifications, and structure-activity relationships of piperine and its derivatives.

Citation: Han, J.; Zhang, S.; He, J.; Li, T. Piperine: Chemistry and Biology. *Toxins* **2023**, *15*, 696. https://doi.org/10.3390/toxins15120696

Received: 26 September 2023
Revised: 17 November 2023
Accepted: 17 November 2023
Published: 12 December 2023

1. Introduction

Natural alkaloids are a huge library of promising lead compounds, exhibiting a variety of biological activities, which can provide multiple strategies for the development of drugs and pesticides. For instance, camptothecin, a well-known antitumor agent first isolated from *Camptotheca acuminata* Decne. in the mid-1960s, belongs to quinoline alkaloids [1,2]. The botanical products were utilized as pesticides to prevent pests in ancient China as early as the 7–5th centuries BC [3]. Nowadays, industrial chemical pesticides still occupy the dominant position of pesticides, but their high toxicity and environmental pollution have aroused many controversies among the public worldwide. Thus, plant secondary metabolites have become a major focus of research due to their potential application in developing new pesticides. Since 1985, neem-based insecticide Margosan-O, the first commercial pesticide with azadirachtin as the main ingredient, has been approved for registration in the United States, which triggered global enthusiasm for research on natural-based products from plants [4,5]. Plant-derived pesticides usually have the characteristics that their constituents are formed over the long period evolution process in nature and possess an integrated degradation mechanism. Due to their unique properties, they are difficult to accumulate and do not easily harm crops or promote resistance. It is estimated that more than 400,000 species of bioactive compounds in plants have been found, nevertheless, only 10% of the plant species have been investigated. Therefore, plant-derived products have a wide application prospect in the field of agriculture for the management of pests [6].

Black pepper (*Piper nigrum* L.), a family member of Piperaceae, is considered one of the most valuable spices and a potential candidate in natural product research, widely cultivated in lots of tropical and subtropical districts [7,8]. In addition, *P. nigrum* is acknowledged as the king of spices and consists of diverse bioactive compounds, such as sterols, fatty acids, terpenes, amides, and other phytoconstituents with the characteristics of various biological activities [9]. Piperine (**1**, Figure 1) is one of the major alkaloids isolated from the black pepper, which also occurs in the ripe fruits of *Piper longum* L. and the roots of *Piper sarmentosum* Roxb. [10,11]. The pepper processing industry participates in a huge number of various wastes that contain lots of piperine. To effectively utilize the by-products, people investigated the conditions of pressure and temperature on the method of supercritical CO_2 (SC-CO_2) extraction for two steps (100 bar, 60 °C for 1 h and 300 bar, 60 °C for 2 h) to obtain piperamide piperine in a gentle and efficient way [12]. A recent study reported that PFPE-CH, a dietary supplement made by mixing a low piperine fractional *Piper nigrum* extract (PFPE) with cold-pressed coconut oil and honey in distilled water, can help decrease the risk of tumor formation and reduce the side effects of chemotherapeutic drugs during breast cancer treatment. This is promising news for those undergoing treatment for breast cancer [13]. In the early 1970s, a piperine analogue Ilepcimide was originally extracted from a Chinese folk remedy, which was discovered as a safe and effective antiepileptic drug through structural characterization. In addition, the hospital of Peking University (Beijing, China) has been clinically implemented in more than 100,000 patients, and the results showed that the effective rate of Ilepcimide was 95.6% [14,15]. By 2020, the actual cultivated area of pepper in Yunnan Province had reached 39.4 square kilometers, the yield was 1070.8 tons, and the output values had achieved 42.8 million RMB [16]. The piperine molecular contains a dioxymethylene ring, an aliphatic olefin chain, and an amide group. Piperine and its derivatives possess many biological activities, including anticancer [17], antitumor [18], antiviral [19], anti-inflammatory [20], antimalarial [21], antioxidant [22,23], anti-Alzheimer's disease [24–26], and anti-Parkinson disease properties [27]. The characteristics of the structure of piperine allow for modification at multiple sites so as to obtain more candidates with better activities, which are widely used in the agricultural field. For instance, Zhang et al. synthesized a series of bisamide-type piperine derivatives and evaluated them for insecticidal activity against *Plutella xylostella* (L.). The study results revealed that most of the desired compounds displayed better insecticidal activity compared to piperine. In particular, the molecular docking results indicated that a synthetic compound could act on γ-aminobutyric acid receptors [28]. Recently, our studies synthesized two novel series of ester and oxime ester piperine-type derivatives, some compounds displayed more than 100 times the acaricidal activity of piperine against *Tetranychus cinnabarinus* (Bois.). Moreover, the scanning electron microscope (SEM) demonstrated that their potential acaricidal activities may be related to the destruction of the construction of the cuticle layer crest of *T. cinnabarinus* [29,30]. Wang et al. found that the ester derivative prepared from piperine exhibited particularly significant broad-spectrum fungicidal activity against *Rhizoctonia solani* Kühn, *Fusarium graminearum* Schwabe, *Alternaria tenuis* Nees, *Gloeosporium theae-sinensis* I. Miyake, *Phytophthora capsica* Leonian, and *Phomopsis adianticola* [31].

Generally, with the characteristics of easy modification and lots of bioactivities, piperine and its derivatives have received much attention in the fields of synthetic organic chemistry and medicinal chemistry. In this review, many works concerning piperine and its derivatives have been conducted, we widely summarized the advances in the construction and structural modification of piperine and its derivatives from 2020 to 2023. Meanwhile, the latest biological activities, mechanisms of action, and structure-activity relationships of piperine and its derivatives are also presented.

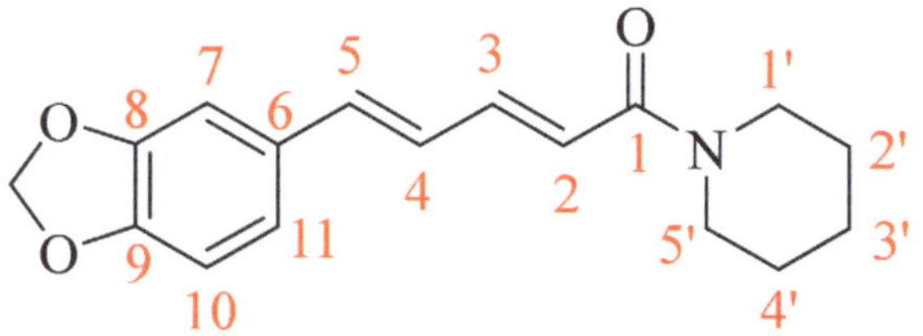

piperine (**1**)

Figure 1. The chemical structure of piperine (**1**).

2. Bioactivities of Piperine and Its Derivatives

2.1. Anticancer Activity

Cancer still poses the biggest danger to human health. For example, breast cancer is an increasing global health challenge. According to the World Health Organization (WHO), in 2020, approximately 2.3 million women were diagnosed with breast cancer and there were 685,000 deaths reported worldwide [32]. Rajarajan et al. reported that the dietary piperine represented a potential candidate that could suppress obesity-associated breast cancer growth and metastasis by regulating the miR-181c-3p/PPARα Axis [33]. Furthermore, Jeong et al. also found that piperine has anticancer properties such as growth inhibition, anti-migration, and anti-invasion of cancer cells [34]. In order to application of piperine derivatives as more potential anticancer drugs, structural modification has received much attention. For example, compound **2** (Figure 2) was evaluated for cytotoxicity and inhibition of TrxR (thioredoxin reductase) activity, paving the way for further exploration of piperine derivatives as TrxR inhibitors [35]. Elimam et al. examined the piperine-based sulfonamide **3** (Figure 2) for its anticancer activity towards the breast MCF-7 cancer cell line. The results indicated that it is a promising lead compound for developing efficient anticancer candidates with potent carbonic anhydrase (CA) inhibitory activity [36]. In addition, to validate the in silico results against triple-negative breast cancer (TNBC) MDA-MB-231, an in vitro vascular endothelial growth factor receptor-2 (VEGFR-2) inhibition assay was conducted. Compound **4** (Figure 2) exhibited powerful inhibitory activity with a half-maximal inhibitory concentration (IC_{50}) value of 231 nM [37]. Pandya et al. found that piperine analogue **5** (Figure 2) may serve as an anticancer therapeutic seeing it affects c-myc oncogene expression via G-quadruplex mediated mechanism [38].

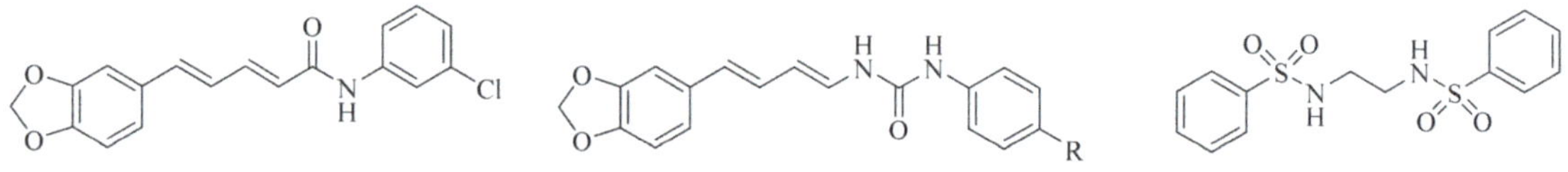

2

3: R = SO_2NH_2;
4: R = Cl.

5

Figure 2. The chemical structures of compounds **2**–**5**.

2.2. Antiviral Activity

The respiratory illness caused by the pandemic H1N1 influenza virus has become a significant global health concern. Mohammed et al. conducted a study in which they screened a piperine derivative **6** (Figure 3) for its antiviral activity and compared it with other strains in vitro on the MDCK cell line. The adsorption assay demonstrated a dose-dependent reduction of viral plaque with an EC_{50} value of 0.33 μM [39]. Over the past five years, the COVID-19 (SARS-CoV-2) epidemic has spread around the world, bringing immeasurable damage to people's lives and health. However, some potential molecules showed promising activities against coronavirus, a published research illustrated that the plant alkaloid piperine could inhibit the vesicle fusion mediated by SARS-CoV-2 peptides and reduce the titer of SARS-CoV-2 progeny in vitro in Vero cells [40]. In addition, largemouth bass virus (LMBV) is a systemic viral pathogen that affects cultivated largemouth bass, causing high mortality rates. Wang et al. investigated the antiviral activity of piperine against LMBV in vitro and in vivo, and the results showed that piperine could act as a therapeutic and preventative drug for further study against LMBV infection [41].

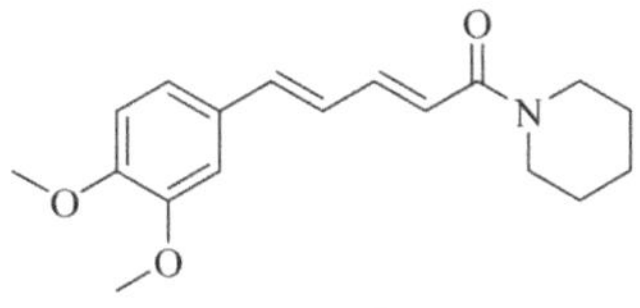
6

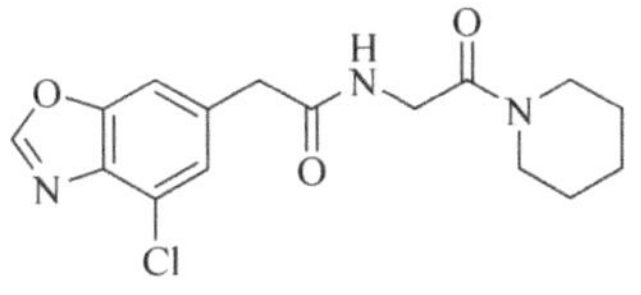
7

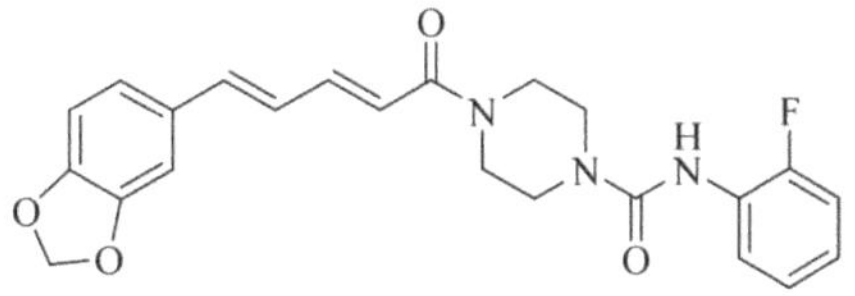
8

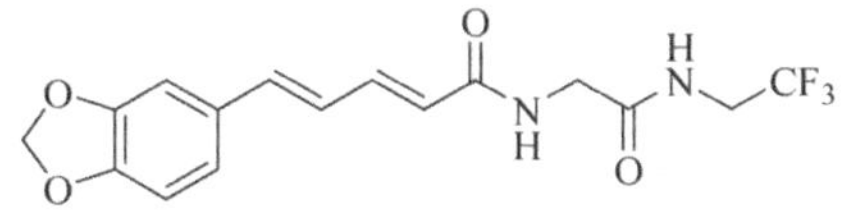
10

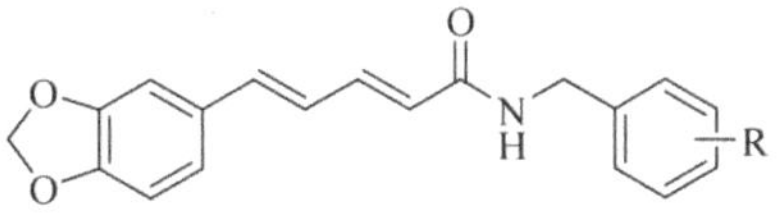
9: R = 3-CF_3; **11**: R = 3-OCH_3; **12**: R = 4-Cl.

Figure 3. The chemical structures of compounds **6–12**.

2.3. Anti-Inflammatory Activity

Ultraviolet (UV) rays from sunlight are one of many environmental insults that harm the skin. Jaisin et al. discovered that piperine may effectively treat skin inflammation caused by UV irradiation [42]. Acute pancreatitis (AP) is a common acute abdominal disease characterized by pancreatic acinar cell death and inflammation. Huang et al. confirmed that piperine can target the endoplasmic reticulum autophagy (ER-phagy), providing a new insight into the pharmacological mechanism of piperine in treating AP [43]. Psoriasis is a common chronic inflammatory skin disease that is prone to relapse and difficult to cure. Studies have shown that piperine can help alleviate psoriasis by reducing epidermal hyperplasia, inflammatory cell infiltration, and the expression of psoriasis-characteristic cytokines, chemokines, and proteins in IMQ-induced psoriasiform dermatitis. Therefore, piperine has the potential to become an effective agent for psoriasis and may provide new strategies for clinical intervention [44]. Additionally, sciatica is a kind of combined pain caused by stimulation and compression of various factors, resulting in stabbing, burning, and dull pain along the route of the sciatic nerve and in the surrounding areas, which brings great physical and psychological pain to patients. Wang et al. confirmed the regulatory relationship between miR-520a and p65. In addition, they investigated the impact of miR-520a/P65 on cytokine levels following piperine stimulation to determine its therapeutic role in sciatica. As a result, they found that piperine can help alleviate pain. Specifically, piperine can promote the expression of miR-520a, which directly targets and inhibits the expression of P65, down-regulate pro-inflammatory factors IL-1β and TNF-α, while up-regulating the effects of anti-inflammatory factors IL-10 and TGF-β1. As a result, piperine may as a treatment for sciatica [45]. Duan et al. suggested that piperine may have anti-inflammatory properties by regulating the key factors of the NF-κB and MAPK signaling pathways [46]. Yang et al. developed a novel piperine derivative **7** (Figure 3) and demonstrated that it exhibited potent therapeutic effects against neuroinflammation, which might be partly attributed to its inhibitory activity on kelch-like ECH-associated protein (Keap1)-nuclear factor erythroid-2-related factor 2 (Nrf2) protein-protein interaction [47]. Tian et al. synthesized a potent inhibitor **8** (Figure 3) of fatty acid amide hydrolase (FAAH) with an IC_{50} value of 0.65 μM. And the inhibitor was found to attenuate the lipopolysaccharide (LPS)-induced activation of BV2 cells, showing a significant anti-inflammatory activity [48].

2.4. Insecticidal Activity

In 2022, Oliveira et al. found that piperine loaded into nanostructured systems might be an effective drug to improve larvicidal activity against *Aedes aegypti* L. [49]. Yang et al. identified that compound **9** (Figure 3) was the most effective multichitinase inhibitor and exhibited higher insecticidal activity against *Ostrinia furnacalis* (Guenée) (Asian corn borer) than dual- or single-chitinase inhibitors. Results of molecular mechanism studies showed that compound **9** can interact with two conserved TRP and TYR of three chitinases in identical ways through hydrogen bonds, hydrophobic, and π-π interactions. Furthermore, the microinjection experiment revealed that the agent displayed significant sublethal effects against *O. furnacalis* by regulating its growth and development [50]. Zhang et al. synthesized a series of piperine derivates containing a linear bisamide. Among them, compound **10** (Figure 3) gave rise to 90% mortality at 1.0 mg/mL concentration against *P. xylostella* [28]. In order to investigate the effects of potential trehalase inhibitors in *Spodoptera frugiperda* (Smith), compounds **11** (Figure 3) and **12** (Figure 3) were synthesized by Zhong et al. The results showed that compound **12** significantly reduced trehalase activity. Additionally, compound **11** not only can reduce membraned-bound trehalase activity, but also inhibit the expression of *SfTRE2*, *SfCHS2*, and *SfCHT*, thus affecting the chitin metabolism, providing a theoretical basis for the application of trehalase inhibitors in the control of agricultural pests [51].

2.5. Antibacterial and Antifungal Activities

A series of piperine amide derivatives were synthesized by Sivashanmugam et al. Of all the derivates, compounds **13** (Figure 4) and **14** (Figure 4) worked exceptionally well against Gram-negative bacteria (*Escherichia coli* and *Acinetobacter baumannii*) and Gram-positive bacteria (*Staphylococcus aureus*, *Escherichia faecalis*, and *Staphylococcus epidermidis*) [52]. Das et al. found that piperine exhibited potent antibiofilm activity against *Pseudomonas aeruginosa* by accumulating reactive oxygen species, affecting cell surface hydrophobicity, and quorum sensing. This research suggested that piperine can effectively disrupt the biofilm formation of *P. aeruginosa*, offering a sustainable solution for protecting public health [53]. The emergence and rapid spread of multidrug-resistant (MDR) bacteria, such as *Vibrio cholerae*, is a major global public health concern. Piperine has been found to show a dose-dependent bactericidal effect on *V. cholerae* growth, regardless of their biotypes and serogroups at the concentrations of 200 and 300 μg/mL, respectively. It also can inhibit the growth of multidrug-resistant (MDR) strains of *P. aeruginosa* and *E. coli* isolated from poultry, and enterohemorrhagic/enteroaggregative *E. coli* O104 in 200 μg/mL. The results demonstrated that piperine has antimicrobial properties against pathogenic bacteria, including MDR strains, making it a potential therapeutic and preventative agent against infections [54]. Souza, Jr. et al. synthesized the compound **15** (Figure 4) and evaluated its antifungal activity against Candida, Trichophyton, and Microsporum strains. As a result, compound **15** exhibited 70% inhibition in seven tested strains, such as *Candida albicans* ATCC 76645, LM-111, LM-122 and *Candida krusei* LM-656, LM-13 and *Microsporum canis* LM-12, and *Microsporum gypseum* LM-512, with a minimum inhibitory concentration (MIC) ranging from 1.23–2.46 μmol/mL and a minimum fungicide concentration (MFC) ranging from 9.84–19.68 μmol/mL [55].

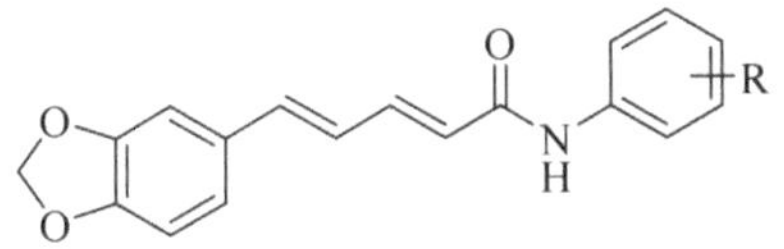

13: R = 2,4,6-CH_3; **14**: R = 4-NO_2; **16**: R = H;
17: R = 2,4-OCH_3; **18**: R = 2,5-OCH_3.

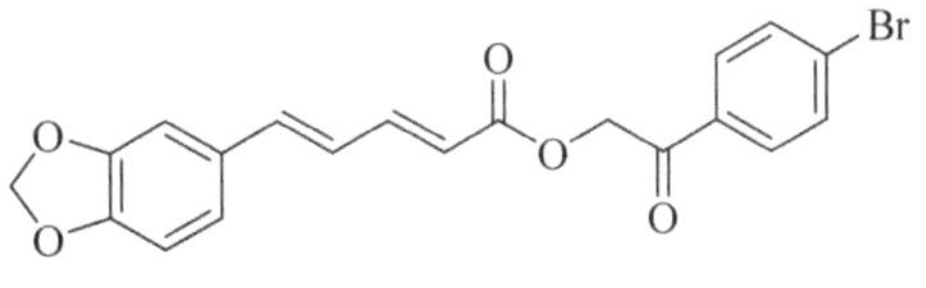

15

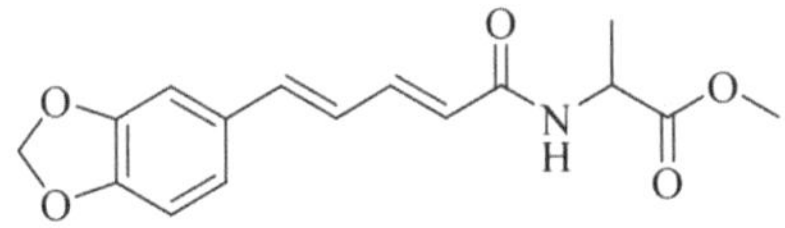

19

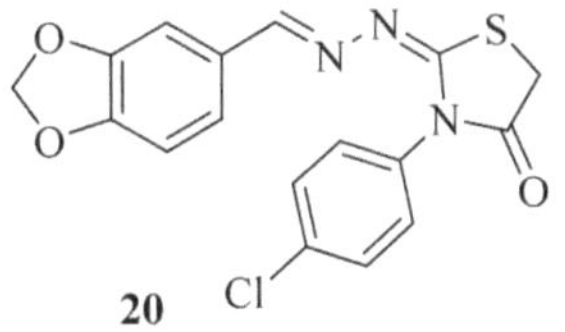

20

Figure 4. The chemical structures of compounds **13**–**20**.

2.6. Other Activities

A series of N-aryl amide derivatives of piperine (**16**–**18**, Figure 4) were prepared by semi-synthesis, and these compounds were examined for their antitrypanosomal, antimalarial, and anti-SARS-CoV-2 main protease activities. Among them, compound **18** exhibited the most robust biological activities with no cytotoxicity against mammalian cell lines Vero and Vero E6, its IC_{50} values for antitrypanosomal activity against Trypanosoma brucei rhodesiense was 15.46 ± 3.09 μM, and its antimalarial activity against the 3D7 strain of Plasmodium falciparum was 24.55 ± 1.91 μM, which were 4-fold and 5-fold higher than that of piperine, respectively. Furthermore, compound **18** inhibited the activity of 3C-like main protease ($3CL^{Pro}$) toward anti-SARS-CoV-2 activity with the IC_{50} value of 106.9 ± 1.2 μM. Docking and molecular dynamic simulation indicated that the potential binding of compound **18** in the $3CL^{Pro}$ active site had improved binding interaction and stability [21]. Peroxisome proliferator-activated receptor γ (PPARγ) plays a key role in glucose, which is a ligand-mediated transcription factor. The lipid homeostasis always serves as a pharmacological target for new drug discovery and development. Wang et al. synthesized and evaluated some compounds for their agonistic activities of PPARγ. In particular, compound **19** (Figure 4) presented itself as a potential PPARγ agonist with an IC_{50} value of 2.43 μM, and the molecular docking studies indicated that compound **19** stably interacts with the amino acid residues of the PPARγ complex active site [56]. Piperine derivate **20** (Figure 4) containing benzodioxole molecule was identified as the promising antiparasitic candidate against Leishmania amazonensis [57]. Hsieh et al. investigated the protective effects of piperine on nerve growth factor (NGF) signaling in a kainic acid (KA) rat model of excitotoxicity. The results showed that piperine can protect hippocampal neurons against KA-induced excitotoxicity by enhancing the NGF/TrkA/Akt/GSK3β signaling pathways [58]. Alsareii et al. conducted an in vivo study and histopathological examination, which revealed early and intrinsic healing of wounds with the piperine-containing bioactive hydrogel system compared to the bioactive hydrogel system without piperine. These findings established that the piperine-containing bioactive hydrogel system is a promising therapeutic approach for wound healing applications [59].

3. Structural Modifications of Piperine and Its Derivatives

3.1. Structural Modifications at the Dioxymethylene Ring or the Aliphatic Olefin Chain of Piperine

As described in Schemes 1 and 2, Li et al. and Lv et al. regio- and stereo-selectively synthesized a series of piperine-type ester derivates **23a**–**23z** and **23a′**–**23l′**, and oxime ester derivates **25a**–**25z** and **25a′**–**25h′**, respectively, by using the Vilsmeier–Haack–Arnold (VHA) reaction. Meanwhile, as shown in Scheme 3, by changing the substituent groups of dioxymethylene ring, compounds **33a–33i** were also prepared by Lv et al. All the synthetic compounds were evaluated for their acaricidal activities against T. cinnabarinus, among them, compounds **23e**, **23f**, **23u**, **23v**, **25f**, **25l**, **25u**, and **25v** showed significant acaricidal activities with the LC_{50} values ranging from 0.12 to 0.19 mg/mL (Table 1), which were comparable to that of the commercial acaricidal agent spirodiclofen (LC_{50}: 0.12 mg/mL), and displayed almost 100-fold higher acaricidal activities than piperine (LC_{50}: 14.20 mg/mL) [28,29,60]. As shown in Scheme 4, Gu et al. used the catalyst **RhH-1** to reduce the aliphatic olefin chain of piperine under a mild condition with a high yield to obtain analogue **34** [61].

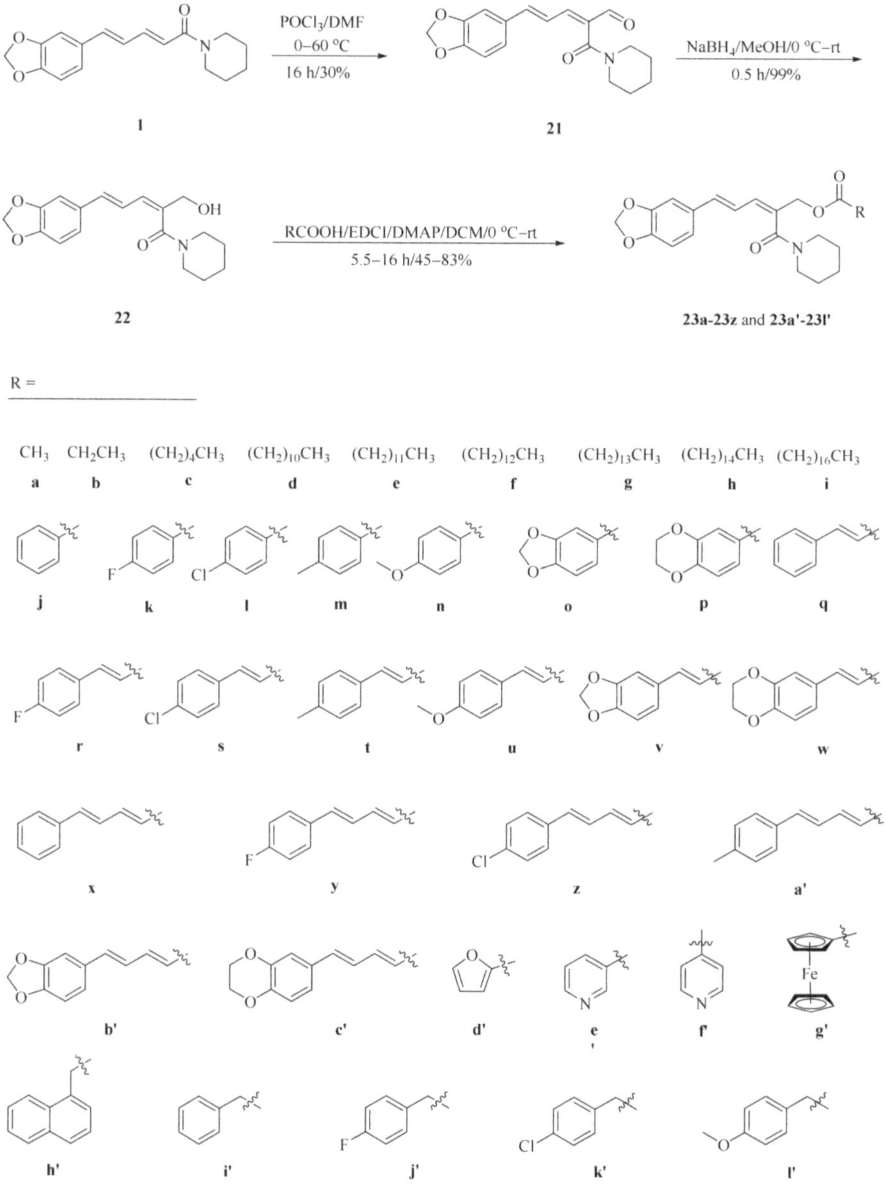

Scheme 1. Synthesis of piperine ester derivates **23a–23z** and **23a′–23l′**.

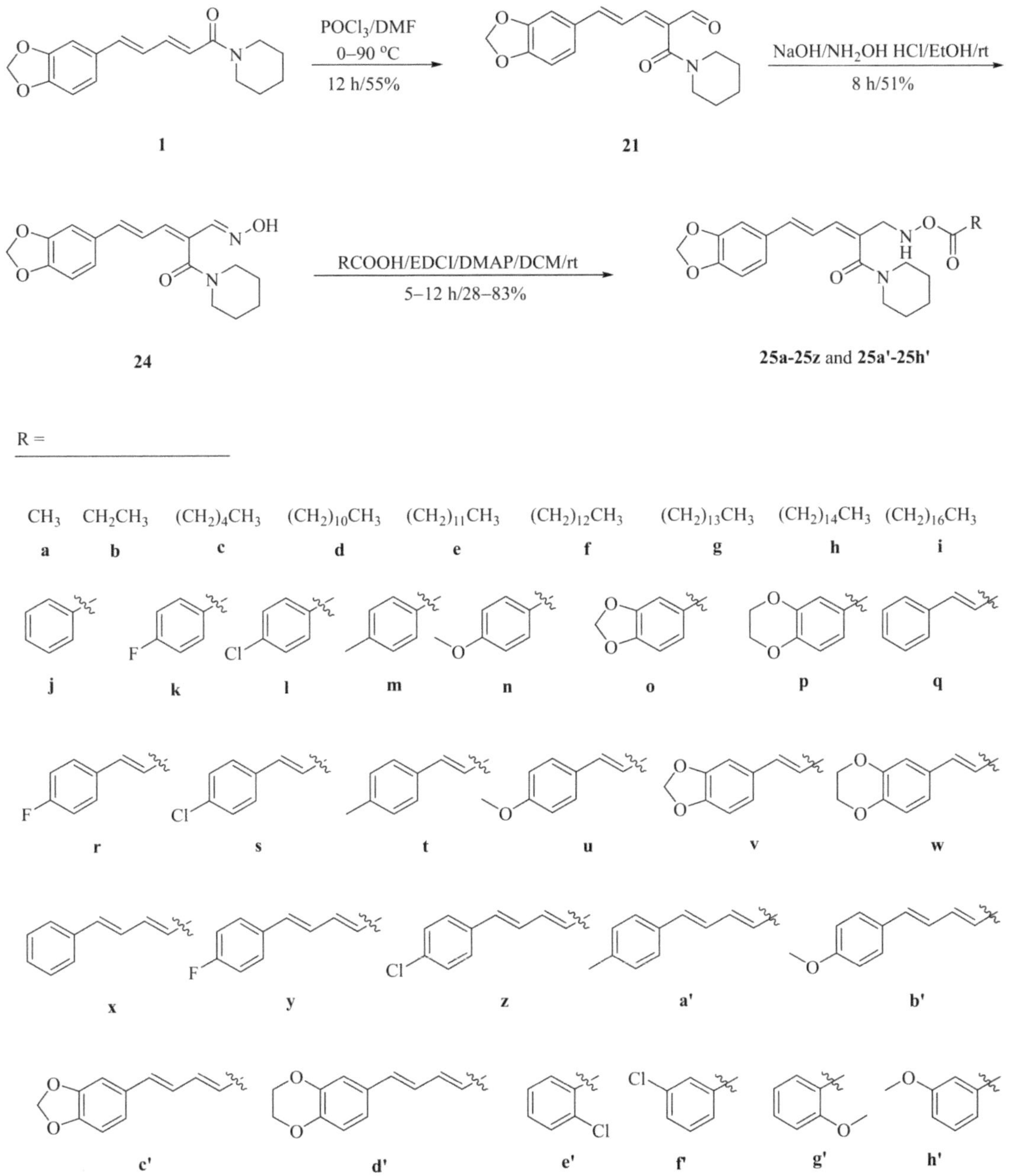

Scheme 2. Synthesis of piperine oxime ester derivates **25a–25z** and **25a′–25h′**.

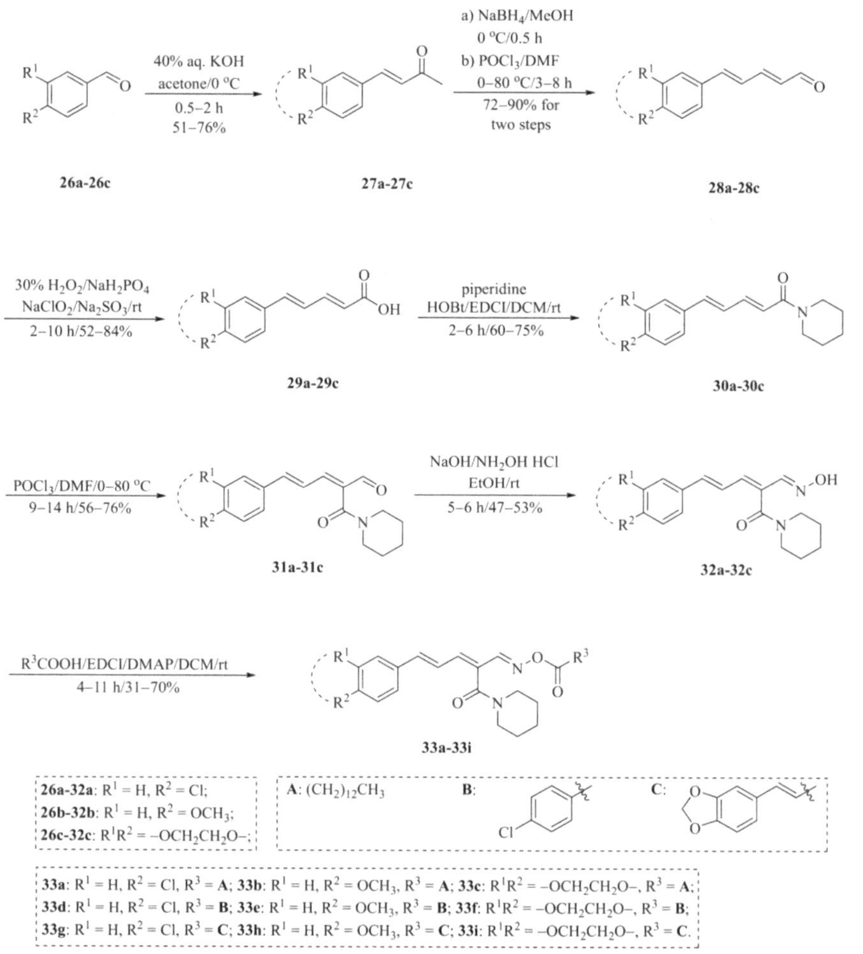

Scheme 3. Synthesis of piperine analogs type oxime ester derivates **33a–33i**.

Table 1. LC_{50} values of some potent compounds against T. cinnabarinus at 72 h.

Compound	LC_{50} (mg/mL)
1	14.20 [29]
23e	0.16 [29]
23f	0.12 [29]
23u	0.18 [29]
23v	0.16 [29]
25f	0.14 [28]
25l	0.16 [28]
25u	0.19 [28]
25v	0.13 [28]
spirodiclofen [a]	0.12 [29]

[a] Spirodiclofen: a commercial acaricide.

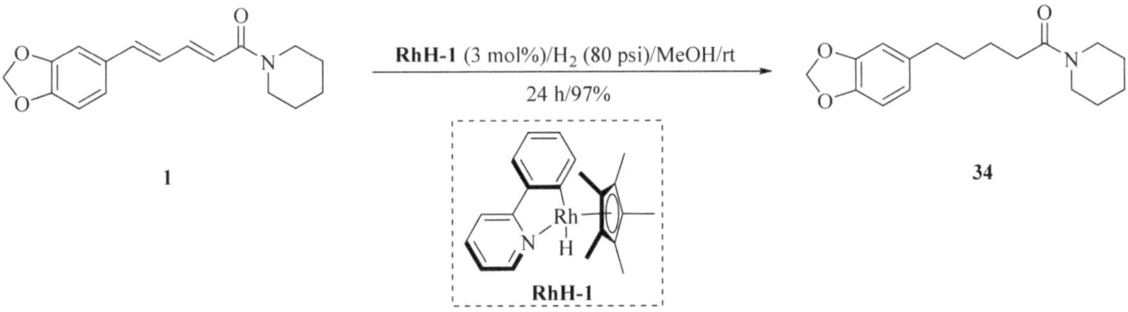

Scheme 4. Synthesis of piperine analogue **34**.

As illustrated in Scheme 5, Luo et al. synthesized four piperine derivates **35** (4R,5R), **36** (4S,5S), **37** (4S,5R), and **38** (4R,5S), which were established by NMR, optical rotation, and CD spectra [62]. As demonstrated in Scheme 6, the sample amine groups were introduced at the aliphatic olefin chain of piperine through a trisulfur-radical-anion-triggered C(sp^2)-H amination of α,β-unsaturated carbonyl to obtain derivate **39** [63]. As presented in Scheme 7, Wojtowicz-Rajchel et al. synthesized five novel corresponding cycloadducts **41–45** in moderate yields by the reaction of prochiral N-alkyltrifluoromethyl-methylene nitrones with piperine under non-catalyzed condition [64].

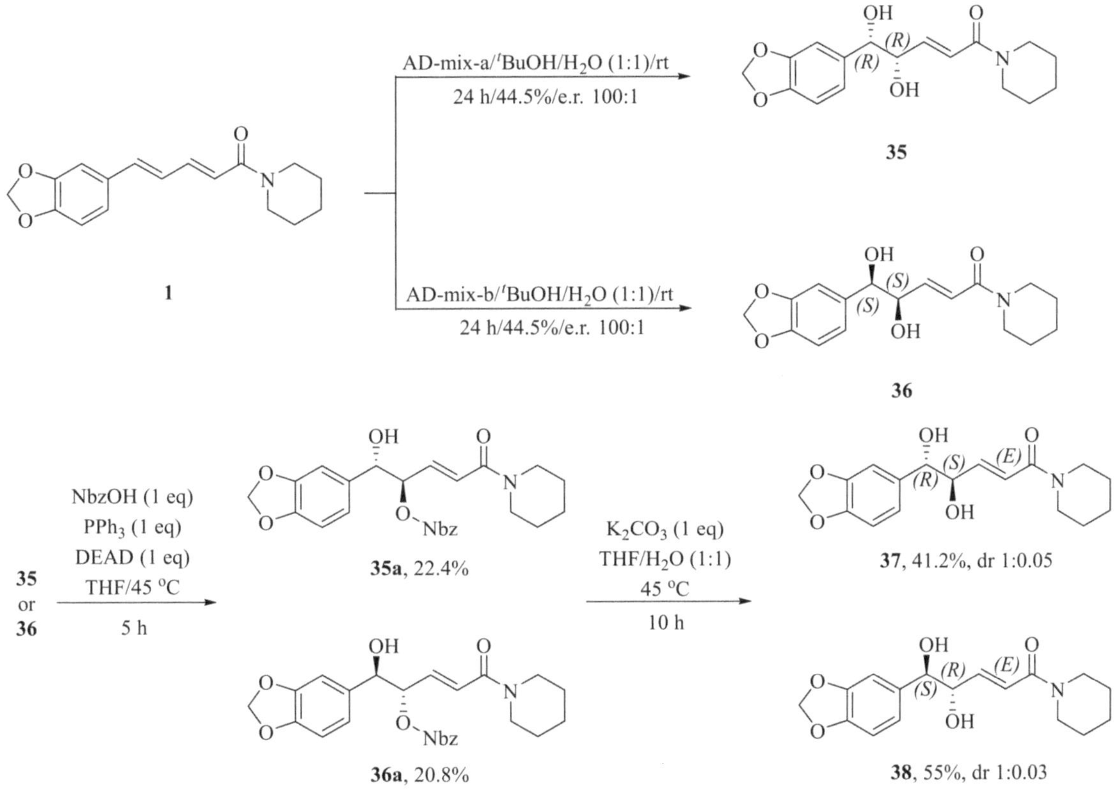

Scheme 5. Synthesis of piperine derivates **35–38**.

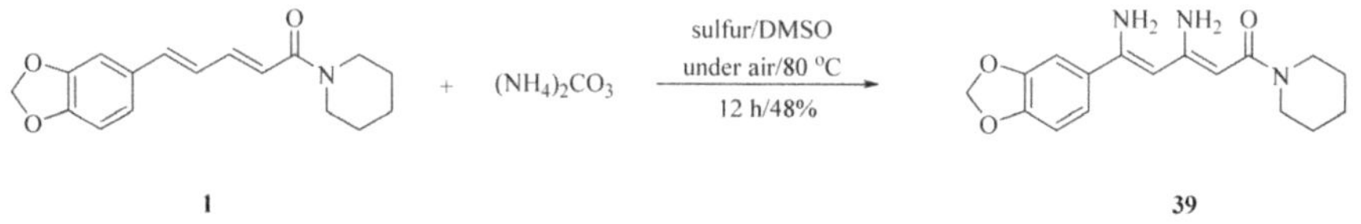

Scheme 6. Synthesis of piperine derivate **39**.

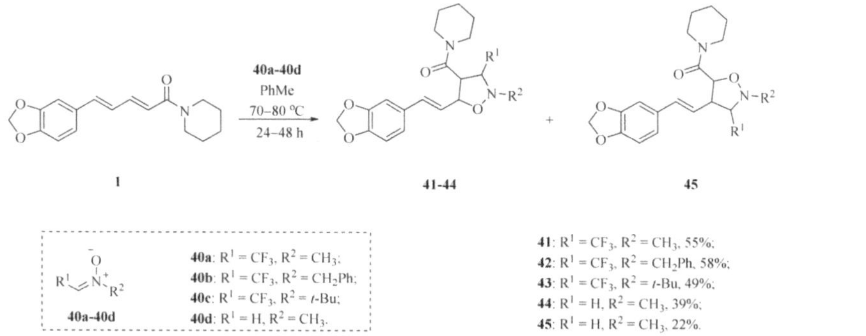

Scheme 7. Synthesis of piperine derivates **41–45**.

3.2. Structural Modifications at the Amide Group of Piperine

As shown in Scheme 8 and Table 2, Tantawy et al. designed and synthesized a series of piperine-based dienehydrazide derivatives **49a–49u** and evaluated their insecticidal activities against third-instar larval of Culex pipiens L. Among all synthetic derivates, compounds **49a, 49b, 49f, 49g, 49m, 49n, 49o, 49p**, and **49u** displayed better activities than piperine and deltamethrin (a commercial positive control). Molecular modeling revealed several interactions between derivates and acetylcholinesterase (AChE) substrate binding sites responsible for binding and inhibition [65]. As shown in Scheme 9, twenty-two piperine derivates **2, 52a–52l**, and **53a–53i** were synthesized by Zhong et al. and evaluated for their anticancer properties [34]. As shown in Scheme 10, a series of novel piperine derivates **56a–56z, 56a′–56b′**, and **59a–59b** containing a linear bisamide were synthesized and evaluated for their insecticidal activities against *P. xylostella* [50].

Table 2. LC_{50} values of some potent compounds against 3rd larval instar of C. pipiens [65].

Compound	LC_{50} (mg/mL)
1	0.357
46	0.398
48	0.421
49a	0.139
49b	0.216
49f	0.146
49g	0.153
49m	0.221
49n	0.094
49o	0.209
49p	0.128
49u	0.174
deltamethrin [a]	1.457

[a] Deltamethrin: a commercial insecticide.

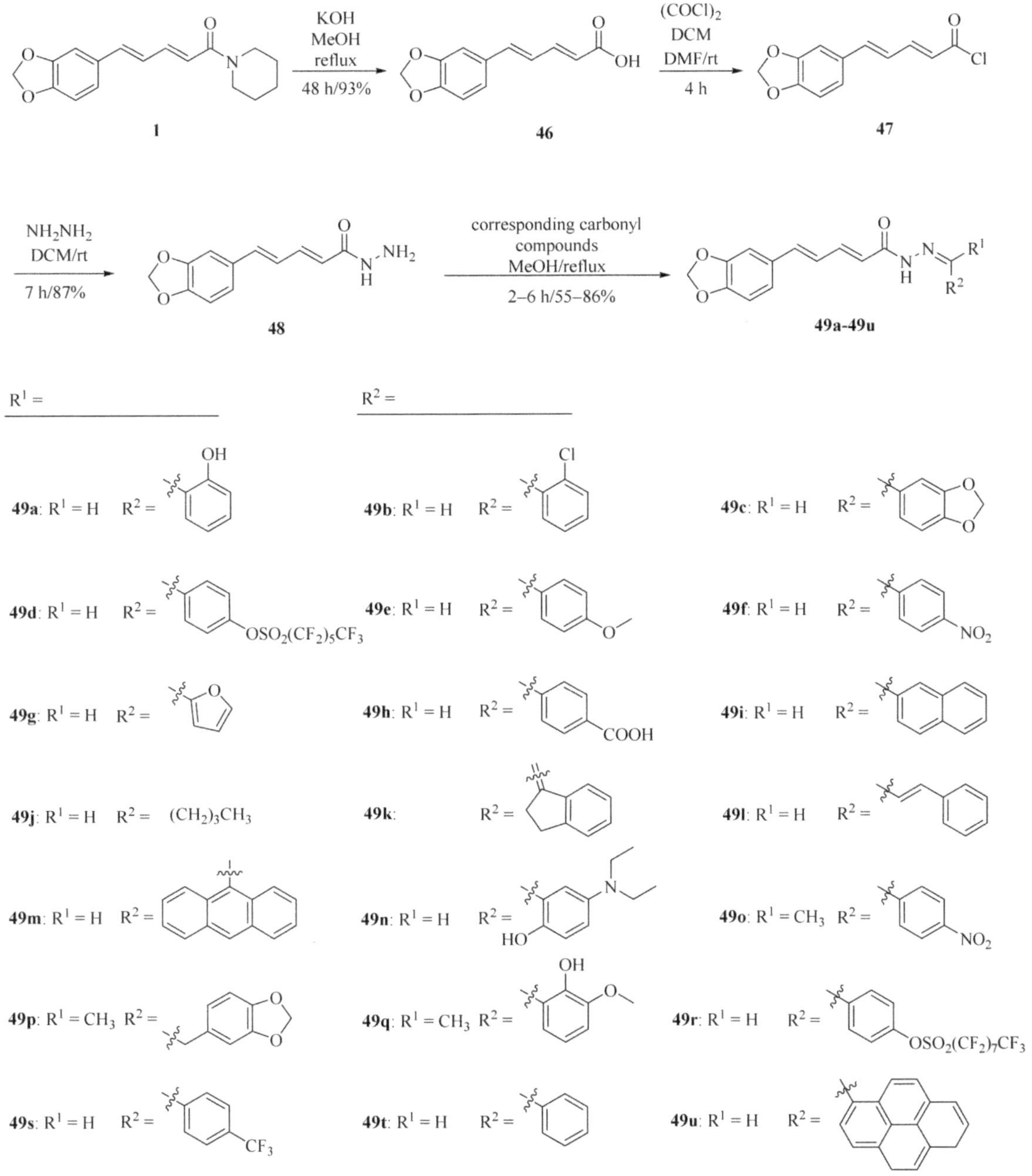

Scheme 8. Synthesis of piperine derivates **49a–49u**.

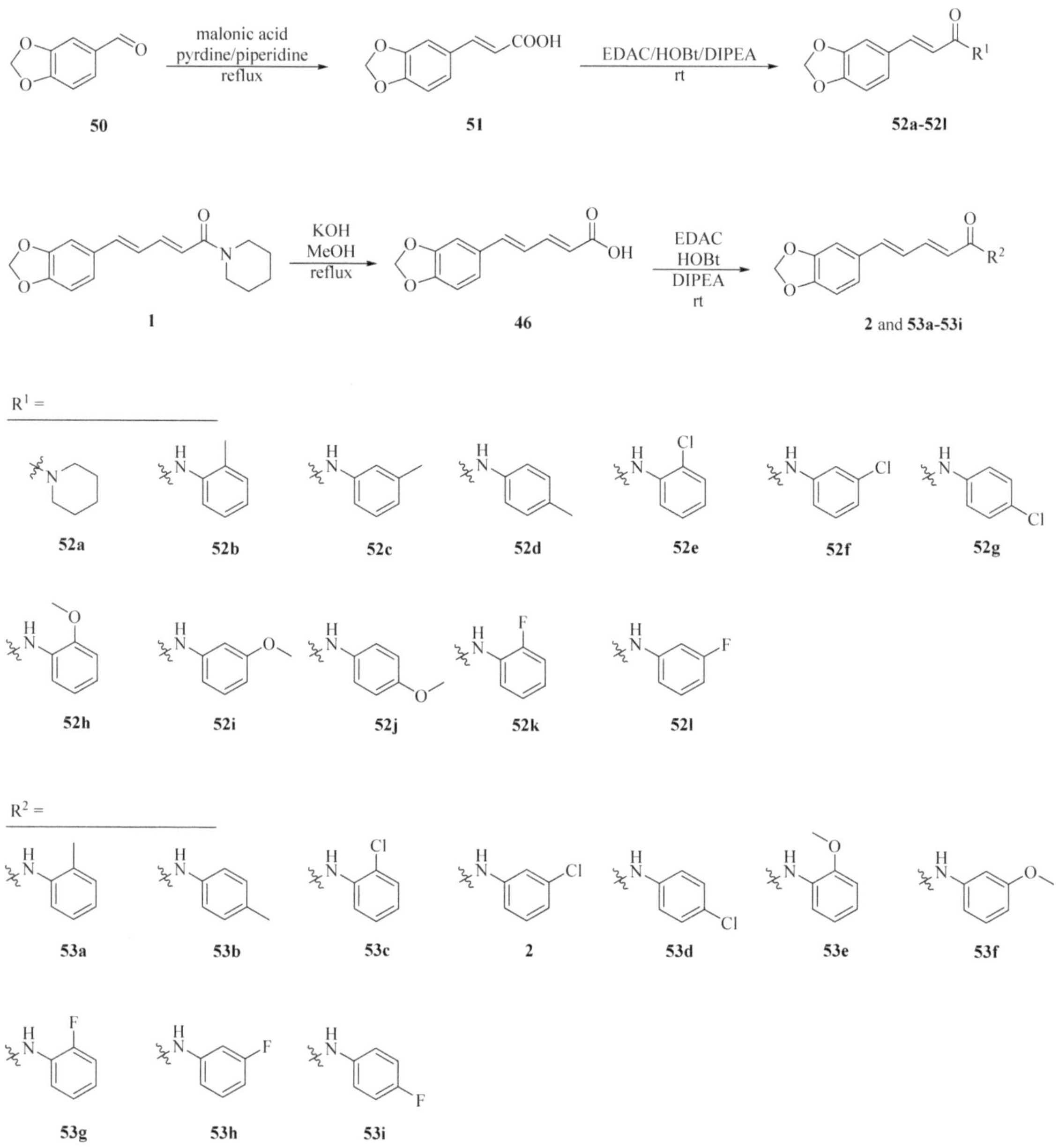

Scheme 9. Synthesis of piperine derivates **2**, **52a–52l**, and **53a–53i**.

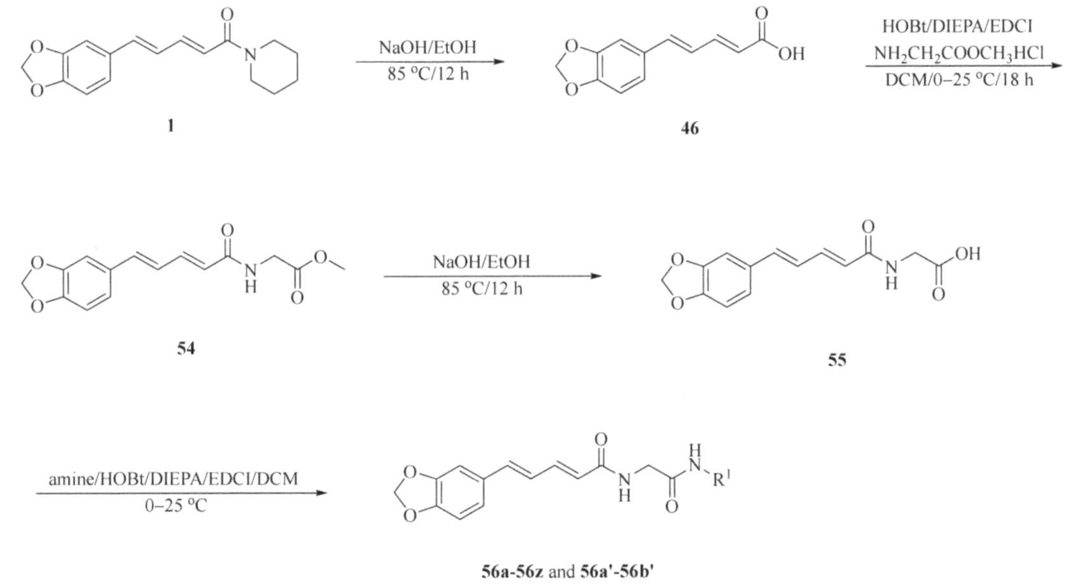

56a: R^1 = Ph;	**56h**: R^1 = 3,4,5-triCH_3-Ph;	**56o**: R^1 = 3-benzyloxy-Ph;	**56v**: R^1 = 2-Cl-PhCH_2;
56b: R^1 = 2-CH_3-Ph;	**56i**: R^1 = 2-F-Ph;	**56p**: R^1 = 4-benzyloxy-Ph;	**56w**: R^1 = CH_2CH_2-Ph;
56c: R^1 = 3-CH_3-Ph;	**56j**: R^1 = 3-F-Ph;	**56q**: R^1 = 2,6-diF-benzyloxy-Ph;	**56x**: R^1 = $CH_2CH_2CH_2$-Ph;
56d: R^1 = 4-CH_3-Ph;	**56k**: R^1 = 4-F-Ph;	**56r**: R^1 = 4-CF_3-benzyloxy-Ph;	**56y**: R^1 = 2-naphthalene;
56e: R^1 = 4-*t*Bu-Ph;	**56l**: R^1 = 3-Cl-Ph;	**56s**: R^1 = 2-benzyloxy-Py;	**56z**: R^1 = 3-benzo[d][1,3]dioxole;
56f: R^1 = 3,5-diCH_3-Ph;	**56m**: R^1 = 3-CH_3CO-Ph;	**56t**: R^1 = 4-PhO-Ph;	**56a'**: R^1 = 5-1-methylindole;
56g: R^1 = 3-ethynyl-Ph;	**56n**: R^1 = 4-CH_3S-Ph;	**56u**: R^1 = Bn;	**56b'**: R^1 = CH_2CF_3.

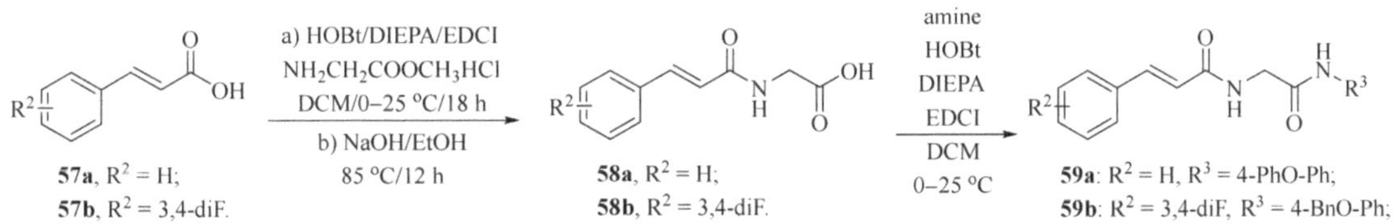

Scheme 10. Synthesis of piperine derivates **56a–56z**, **56a'–56b'**, and **59a–59b**.

Human Cytochrome P450 2J2 (CYP2J2) plays an important role in metabolizing polyunsaturated fatty acids (PUFAs). As described in Scheme 11, a series of piperine derivatives **62a–62k** were designed and synthesized based on the underlying interactions of piperine with CYP2J2. Among them, compounds **62j** and **62k** were developed as much stronger inhibitors and their inhibition activities increased approximately 10-fold higher than piperine with the IC_{50} values of 40 and 50 nM, respectively (Table 3) [66].

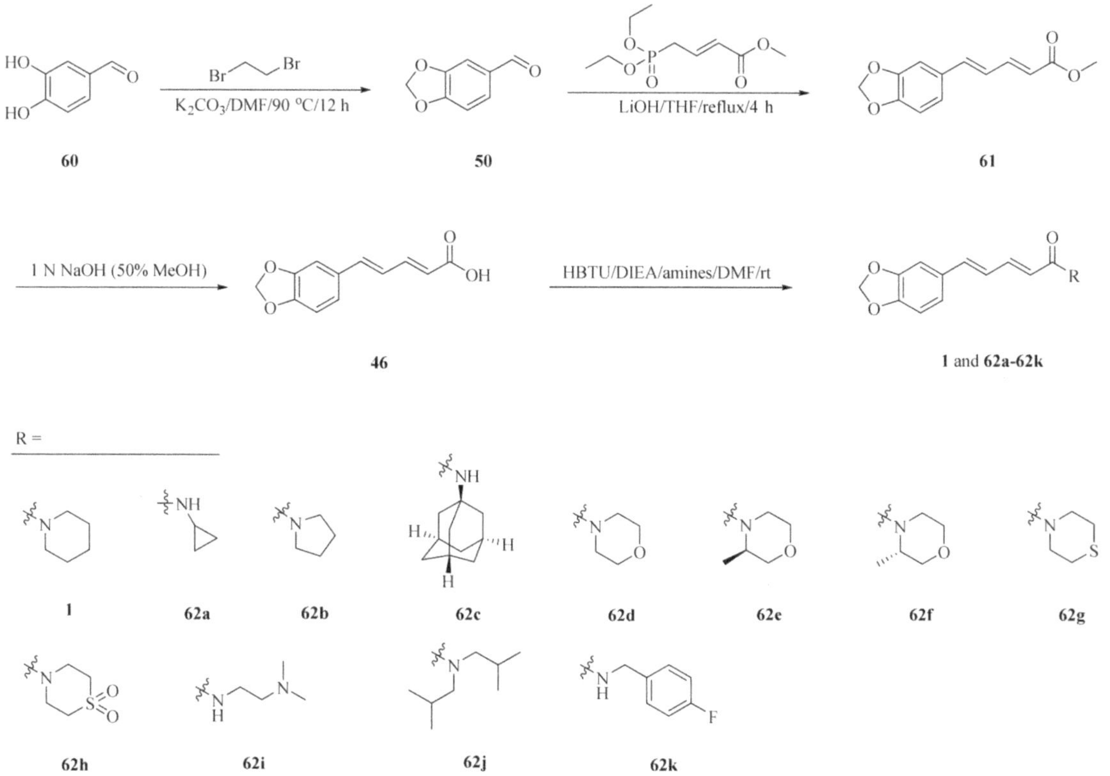

Scheme 11. Synthesis of piperine (1) and its derivatives 62a–62k.

Table 3. The CYP2J2 inhibitory activities of compounds 62a–62k [66].

Compound	Inhibitory Activity (μM)
1	0.44 ± 0.05
62a	4.72 ± 0.73
62b	1.58 ± 0.22
62c	9.33 ± 1.06
62d	11.98 ± 1.35
62e	4.66 ± 0.56
62f	2.25 ± 0.56
62g	0.75 ± 0.08
62h	1.24 ± 0.45
62i	11.81 ± 1.47
62j	0.04 ± 0.01
62k	0.05 ± 0.01

4. Mechanisms of Action of Piperine and Its Derivatives

The natural product piperine (1) and its derivates exhibit wide biological activity in the fields of medicine and agriculture. For example, piperine and its derivates have anticancer properties such as growth-inhibition, anti-migration, and anti-invasion of cancer cells by regulating the miR-181c-3p/PPARα Axis [32] and inhibiting thioredoxin reductase and carbonic anhydrase [34,35]. In addition, piperine can target endoplasmic reticulum autophagy (ER-phagy) in treating acute pancreatitis [42]. On the other hand, the insect chitinase OfChtI from the agricultural pest O. furnacalis is a promising target for green insecticide design. Han et al. first found that piperine can inhibit the insect chitinase from O. furnacalis. Piperine derivates **63a–63f** (Figure 5) were designed and synthesized by introducing a butenolide scaffold into the lead compound piperine. The results of the enzymatic activity assay revealed that the synthetic compounds (K_i = 1.03–2.04 μM) were approximately 40–80 times more effective in inhibiting OfChtI than the lead compound piperine (K_i = 81.45 μM). The inhibitory mechanism demonstrated that the introduced butenolide skeleton improved the binding affinity to OfChtI [67].

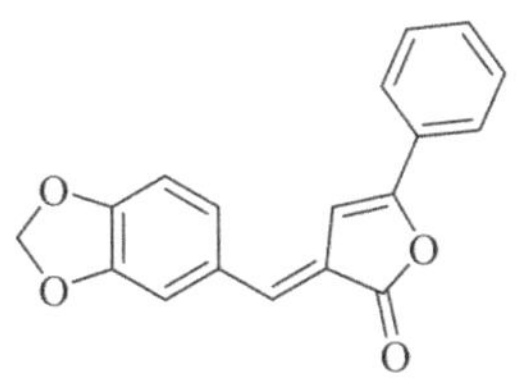

63a

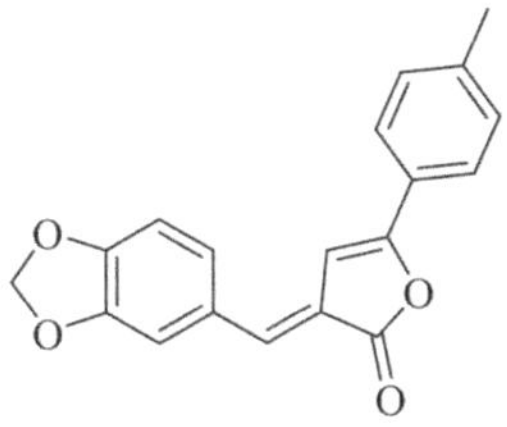

63b

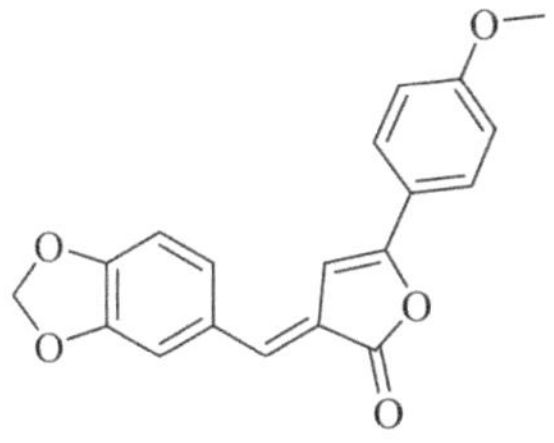

63c

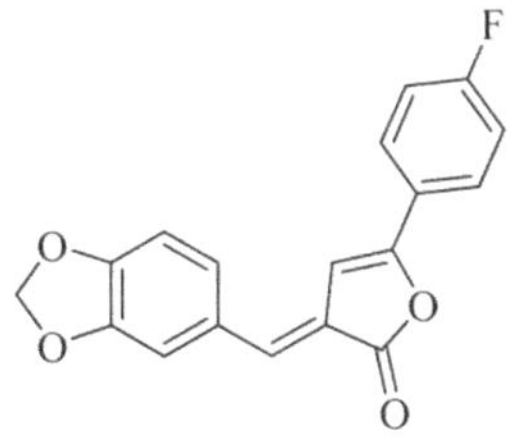

63d

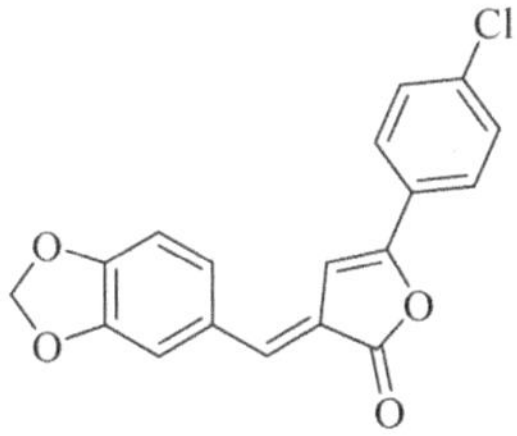

63e

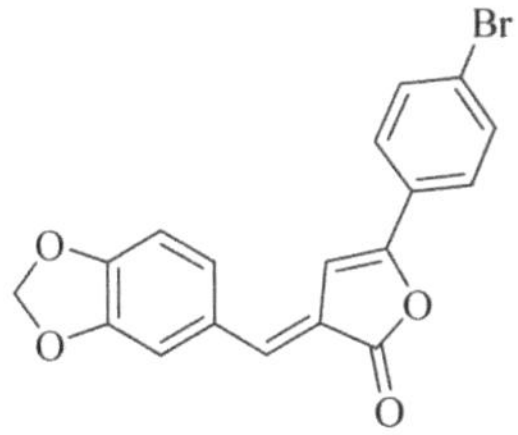

63f

Figure 5. The chemical structures of compounds **63a–63f**.

5. Structure-Activity Relationships of Piperine and Its Derivatives

The SARs analysis of piperine and its derivatives are described in Figure 6, and the detailed descriptions are as follows: (i) introduction of hydroxyl groups at C-8 and C-9 positions can obtain a potent antiviral candidate [38]. Replacing the dioxymethylene ring with a 2-oxazoline heterocyclic ring and introducing a Cl atom at the C-10 position can produce an anti-inflammatory agent, which has potent therapeutic effects against neuroinflammation [46]; (ii) introduction of ester and oxime ester groups at C-2 position of piperine is important for improving acaricidal activity. In particular, the long aliphatic chain esters or oxime esters, and a very crucial prerequisite is to retain the dioxymethylene ring [28,29,60]; (iii) introduction of the dienehydrazide groups can obtain potent insecticidal compounds against third-instar larval of *C. pipiens* [65]. The introduction of different substituted amides is beneficial for anticancer activity and can obtain a potential inhibitor against CYP2J2 [34,67]. Piperine derivates containing a linear bisamide exhibited significant insecticidal activity against *P. xylostella*, and they can be further studied as lead pesticidal agents [50].

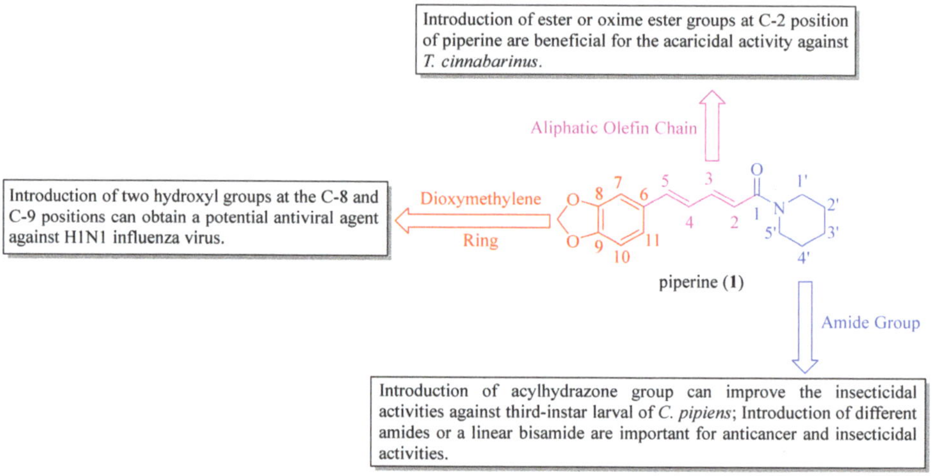

Figure 6. The structure-activity relationships of piperine and its derivatives.

6. Conclusions

In recent years, research and development of plant-derived pesticides in China have been steadily improving. The commercialization of plant-derived pesticides should capitalize on their benefits and prioritize sustainability. In the future, plant-derived pesticides will play a significant role in food security and the agricultural field for improving the local economic development. This review has summarized the recent developments from 2020 to 2023 on biological activities, structural modifications, and structure-activity relationships of piperine and its derivatives, in addition to their mechanisms of action. The structural characteristics of piperine implied that it had various sites for structural modifications, making it a high-value-added lead compound. It is prospective that this paper can provide essential information and proposals for further design and development of novel piperine derivatives as potent natural-product-based drugs and pesticides for improving the local economic development in the future.

Author Contributions: All persons who have made substantial contributions to present work are named in the manuscript. J.H. (Jin Han), T.L., S.Z. and J.H. (Jun He) designed the work, analyzed the data, and wrote and revised the paper. All authors have read and agreed to the published version of the manuscript.

Funding: This research received no external funding.

Conflicts of Interest: The authors declare no conflict of interest.

Abbreviations

TrxR	Thioredoxin reductase
VEGFR	Vascular endothelial growth factor receptors
TNF-α	Tumor necrosis factor-α
TGF-β	Transforming growth factor-β
NF-κB	Nuclear factor-κB
MAPK	Mitogen-activated protein kinase
LC_{50}	Lethal concentration
DMF	*N,N*-Dimethylformamide
t-Bu	*tert*-Butyl
EDCI	1-(3-Dimethylaminopropyl)-3-ethylcarbodiimide hydrochloride
HOBt	1-Hydroxybenzotriazole
DMAP	4-Dimethylaminopyridine

References

1. Lazareva, N.F.; Baryshok, V.P.; Lazarev, I.M. Silicon-containing analogs of camptothecin as anticancer agents. *Arch. Pharm.* **2018**, *351*, e1700297. [CrossRef] [PubMed]
2. Pizzolato, J.F.; Saltz, L.B. The camptothecins. *Lancet* **2003**, *361*, 2235–2242. [CrossRef] [PubMed]
3. Zhang, X.; Ma, Z.Q.; Feng, J.T.; Wu, H.; Han, L.R. Review on research and development of botanical pesticides. *Chin. J. Biol. Control* **2015**, *31*, 685–698.
4. Tunce, C.; Aliniazee, M.T. Acute and chronic effects of neem on *Myzocallis coryli* (Homoptera: Aphididae). *Int. J. Pest Manag.* **1998**, *44*, 53–58. [CrossRef]
5. Zhang, Z.W.; Xi, H.C.; Chang, W.C.; Huang, L.L.; Chen, X. Current situation of commercialized application of plant-derived pesticides in China and suggestions for industrial development. *World Pestic.* **2020**, *42*, 6–15.
6. Guo, Y.J.; Han, J.Y.; Li, Z.Q.; Yang, S.B. Research and application of plant-derived pesticides. *Heilongjiang Agric. Sci.* **2019**, *4*, 131–133.
7. Yu, L.; Hu, X.; Xu, R.; Ba, Y.; Chen, X.; Wang, X.; Cao, B.; Wu, X. Amide alkaloids characterization and neuroprotective properties of *Piper nigrum* L.: A comparative study with fruits, pericarp, stalks and leaves. *Food Chem.* **2022**, *368*, 130832. [CrossRef]
8. Zhu, F.; Mojel, R.; Li, G. Physicochemical properties of black pepper (*Piper nigrum*) starch. *Carbohyd. Polym.* **2018**, *181*, 986–993. [CrossRef]
9. Al-Khayri, J.M.; Upadhya, V.; Pai, S.R.; Naik, P.M.; Al-Mssallem, M.Q.; Alessa, F.M. Comparative quantification of the phenolic compounds, piperine content, and total polyphenols along with the antioxidant activities in the *Piper trichostachyon* and *P. nigrum*. *Molecules* **2022**, *27*, 5965. [CrossRef]
10. Guo, Z.; Xu, J.; Xia, J.; Wu, Z.; Lei, J.; Yu, J. Anti-inflammatory and antitumour activity of various extracts and compounds from the fruits of *Piper longum* L. *J. Pharm. Pharmacol.* **2019**, *71*, 1162–1171. [CrossRef]
11. Ee, G.C.L.; Lim, C.M.; Lim, C.K.; Rahmani, M.; Shaari, K.; Bong, C.F.J. Alkaloids from *Piper sarmentosum* and *Piper nigrum*. *Nat. Prod. Res.* **2009**, *23*, 1416–1423. [CrossRef] [PubMed]
12. Luca, S.V.; Kittl, T.; Minceva, M. Supercritical CO_2 extraction of spices: A systematic study with focus on terpenes and piperamides from black pepper (*Piper nigrum* L.). *Food Chem.* **2023**, *406*, 135090. [CrossRef] [PubMed]
13. Mad-adam, N.; Madla, S.; Lailerd, N.; Hiransai, P.; Graidist, P. *Piper nigrum* extract: Dietary supplement for reducing mammary tumor incidence and chemotherapy-induced toxicity. *Foods* **2023**, *12*, 2053. [CrossRef]
14. Wood, A.J.L.; Weise, N.J.; Frampton, J.D.; Dunstan, M.S.; Hollas, M.A.; Derrington, S.R.; Lloyd, R.C.; Quaglia, D.; Parmeggiani, F.; Leys, D.; et al. Adenylation activity of carboxylic acid reductases enables the synthesis of amides. *Angew. Chem. Int. Ed.* **2017**, *56*, 14498–14501. [CrossRef] [PubMed]
15. Wang, L.; Zhao, D.Y.; Zhang, Z.H.; Zuo, C.H.; Zhang, Y.; Pei, Y.Q.; Lo, Y.Q. Trial of antiepilepsirine (AES) in children with epilepsy. *Brain Dev.* **1999**, *21*, 36–40. [CrossRef] [PubMed]
16. Shen, S.B. Pepper-the characteristic industry in Yunnan Province. *China Rural. Sci. Technol.* **2020**, *304*, 74–75.
17. Chaudhari, V.S.; Gawali, B.; Saha, P.; Naidu, V.G.M.; Murty, U.S.; Banerjee, S. Quercetin and piperine enriched nanostructured lipid carriers (NLCs) to improve apoptosis in oral squamous cellular carcinoma (FaDu cells) with improved biodistribution profile. *Eur. J. Pharmacol.* **2021**, *909*, 174400. [CrossRef]
18. Qi, Y.B.; Yang, W.; Si, M.; Nie, L. Wnt/β-catenin signaling modulates piperine-mediated antitumor effects on human osteosarcoma cells. *Mol. Med. Rep.* **2020**, *21*, 2202–2208. [CrossRef]
19. Amperayani, K.R.; Varadhi, G.; Oruganti, B.; Parimi, U.D. Molecular dynamics and absolute binding free energy studies of piperine derivatives as potential inhibitors of SARS-CoV-2 main protease. *J. Biomol. Struct. Dyn.* **2023**. [CrossRef]
20. Priscilla, J.; Arul Dhas, D.; Hubert Joe, I.; Balachandran, S. Spectroscopic, quantum chemical, hydrogen bonding, reduced density gradient analysis and anti-inflammatory activity study on piper amide alkaloid piperine and wisanine. *J. Mol. Struct.* **2021**, *1225*, 129146. [CrossRef]
21. Wansri, R.; Lin, A.C.K.; Pengon, J.; Kamchonwongpaisan, S.; Srimongkolpithak, N.; Rattanajak, R.; Wilasluck, P.; Deetanya, P.; Wangkanont, K.; Hengphasatporn, K.; et al. Semi-synthesis of *N*-aryl amide analogs of piperine from *Piper nigrum* and evaluation of their antitrypanosomal, antimalarial, and anti-SARS-CoV-2 main protease activities. *Molecules* **2022**, *27*, 2841. [CrossRef] [PubMed]
22. Hu, X.; Wu, D.; Tang, L.; Zhang, J.; Zeng, Z.; Geng, F.; Li, H. Binding mechanism and antioxidant activity of piperine to hemoglobin. *Food Chem.* **2022**, *394*, 133558. [CrossRef] [PubMed]
23. Dhiman, P.; Malik, N.; Khatkar, A. Natural based piperine derivatives as potent monoamine oxidase inhibitors: An in silico ADMET analysis and molecular docking studies. *BMC Chem.* **2020**, *14*, 12. [CrossRef] [PubMed]
24. Nazifi, M.; Oryan, S.; Esfahani, D.E.; Ashrafpoor, M. The functional effects of piperine and piperine plus donepezil on hippocampal synaptic plasticity impairment in rat model of Alzheimer's disease. *Life Sci.* **2021**, *265*, 118802. [CrossRef]
25. Yang, X.; Zhi, J.; Leng, H.; Chen, Y.; Gao, H.; Ma, J.; Ji, J.; Hu, Q. The piperine derivative HJ105 inhibits $A\beta_{1\text{-}42}$-induced neuroinflammation and oxidative damage via the Keap1-Nrf2-TXNIP axis. *Phytomedicine* **2021**, *87*, 153571. [CrossRef]
26. Jaipea, S.; Saehlim, N.; Sutcharitruk, W.; Athipornchai, A.; Ingkaninan, K.; Saeeng, R. Synthesis of piperine analogues as AChE and BChE inhibitors for the treatment of Alzheimer's disease. *Phytochem. Lett.* **2023**, *53*, 216–221. [CrossRef]
27. Li, R.; Lu, Y.; Zhang, Q.; Liu, W.; Yang, R.; Jiao, J.; Liu, J.; Gao, G.; Yang, H. Piperine promotes autophagy flux by P2RX4 activation in *SNCA*/α-synuclein-induced Parkinson disease model. *Autophagy* **2022**, *18*, 559–575. [CrossRef]

28. Zhang, C.; Tian, Q.; Li, Y. Design, synthesis, and insecticidal activity evaluation of piperine derivatives. *Front. Chem.* **2022**, *10*, 973630. [CrossRef]
29. Lv, M.; Li, S.; Wen, H.; Wang, Y.; Du, J.; Xu, H. Expedient discovery of novel oxime ester derivatives of piperine/piperine analogs as potent pesticide candidates and their mode of action against *Tetranychus cinnabarinus* Boisduval. *Pest Manag. Sci.* **2023**, *79*, 3459–3470. [CrossRef]
30. Li, T.; Lv, M.; Wen, H.; Wang, J.; Wang, Z.; Xu, J.; Fang, S.; Xu, H. High value-added application of natural plant products in crop protection: Construction and pesticidal activities of piperine-type ester derivatives and their toxicology study. *J. Agric. Food Chem.* **2022**, *70*, 16126–16134. [CrossRef]
31. Wang, J.; Wang, W.; Xiong, H.; Song, D.; Cao, X. Natural phenolic derivatives based on piperine scaffold as potential antifungal agents. *BMC Chem.* **2020**, *14*, 24. [CrossRef] [PubMed]
32. Coles, C.E.; Anderson, B.O.; Cameron, D.; Cardoso, F.; Horton, R.; Knaul, F.M.; Mutebi, M.; Lee, N.; Abraham, J.E.; Anderson, B.O.; et al. The Lancet Breast Cancer Commission: Tackling a global health, gender, and equity challenge. *Lancet* **2022**, *399*, 1101–1103. [CrossRef] [PubMed]
33. Rajarajan, D.; Natesh, J.; Penta, D.; Meeran, S.M. Dietary piperine suppresses obesity-associated breast cancer growth and metastasis by regulating the miR-181c-3p/*PPARα* Axis. *J. Agric. Food Chem.* **2021**, *69*, 15562–15574. [CrossRef] [PubMed]
34. Jeong, J.H.; Ryu, J.H.; Lee, H.J. In vitro inhibition of *Piper nigrum* and piperine on growth, migration, and invasion of PANC-1 human pancreatic cancer cells. *Nat. Prod. Commun.* **2021**, *16*, 1–8. [CrossRef]
35. Zhong, M.; Chen, L.; Tao, Y.; Zhao, J.; Chang, B.; Zhang, F.; Tu, J.; Cai, W.; Zhang, B. Synthesis and evaluation of piperine analogs as thioredoxin reductase inhibitors to cause oxidative stress-induced cancer cell apoptosis. *Bioorg. Chem.* **2023**, *138*, 106589. [CrossRef] [PubMed]
36. Elimam, D.M.; Elgazar, A.A.; Bonardi, A.; Abdelfadil, M.; Nocentini, A.; El-Domany, R.A.; Abdel-Aziz, H.A.; Badria, F.A.; Supuran, C.T.; Eldehna, W.M. Natural inspired piperine-based sulfonamides and carboxylic acids as carbonic anhydrase inhibitors: Design, synthesis and biological evaluation. *Eur. J. Med. Chem.* **2021**, *225*, 113800. [CrossRef] [PubMed]
37. Elimam, D.M.; Elgazar, A.A.; El-Senduny, F.F.; El-Domany, R.A.; Badria, F.A.; Eldehna, W.M. Natural inspired piperine-based ureas and amides as novel antitumor agents towards breast cancer. *J. Enzym. Inhib. Med. Chem.* **2022**, *37*, 39–50. [CrossRef]
38. Pandya, N.; Kumar, A. Piperine analogs arrest *c-myc* gene leading to downregulation of transcription for targeting cancer. *Sci. Rep.* **2021**, *11*, 22909. [CrossRef]
39. Mohammed, A.; Velu, A.B.; Al-Hakami, A.M.; Meenakshisundaram, B.; Esther, P.; Abdelwahid, S.A.; Irfan, A.; Prasanna, R.; Anantharam, D.; Harish, C.C. Novel piperine compound AB05 (N-5-(3,4-dimethoxyphenyl)-2E,4E pentadienylpiperidine) inhibits H1N1 influenza virus propagation in vitro. *Trop. Biomed.* **2020**, *37*, 1062–1073.
40. Shekunov, E.V.; Efimova, S.S.; Yudintceva, N.M.; Muryleva, A.A.; Zarubaev, V.V.; Slita, A.V.; Ostroumova, O.S. Plant alkaloids inhibit membrane fusion mediated by Calcium and fragments of MERS-CoV and SARS-CoV/SARS-CoV-2 fusion peptides. *Biomedicines* **2021**, *9*, 1434. [CrossRef]
41. Wang, M.; Yang, B.; Ren, Z.; Liu, J.; Lu, C.; Jiang, H.; Ling, F.; Wang, G.; Liu, T. Inhibition of the largemouth bass virus replication by piperine demonstrates potential application in aquaculture. *J. Fish Dis.* **2023**, *46*, 261–271. [CrossRef] [PubMed]
42. Jaisin, Y.; Ratanachamnong, P.; Wongsawatkul, O.; Watthammawut, A.; Malaniyom, K.; Natewong, S. Antioxidant and anti-inflammatory effects of piperine on UV-B-irradiated human HaCaT keratinocyte cells. *Life Sci.* **2020**, *263*, 118607. [CrossRef] [PubMed]
43. Huang, W.; Zhang, J.; Jin, W.; Yang, J.; Yu, G.; Shi, H.; Shi, K. Piperine alleviates acute pancreatitis: A possible role for FAM134B and CCPG1 dependent ER-phagy. *Phytomedicine* **2022**, *105*, 154361. [CrossRef] [PubMed]
44. Lu, H.; Gong, H.; Du, J.; Gao, W.; Xu, J.; Cai, X.; Yang, Y.; Xiao, H. Piperine ameliorates psoriatic skin inflammation by inhibiting the phosphorylation of STAT3. *Int. Immunopharmacol.* **2023**, *119*, 110221. [CrossRef]
45. Yu, J.W.; Li, S.; Bao, L.D.; Wang, L. Piperine treating sciatica through regulating inflammation and MiR-520a/P65 pathway. *Chin. J. Nat. Med.* **2021**, *19*, 412–421. [CrossRef]
46. Duan, Z.; Xie, H.; Yu, S.; Wang, S.; Yang, H. Piperine derived from *Piper nigrum* L. inhibits LPS-induced inflammatory through the MAPK and NF-κB signalling pathways in RAW264.7 Cells. *Foods* **2022**, *11*, 2990. [CrossRef]
47. Yang, X.; Ji, J.; Liu, C.; Zhou, M.; Li, H.; Ye, S.; Hu, Q. HJ22, a novel derivative of piperine, attenuates ibotenic acid-induced cognitive impairment, oxidativestress, apoptosis and inflammation via inhibiting the protein-protein interaction of Keap1-Nrf2. *Int. Immunopharmacol.* **2020**, *83*, 106383. [CrossRef]
48. Tian, M.; Tian, Z.; Yao, D.; Ning, J.; Deng, S.; Feng, L.; Huo, X.; Tian, X.; Zhang, B.; Wang, C.; et al. A NIR fluorescent probe for fatty acid amide hydrolase bioimaging and its application in development of inhibitors. *J. Mater. Chem. B* **2021**, *9*, 6460–6465. [CrossRef] [PubMed]
49. de Oliveira, J.G.; Pilz-Júnior, H.L.; de Lemos, A.B.; da Silva da Costa, F.A.; Fernandes, M.; Gonçalves, D.Z.; Variza, P.F.; de Moraes, F.M.; Morisso, F.D.P.; Magnago, R.F.; et al. Polymer-based nanostructures loaded with piperine as a platform to improve the larvicidal activity against *Aedes aegypti*. *Acta Trop.* **2022**, *230*, 106395. [CrossRef] [PubMed]
50. Jiang, Z.; Shi, D.; Li, H.; He, D.; Zhu, K.; Li, J.; Zi, Y.; Xu, Z.; Huang, J.; Duan, H.; et al. Rational design and identification of novel piperine derivatives as multichitinase inhibitors. *J. Agric. Food Chem.* **2022**, *70*, 10326–10336. [CrossRef]

51. Zhong, F.; Yu, L.; Jiang, X.; Chen, Y.; Wang, S.; Chao, L.; Jiang, Z.; He, B.; Xu, C.; Wang, S.; et al. Potential inhibitory effects of compounds ZK-PI-5 and ZK-PI-9 on trehalose and chitin metabolism in *Spodoptera frugiperda* (J. E. Smith). *Front. Physiol.* **2023**, *14*, 1178996. [CrossRef] [PubMed]
52. Sivashanmugam, A.; Velmathi, S. Synthesis and characterization of piperine amide analogues: Their in-silico and invitro analysis as potential antibacterial agents. *Results Chem.* **2022**, *4*, 100369. [CrossRef]
53. Das, S.; Paul, P.; Dastidar, D.G.; Chakraborty, P.; Chatterjee, S.; Sarkar, S.; Maiti, D.; Tribedi, P. Piperine exhibits potential antibiofilm activity against *Pseudomonas aeruginosa* by accumulating reactive oxygen species, affecting cell surface hydrophobicity and quorum sensing. *Appl. Biochem. Biotech.* **2023**, *195*, 3229–3256. [CrossRef] [PubMed]
54. Manjunath, G.B.; Awasthi, S.P.; Zahid, M.S.H.; Hatanaka, N.; Hinenoya, A.; Iwaoka, E.; Aoki, S.; Ramamurthy, T.; Yamasaki, S. Piperine, an active ingredient of white pepper, suppresses the growth of multidrug-resistant toxigenic *Vibrio* cholerae and other pathogenic bacteria. *Lett. Appl. Microbiol.* **2022**, *74*, 472–481. [CrossRef] [PubMed]
55. Souza, J.S., Jr.; Martins, E.P.S.; Souza, H.D.S.; de Oliveira, R.F.; Alves, F.S.; Lima, E.O.; Cordeiro, L.V.; Trindade, E.O.; Lira, B.F.; Rocha, G.B.; et al. Synthesis, spectroscopic characterization, DFT calculations and preliminary antifungal activity of new piperine derivatives. *J. Braz. Chem. Soc.* **2021**, *32*, 490–502. [CrossRef]
56. Wang, Y.; Yao, Y.; Liu, J.; Wu, L.; Liu, T.; Cui, J.; Lee, D.Y.W. Synthesis and biological activity of piperine derivatives as potential *PPAR*γ agonists. *Drug Des. Dev. Ther.* **2020**, *14*, 2069–2078. [CrossRef]
57. Silva, W.L.; de Andrade, F.H.D.; Lins, T.B.; da Silva, A.L.; da Cruz Amorim, C.A.; dos Santos Lima, M.J.; da Silva, P.C.D.; Vilela, W.T.; Nascimento, P.H.d.B.; de Oliveira, J.F.; et al. Synthesis, thermal behavior and biological evaluation of benzodioxole derivatives as potential cytotoxic and antiparasitic agents. *Med. Chem. Res.* **2023**, *32*, 944–956. [CrossRef]
58. Hsieh, T.Y.; Chang, Y.; Wang, S.J. Piperine provides neuroprotection against kainic acid-induced neurotoxicity via maintaining NGF signalling pathway. *Molecules* **2022**, *27*, 2638. [CrossRef]
59. Alsareii, S.A.; Ahmad, J.; Umar, A.; Ahmad, M.Z.; Shaikh, I.A. Enhanced in vivo wound healing efficacy of a novel piperine-containing bioactive hydrogel in excision wound rat model. *Molecules* **2023**, *28*, 545. [CrossRef]
60. Li, T.; Lv, M.; Wen, H.; Wang, Y.; Thapa, S.; Zhang, S.; Xu, H. Synthesis of piperine-based ester derivatives with diverse aromatic rings and their agricultural bioactivities against *Tetranychus cinnabarinus* Boisduval, *Aphis citricola* Van der Goot, and *Eriosoma lanigerum* Hausmann. *Insects* **2023**, *14*, 40. [CrossRef]
61. Gu, Y.; Norton, J.R.; Salahi, F.; Lisnyak, V.G.; Zhou, Z.; Snyder, S.A. Highly selective hydrogenation of C=C bonds catalyzed by a Rhodium hydride. *J. Am. Chem. Soc.* **2021**, *143*, 9657–9663. [CrossRef] [PubMed]
62. Luo, J.; Xiang, J.Y.; Yuan, H.Y.; Wu, J.Q.; Li, H.Z.; Shen, Y.H.; Xu, M. Isolation, synthesis and absolute configuration of 4,5-dihydroxypiperines improving behavioral disorder in $AlCl_3$-induced dementia. *Bioorg. Med. Chem. Lett.* **2021**, *42*, 128057. [CrossRef] [PubMed]
63. Nguyen, K.X.; Pham, P.H.; Nguyen, T.T.; Yang, C.H.; Pham, H.T.B.; Nguyen, T.T.; Wang, H.; Phan, N.T.S. Trisulfur-radical-anion-triggered C(sp^2)-H amination of electron-deficient alkenes. *Org. Lett.* **2020**, *22*, 9751–9756. [CrossRef] [PubMed]
64. Wójtowicz-Rajchel, H.; Kaźmierczak, M. Chemo-, regio-, and stereoselectivity in 1,3-dipolar cycloaddition of piperine with nitrones. A cycloadditive route to aminoalcohols. *New J. Chem.* **2020**, *44*, 6015–6025. [CrossRef]
65. Tantawy, A.H.; Farag, S.M.; Hegazy, L.; Jiang, H.; Wang, M.Q. The larvicidal activity of natural inspired piperine-based dienehydrazides against *Culex pipiens*. *Bioorg. Chem.* **2020**, *94*, 103464. [CrossRef]
66. Tian, X.; Zhou, M.; Ning, J.; Deng, X.; Feng, L.; Huang, H.; Yao, D.; Ma, X. The development of novel cytochrome P450 2J2 (CYP2J2) inhibitor and the underlying interaction between inhibitor and CYP2J2. *J. Enzym. Inhib. Med. Ch.* **2021**, *36*, 737–748. [CrossRef]
67. Han, Q.; Wu, N.; Li, H.L.; Zhang, J.Y.; Li, X.; Deng, M.F.; Zhu, K.; Wang, J.E.; Duan, H.X.; Yang, Q. A piperine-based scaffold as a novel starting point to develop inhibitors against the potent molecular target *Of*ChtI. *J. Agric. Food Chem.* **2021**, *69*, 7534–7544. [CrossRef]

MDPI AG
Grosspeteranlage 5
4052 Basel
Switzerland
Tel.: +41 61 683 77 34

Toxins Editorial Office
E-mail: toxins@mdpi.com
www.mdpi.com/journal/toxins

www.ingramcontent.com/pod-product-compliance
Lightning Source LLC
LaVergne TN
LVHW072352090526
838202LV00019B/2528
* 9 7 8 3 7 2 5 8 2 6 9 9 5 *